BEARD'S MASSAGE

FOURTH EDITION

BEARD'S MASSAGE

FOURTH EDITION

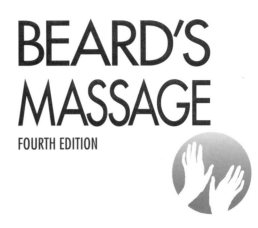

Giovanni De Domenico
  Grad Dip (Physiotherapy), Dip TP, MSc, PhD,
  MCSP, MAPA, MCPA
Professor and Chair
Department of Physical Therapy
College of Allied Health Professions
University of South Alabama
Mobile, Alabama

Elizabeth C. Wood, MA, MS, RPT
Associate Professor Emeritus
Programs in Physical Therapy
Northwestern University Medical School
Chicago, Illinois

W.B. SAUNDERS COMPANY
A Division of Harcourt Brace & Company
Philadelphia   London   Toronto   Montreal   Sydney   Tokyo

W.B. SAUNDERS COMPANY
A Division of Harcourt Brace & Company

The Curtis Center
Independence Square West
Philadelphia, Pennsylvania 19106

Library of Congress Cataloging-in-Publication Data

De Domenico, Giovanni.
    Beard's massage.—4th ed. / Giovanni De Domenico, Elizabeth C. Wood.

      p.   cm.

    Previous ed. entered under Beard.

    Includes bibliographical references and index.

    ISBN 0–7216–6234–X

    1. Massage therapy.   I. Wood, Elizabeth C.   II. Beard, Gertrude.
Beard's massage.   III. Title.
    [DNLM: 1. Massage.   WB 537 D278b 1997]

RM721.B4 1997

615.8′22—dc20

DNLM/DLC   96–14136

BEARD'S MASSAGE   ISBN 0–7216–6234–X

Printed in the United States of America.

Last digit is the print number: 9   8   7   6   5   4   3   2   1

This book is dedicated to the memory of
GERTRUDE BEARD, RN, RPT
and
to all those who seek to learn the skills and benefits of this ancient art

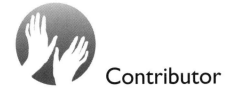

Contributor

Colleen Liston, AUA, Grad Dip (Physiotherapy), Grad Dip Hlth Sc, MSc, PhD

Associate Professor and Supervisor of Higher Degrees, School of Physiotherapy, Curtin University of Technology, Perth, Western Australia, Australia

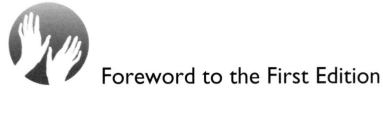

Foreword to the First Edition

There are some things in every man's life that have a great effect upon his future success and the success of some of the people around him. One of these things happened to me when a physical therapist named Gertrude Beard came to Chicago shortly after the First World War, after she was discharged from the Army.

Miss Beard was taken onto the staff of Wesley Hospital immediately and started work on my patients, most of them workers who had been injured at the stockyards. She worked in a place called the "bath department," which consisted of one shower, one Scotch douche, a table and a couple of sinks. She and the patients had to sit on stools, and no one in the hospital took her appearance with any great degree of hope that she was going to do anything that had not been done before. At that time (1919–1920) physical therapy, in my experience, was something to do when you couldn't think of anything else to do to get rid of the patient.

Miss Beard had made a study of what was not considered a very great science at that time, and went on to develop physical therapy techniques which have brought help to many patients who would never have recovered had it not been for her efforts.

In 1927 she became the technical director of Northwestern University's new school of physical therapy. She and her teaching colleagues have taught more than five hundred physical therapists the techniques and principles of physical therapy since that date. The story of their work is worth noting—a story of devoted, dedicated persons who believe in what they know, and who continue to educate doctors and patients as well as students in the benefits of physical therapy and especially massage.

Massage has often been neglected in favor of other physical measures which can be used more easily. Massage requires skilled use of the hands and brain for its curative effects—producing or regaining elasticity of tissues, stimulating blood supply, giving the patient confidence and at the same time giving him encouragement and psychological stimulation to use the part that is disabled—and no machine can substitute. There is a psychology that goes along with any form of medical treatment, and if the physical therapist is not using his or her powers of encouragement to get the patient to do what he should do, then he or she is not doing a job in whatever is being done.

In my opinion massage is one of the things that can be neglected, misused, paid for and thrown out the window without accomplishing what it should unless it is understood and properly applied. This book presents a clear picture of techniques and the principles upon which they are based. The text is well written and illustrated and should be read and reread by the doctor and the physical therapist to the ever-lasting benefit of the patient's recovery.

PAUL B. MAGNUSON, M.D.
Professor of Bone and Joint Surgery,
Emeritus, Northwestern University
Medical School
Founder and Honorary Chairman,
Rehabilitation Institute of Chicago
Former Chief Medical Director,
Veterans Administration

May 1964

Preface

The basic principles and techniques of soft tissue massage have changed very little with the passage of time. In an age of high technology in medicine and indeed all aspects of modern life, soft tissue massage continues to provide a direct link with the cultural and medical practices of our ancestors. The increasing movement toward a more holistic approach to the management of disease and the promotion of wellness will ensure a place for this ancient art in the twenty-first century and well beyond.

The third edition of *Beard's Massage* was the culmination of important contributions from many sources. These contributors added significantly to the text, and the success of the book is a tribute to the importance of their work. The fourth edition of *Beard's Massage* continues to emphasize Gertrude Beard's (1887–1971) major contribution to the previous editions of the book as senior author of the first edition. The retention of the dedication to her from the first edition's Foreword by Dr. Paul B. Magnuson (1884–1968) continues to honor these two pioneers in physical therapy and rehabilitation over a period of some 50 years.

The fourth edition marks a significant rearrangement of material from previous editions. In particular, the photographs are a major added feature. Most are new to this edition and were taken by Carl Moss of M & A Studios in Mobile, Alabama. The obvious professionalism of these photographs is a fine tribute to the photographer, and grateful thanks are extended to him and all those involved at the studio. Of course, without the assistance of the models, the photographs would not have turned out so well. Sincere thanks are extended to Kristie Love and Ron Lassiter for their important contribution to this work. Significant contributions to the preparation of the final manuscript were also made by Thelma Topper and Mavis Jarrell, for which grateful thanks are extended.

The techniques described in this text continue to follow the basic Swedish remedial massage system. Each of the basic massage strokes is described in some detail, with many photographic examples. This will enable therapists to develop their own massage sequences, properly based on the needs of the patient. As an important guide to planning sequences of massage strokes, chapters 5 and 6 on general and local massage techniques continue to follow quite closely the methods described in the third edition.

Three new chapters consider massage systems from a number of different traditions. These important contributions were written by Colleen Liston of the School of Physiotherapy at Curtin University in Perth, Western Australia. Dr. Liston has provided the reader with a condensed view of several different massage concepts, and these will help the reader to a wider understanding of the subject. The material in these chapters is intended to provide only an outline of the subject areas, since a complete examination of each concept is well beyond the scope of the present text.

This book is intended for those students pursuing a serious study of soft tissue massage. The material is arranged to facilitate such study, but of course it is recognized that effective massage cannot be learned entirely from a textbook. Only close guidance from an experienced teacher will ensure that the student reaches the appropriate level of competence in what is, after all, a finely tuned motor skill on the part of the therapist. This text does not pretend to be sufficient in itself, but it does provide the background information and concepts necessary to give the theoretical framework for the subject area, along with the basic elements of the practical techniques for soft tissue massage. Together with an experienced teacher and sufficient clinical practice, the student should expect to be able to reach high levels of competence.

Although massage as a specific treatment in its own right is not used a great deal in modern rehabilitation practice, various techniques are extremely useful as part of an overall treatment plan for many conditions. Experience over many years strongly suggests that a significant study of soft tissue massage is one of the very best ways of developing sensitivity and competence in using the hands. As such, significant training in soft tissue massage should be seen as a fundamental part of the preparation of a number of health care professionals.

GIOVANNI De DOMENICO
ELIZABETH C. WOOD

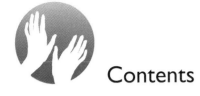

Contents

Part I

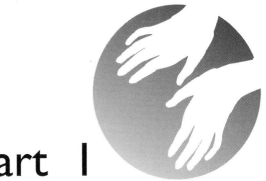

General
Principles

Chapter 1

Historical Perspectives

The modern French words *masser* (verb) and *massage* (noun) could have derived from any of three original roots, namely the Hebrew word *mashesh*, the Arabic word *mass*, or the Greek word *massin*. Although obviously French in origin, *masseur* (male) and *masseuse* (female) have come into the English language to denote those who practice massage. By the early 1780s the word *massage* was used in India, and it appeared in most European cultures around 1800.

Massage is mentioned as a form of treatment in the very earliest medical records, and its use persisted down through recorded history. Writings of physicians, philosophers, poets, and historians show that some form of rubbing or anointing was used from the most ancient of times in cultures all around the world. The history of massage is large and complex. In this chapter we present a broad overview of its chronology and a more detailed review of a number of the important aspects of massage.

AN OVERVIEW OF THE HISTORY OF MASSAGE

Prehistoric Times

Although there is little direct evidence that massage was practiced as a healing art in prehistoric times, it seems very likely that it was. There is a certain instinctive quality to the use of the hands in a rubbing and squeezing motion that is both soothing and comforting. Indeed, one sees that many animal species, especially primates, use grooming behavior and, although it is not necessarily therapeutic, it is certainly part of the behavioral repertoire of many species. In short, touching as an activity had its genesis at the very earliest point in human evolution. It is not too great a leap of faith to believe that some forms of manual massage techniques were in regular use then, together with the application of various medicinal compounds derived from plants, animal sources, and inorganic materials.

Although such ancient cultures had little if any recorded history, massage techniques almost certainly were part of their "medical culture." Certainly, prehistoric humans were capable of practicing quite sophisticated medicine, including brain surgery. The well-known prehistoric practice of removing small circles of bone from the skull, called *trephining* (or *trepanning*), clearly shows that the practitioners of the day were quite capable of very complex medical tasks (Broca, 1876; Prunieres, 1874). Not only were they able to make holes in the skulls of their "patients," but these latter-day surgeons were able to do this more than once in a given person. In addition, the anthropologists' findings clearly show that many people survived the procedure. One cannot help but believe that a culture capable of this level of surgical practice must long before have discovered the considerable and obvious benefits of massagelike ministrations.

Ancient History

The use of manual massage techniques in many ancient cultures is well-recorded in extensive written and pictorial records. For example, at the time of Hwang Ti, the Yellow Emperor (died in 2599 B.C.), the great Chinese medical work known as the *Nei Chang* was written (about 2760 B.C.). This work contains detailed descriptions of massagelike procedures and a great many details of their use (Veith, 1949). During the Tang dynasty (A.D. 619–907) four primary kinds of medical practitioners were recognized, physicians, acupuncturists, masseurs, and exorcists; however, following the Sung dynasty (A.D. 960–1279) the use of massage declined greatly. Massage is also described in one of ancient India's first great medical writings, the *Ayur-Veda* books of wisdom (about 1800 B.C.). Most of the great ancient cultures of the world have described in some detail the uses and benefits of massage, which was often combined with other kinds of traditional treatment, particularly bath treatments. The Egyptian, Persian, and

Japanese cultures, in particular, placed great emphasis on the use of massage and these allied treatments.

The ancient Greeks used massage widely to maintain physical health and ensure lasting beauty. Homer described in the *Odyssey* how "war torn" soldiers were massaged back to health. Hippocrates (460–360 B.C.) also wrote on the subject and described many of the uses of massage in medical practice. In discussing treatment following reduction of a dislocated shoulder, Hippocrates said , "And it is necessary to rub the shoulder gently and smoothly. The physician must be experienced in many things, but assuredly also in rubbing; for things that have the same name have not the same effects. For rubbing can bind a joint which is too loose and loosen a joint that is too hard. However, a shoulder in the condition described should be rubbed with soft hands and, above all things, gently; but the joint should be moved about, not violently, but so far as it can be done without producing pain" (Johnson, 1866).

The ancient Greeks, perhaps more than other cultures, are responsible for giving massage such a high level of social acceptance. They established very elaborate bathhouses where exercise, massage, and bathing were available, but the patrons were lovers of luxury rather than seekers of health. They were very much the playgrounds of the rich and powerful. Ordinary citizens were not so fortunate.

The Romans inherited much of the tradition of massage from the Greeks, and it was widely used, especially in conjunction with hot baths. Galen (A.D. 131–201), the most famous physician in the Roman Empire, wrote extensively on the topic of massage and described several different ways in which it could be administered (Green, 1951). Julius Caesar (100 B.C.) is said to have had himself "pinched" all over as a cure for a complaint similar to neuralgia. The influence of Galen on all aspects of medical thinking cannot be overstated; it is probably because of him that massage and its allied treatments survived long past the fall of Rome. Galen strongly recommended that in preparation for impending combat, gladiators be rubbed all over until their skin was red. The use of massage continued, and it was not until the early part of the Middle Ages that it fell into some decline in Europe and Asia. This era was the "Dark Ages," when many aspects of ancient culture and practice were abandoned.

Modern History of Medical Massage (European, Mainly British)

Much of ancient culture and tradition in medicine and science was lost through the Middle Ages, and it was not until the sixteenth century that some of the older methods of medical practice were again used. Advances in the study of anatomy and physiology enabled scientists of the time to understand more about the effects and uses of some of these more ancient traditions. Ambroise Pare (1518–1590),

the famous French surgeon, was among the earliest writers to consider and discuss the effects of massage. Pare was particularly interested in the use of friction and general massage movements to treat patients who had dislocated a joint.

Harvey's discovery of the circulation of the blood in 1628 did much to enhance acceptance of massage as a therapeutic measure. Despite these seemingly important advances, massage treatments did not become popular throughout Europe until the eighteenth century. At that time, two of the more notable exponents of the treatment were German, namely Hoffmann (1660–1742) and Guthsnuths. Another famous physician, who in the 1880s claimed that massage could be a very useful treatment, particularly to the soft tissues following fracture, was the famous French physician Just Lucas-Championnière (1843–1913). In the late 1890s Sir William Bennett was impressed with Lucas-Championnière's work and began what was then a revolutionary treatment using massage at St. George's Hospital in London, England. Other authors also strongly advocated massage for a variety of soft tissue problems, especially writer's cramp (Robins, 1885; de Watteville, 1885a, b).

The era of modern massage is usually said to have begun during the early 1800s, when a wide variety of authors were advocating massage and developing their own systems. A famous thesis by Estradere in 1886 was an important contribution to the developing science of massage (Estradere, 1886).

Arguably, the most famous and enduring influence on massage is the contribution made by Pehr Henrik Ling (1776–1839). Ling developed his own style of massage and exercises, which later gained international recognition (Swedish Remedial Massage and Exercise). Ling was a fencing instructor, and in 1805 he was appointed gymnastics and fencing master to the University of Lund, in Sweden. He designed a system of his own that consisted of four types of gymnastics: educational, military, medical, and esthetic. In 1813 he founded the Central Institute of Gymnastics in Stockholm, and he taught there until his death in 1839. Much of Ling's work was published after his death, mainly owing to the efforts of his students and colleagues (Kellgren, 1890). He gained international recognition for the terminology that bears his name, and in many cases modifications of his basic concepts of exercise have been used throughout the world. In more recent times, however, many of Ling's original ideas faded from popularity, but his work remains a very important influence in the early development of the profession of physical therapy (physiotherapy).

In Holland, Johann Mezger (1839–1909) also used massage widely and developed his own style. By 1900, modern medical massage techniques were being used in most parts of the developed world and, of course, continued to be used in more ancient cultures. In England in 1894 a group of four dedicated women founded the Society of Trained Masseuses with the aim of raising the standards of massage and the status of women taking up the work. In 1900 the Society was incorporated by license to the Board of Trade and became known as the Incorporated Society of Trained Masseuses. During World War I membership rose, and by 1920 some 5000 members were practicing. In 1920 the society merged with the Institute of Massage and Remedial Exercises (Manchester). These two bodies were then granted a Royal Charter and became known as the Chartered Society of Massage and Medical Gymnastics (CSMMG). World War II saw the emergence of a young profession, as large numbers of soldiers returned from various parts of the world, and the role of physiotherapy became more and more important. Massage alone became less and less important, however, as other means of rehabilitation were developed. For this reason it was decided that the name of the society would be changed, and in 1943 it became the Chartered Society of Physiotherapy (CSP), which it remains today.

From similar beginnings in many other countries the profession of physical therapy as we now know it developed and branched into most parts of the world, developing differently in each one to accommodate particular needs. Medical massage is rarely used in modern rehabilitation practice as a treatment in its own right, but it is used as part of an overall treatment plan for some patients. It has largely been superseded by other, more active treatments, but it remains one of the most important means of developing hand skills in the therapist. In physical therapy practice, soft tissue massage has developed into many types of manual mobilizing techniques that take the form of a wide variety of manipulations performed on both soft tissues and joint structures. In effect, the skilled use of the hands is still the cornerstone of the profession of physical therapy and is likely to remain so for the forseeable future.

In many older Asian cultures such as China, Japan, and India, massage is still used extensively as part of the "traditional" methods of treatment. Massage as a specific treatment in its own right plays a relatively small role in modern "Western" medicine; however, in recent years in many countries specific massage professionals (massage therapists) have emerged. In this case, the treatment modality is massage itself. Massage techniques are used to promote a general sense of relaxation and wellness. These days, thanks to the resurgence of interest in holistic medicine and very popular concepts of wellness, the general public still has great faith in the laying on of hands; however, such forms of massage need to be differentiated from the medical massage techniques used in other health professions, mainly physical therapy. These more general massage techniques, performed on persons who are otherwise healthy, may be termed "recreational massage." *Collins English Dictionary* defines the word recreation as "refreshment of health or spirits by relaxation and enjoyment." Other major English dictionaries use similar descriptions, and it is in this context that the term recreational massage is intended.

Dorland's Medical Dictionary defines the word "therapeutic" as "that which pertains to the science and art of healing or curing." Clearly intended in this definition is the assumption that there is a health problem that requires healing. For this reason, the term "therapeutic massage" is used to denote a massage treatment intended to facilitate healing when a specific health problem exists.

There are a great many variations of technique used in recreational massage. While many of these techniques certainly feel good to the client, they may have little therapeutic value. Other techniques seem similar to the more therapeutic procedures. Of course, all of these techniques have very considerable psychological value. For this reason, it is helpful to distinguish between recreational massage and therapeutic massage. These two terms are defined next.

Recreational massage may be defined thus:

The use of a variety of manual techniques designed to relieve stress, promote relaxation and general wellness in a person who has no definable health problem.

Therapeutic massage may be defined thus:

The use of a variety of manual techniques designed to promote stress relief and relaxation, mobilize various structures, relieve pain and swelling, prevent deformity and promote functional independence in a person who has a specific health problem.

Another technique that appears to be similar to massage is known as "therapeutic touch." This somewhat controversial technique needs to be clearly differentiated from therapeutic massage. Essentially, although the name implies that touching is involved in the concept, therapeutic touch does not actually require the therapist to touch the patient. The therapist's hands are simply moved over the part to be treated, without actually making contact. Here, the technique is intended to "balance energy fields" around the affected parts (Feltham, 1991; Krieger, 1979, 1981).

Since the primary effects of therapeutic massage are mechanical, a technique that does not have a mechanical component cannot work on the same principles. Others must be invoked to explain its efficacy. Although therapeutic touch is a popular facet of the New Age medicine, it is a long way from enjoying strong scientific acceptance. Paradoxically, this concept is *not* new. Traditional Chinese medicine has many techniques that are very similar to so-called therapeutic touch.

In this text we consider only the theory and practice of therapeutic massage. In this regard, the major influence behind the techniques described comes originally from the Swedish remedial massage tradition. Before describing these techniques in detail, we will describe the history of various aspects of medical massage. This section is self-contained and may be referred to in relative isolation from the rest of the text, since many of the concepts mentioned here will be expanded upon in the remainder of the book. The review focuses on a number of aspects of the practice of massage rather than on a chronologic history. Readers interested in the history of massage from these perspectives are directed to these sources: Beard (1952); Bohm (1918); Bucholz (1917); Cole and Stovell (1991); Despard (1932); Graham (1884, 1913); Henry (1884); Johnson (1866); Kamentz (1960, 1985); Mason (1992); Quintner (1993, 1994); Stockton (1994).

Anyone reviewing the early literature on massage must be impressed with the fact that it does not contain detailed descriptions of the massage strokes themselves. Even in more recent material there is little information on the techniques of massage. Given the great variations in massage techniques used today and, often, the apparent lack of scientific basis for the movements one might wonder how any conclusions can be drawn about their value—or lack of it—in treatment. The paucity of detailed information on techniques and confusion about the meaning of the terms currently in use are considered in the rest of this chapter. It is not a complete account of the history of massage, since only the techniques are considered and the methods compared to determine, if possible, their influence on the development of present-day methods and techniques. This account does not cover every technique that can be found in the literature, only the most common ones. Some techniques that were once popular will not be considered here because they are not used to any great degree today. An excellent example of this is the many different types of nerve manipulation. Once quite popular, these techniques could involve direct stroking, friction, or stretching of the major peripheral nerves (Jabre, 1994; Lace, 1946). It will be interesting to see if in the future these techniques are rediscovered.

DEFINITIONS OF MASSAGE

A comprehensive definition of massage cannot be found in the early medical literature. *Thomas's Medical Dictionary* (1886) offers this description: "Massage, from the Greek, meaning to knead. Signifying the act of shampooing." ("Shampoo" is from the Hindi, meaning "press.") In much of the history of medicine massage and exercises are referred to simultaneously, and in the very early literature little distinction is made between the two. Kleen (1847–1923) of Sweden, who first published a handbook of massage in 1895, claimed to be the first to show clearly that massage is not an exercise therapy (Kleen, 1906, 1921).

William Murrell (1853–1912) of Edinburgh and London, writing at about the same time, was more specific when he defined massage as "the scientific mode of treating certain forms of a disease by systematic manipulations." He limited massage to the amelioration of disease but evidently realized the need for a system for its use. He placed no limit on the means of massage. At the same time, Douglas Graham, of Boston, writing from 1884 to 1918,

wrote of massage as "a term now generally accepted by European and American physicians to signify a group of procedures which are usually done with the hands, such as friction, kneading, manipulations, rolling, and percussion of the external tissues of the body in a variety of ways, either with a curative, palliative, or hygienic object in view." He went much farther than Murrell (in recognizing that the term needed definition) and limited the means to the hand and the surfaces involved to the external tissues, and identified the objectives as being curative, palliative, or hygienic.

Kleen, a contemporary of Graham's, limited the areas involved to the soft tissues. To the hand as a means of administering massage he added ancillary apparatuses. This seems contradictory given that he eliminated the idea that massage is exercise. In this he differed from his early compatriot, Ling.

Albert Hoffa (1859–1907), of Germany, also limited the *means* of massage to the hand but embraced its broad application—to all the "mechanical procedures that can cure illness" (Hoffa, 1897). At about the same time, another German, J. B. Zabludowski (1851–1906), also limited the administration of massage to the hand but specified "skillful hand grasps, skillfully and systematically applied to the body." While limiting the movement to skillful hand grasps, he, like Murrell, recognized the use of systems (Zabludowski, 1903).

C. Herman Bucholz of the United States (Boston) and Germany was as imprecise as any of his predecessors. He did not mention the hand or any other means of administering massage in his recommendations for therapeutic manipulation of the soft tissues. Even James B. Mennell (1880–1957)—whose great contributions have made the science of massage what it is today—gave no formal definition of massage.

In 1932 John S. Coulter (1885–1949) said, "According to the present, generally accepted meaning of the word, massage includes a great number of manipulations of the tissues and organs of the body for therapeutic purposes." In 1952 Gertrude Beard (1887–1971) wrote of massage as "the term used to designate certain manipulations of the soft tissues of the body; these manipulations are most effectively performed with the hands and are administered for the purpose of producing effects on the nervous, muscular, and respiratory systems and the local and general circulation of the blood and lymph" (Beard, 1952).

MASSAGE TERMINOLOGY

A student of the literature in this area must be impressed with the number of different terms used to describe the various techniques of massage. Despite some similarities, there is considerable confusion, and a comparison reveals that few writers have given the same meanings to these terms. A survey of these differences seems useful if one is to be able to interpret correctly any reading of earlier massage techniques and at the same time possess a clear idea of the meanings as they are presently accepted and used in this text. Much of the background information in this area comes from the work of Graham (1884, 1913).

The terms used by the various advocates of massage among the ancient Greeks and Romans from the time of Homer in the ninth century B.C. through the fourth and fifth centuries A.D. used relatively consistent terminology. "Friction," "rubbing," and "anointing" were used most frequently by these writers. Celsus of Rome (25 B.C.–A.D. 50) used, in addition, the term "unction" (Cellsus, 1665). *Anatripsis* and "rubbing" were the terms used by Hippocrates. Later, Galen adopted the term *anatripsis* from Hippocrates but added *"tripsis," "tripsisparaskeu lasthke,"* and *"apotherapeia."* Oribasius (325–403), a Roman who followed Galen a century later, described *apotherapeia* as bathing, friction, and inunction. Other terms used in this period were "pommeling," "squeezing," and "pinching."

There is very little literature on medical practice during the Dark Ages, but the terminology of the earlier period was adopted by the users of massage during the fifteenth, sixteenth, and seventeenth centuries in many European cultures. Among those who strongly advocated the use of massage were the noted French surgeon Ambroise Pare and the famous English physician Thomas Sydenham (1624–1689), who confined their terminology to "friction." Alpinus (1553–1617) of Italy used "rubbing" but added "maxalation," "manipulation," and "pressure"; Frederick Hoffman (1660–1742) of Prussia adopted Galen's term *apotherapeia*. Hieronymus Fabricius (1537–1619), an Italian, seems to be the first to have used the term "kneading," and he also used "rubbing."

In the early part of the nineteenth century there was a definite change in terminology, evidently owing to the influence of Ling. Ling, who has been credited as the originator of the Swedish system of remedial massage, traveled widely all over Europe and incorporated into his system the French terms *effleurage, petrissage, massage à friction,* and *tapotement*. To these he added "rolling," "slapping," "pinching," "shaking," "vibration," and "joint movement" (a specific example of a part of present-day exercise in the classification of massage movements).

Mezger (1839–1909) of Holland used the French terminology exclusively, and William Beveridge (1774–1839) of Scotland seems to have originated use of the term "finger rubbing." Lucas-Championnière of France also used unique terminology: his gentle massage, which he termed "glucokinesis" and "effrayan," influenced the massage techniques used to this day. Blundell (1864) of England used the terms "inunction," "friction," "pressure," and "percussion." In contrast, the terms used by the islanders of Tonga in this same period were *"toogi toogi," "mili,"* and *"fota"*; Hawaiians used the term *lomi-lomi*.

In the early twentieth century, physicians in the United States contributed to the literature of massage. Graham avoided the French terms and listed "friction, kneading, manipulation, rolling, pinching, percussion,

movement, pressure, squeezing" and the very early Italian term, *"maxalation."* In his 1919 book J.H. Kellogg (1852–1943) described different movements, in contrast to some of the English writers of a century earlier (for example, John Grosvenor), who used only "friction."

Murrell of Scotland and England, Kleen of Sweden, Hoffa of Germany, Bucholz of Germany and the United States, and John K. Mitchell (1859–1917) of the United States embraced the French terminology, while Zabludowski of Germany and Mennell of England dropped it almost entirely.

Kleen, Zabludowski, Mitchell, Bucholz, and Mennell gave a rather simple general classification of the terminology with subdivisions of the movements. Mennell's general classification identified stroking, compression, and percussion. McMillan (1925) used effleurage, petrissage, friction, tapotement, and vibration. Louisa Despard (1932), Frances Tappan (1978, 1988), and Lace (1946) use a mixture of French and English terms. Elizabeth Dicke and associates (1978) used both German and English terms to describe specific movements in connective tissue massage.

DESCRIPTION OF MASSAGE MOVEMENTS

There is little description of the individual massage techniques in the early literature. The present analysis has been limited to a description of the movements from information available since the time of Ling, and the terms to those used most commonly today. To understand the meaning of the terms used by various authors, it is helpful to analyze several aspects of the techniques, including direction of the movement, amount of pressure applied, what part of the hand is used to perform the technique, the actual motion that is performed, and the specific tissues of the body to which it is applied.

Petrissage

Several techniques come under the general heading of petrissage (from the French meaning *pressure, to knead*). Essentially, these techniques involve applying pressure to the tissues in a kneading manner. They can be performed with the whole hand, the fingers, or the thumb. They may be performed with either hand or both hands at the same time. When performed with two hands, one hand reinforces the other.

To perform petrissage strokes, Ling grasped the tissues between the thumb and fingers whereas Mitchell (1904), Kellogg (1919), Bucholz (1917), and Mennell (1945) advised that chiefly the palm be used in contact with the tissues. Hoffa and Mennell emphasized that the hand must fit the contour of the tissues. It was Hoffa (1897) who distinguished different types of petrissage, depending on what parts of one or both hands were used to perform the movement.

According to Ling and Murrell, the motion is a rolling one and the skin moves with the fingers, but Hoffa, Mitchell, Kellogg, Despard (1932), Bucholz, and Mennell lifted the mass of tissues and used a squeezing movement. In addition to the rolling, Murrell (1886) added that the tissues are pressed and squeezed, as one would squeeze out a sausage. Bucholz and Mennell recommended that the hand glide over the skin instead of moving the skin along with the hand. Despard and Mennell alternately compressed the tissues between the thumb of one hand and the fingers of the other. Mezger lifted the tissues and kneaded them between the hands. In addition to *lifting* the tissues for petrissage, Despard also described a type of petrissage in which the tissues are grasped and pressed down onto the underlying structures and at the same time squeezed (compression kneading). Murrell and Hoffa stipulated firm pressure, Ling said that it varies, and Mennell prescribed that it should be gentle. Mitchell and Despard alternately tightened and loosened the pressure. Kellogg stated that it must not be so great as to prevent deeper parts from gliding over still deeper structures.

Many authors mentioned that petrissage is applied to muscle groups, individual muscles, or some part of a muscle. Ling mentioned specifically that the skin, subcutaneous tissues, and muscles are grasped. Mitchell was not specific; he mentioned only "tissues." Murrell said "a portion of muscle or other tissue" was manipulated. The direction is described as centripetal by most authors; Hoffa and Mennell made compression transversely to the muscle fibers although the general movement was centripetal, and Bucholz stated that the manipulations might be either centripetal or centrifugal.

Kneading

Only the most recent authors described kneading as a separate technique; earlier ones used the French term *petrissage* to describe the movement, which was very similar in many respects to kneading, as we now understand.

Several authors described petrissage as a kneading movement and made little distinction between the two. Other descriptions of kneading were very similar to those of petrissage. Mennell stated that they resemble each other very closely, the only difference being that petrissage is a picking-up movement with lateral compression whereas in kneading the compression is vertical. Kellogg's concept is opposite to that of Mennell: he stated that the tissues are lifted in kneading but not in petrissage. According to Graham (1913), in kneading the fingers and hand slip on the skin, whereas Kellogg cautioned that the surface of the hand must *not* be allowed to slip across the surface of the skin.

McMillan (1925) used petrissage, or kneading. Graham used kneading on the tissues beneath the skin, whereas Kellogg subdivided kneading as superficial for skin and underlying tissues, and deep for muscles. Graham and Kellogg differed also on direction. Graham stated that movements should be congruent with the return circulation, and Kellogg stated that for superficial kneading the relation to the veins is not important. Mennell began kneading of the limbs at the proximal portion of an area and progressing to the more distal portion. This kneading is performed with the two hands on opposite sides of the limb, the whole palmar surface being in contact with the part. Gentle pressure is then applied, usually as the hands work in opposite directions. He stated that the pressure is gentle, alternating waves of compression and relaxation are applied to a series of points, and the pressure is greatest when the hand is engaged with the "lowest part of the circumference of the circle and least when at the opposite pole."

Friction

Their descriptions of friction betray much confusion among the users of this form of massage. Kleen (1921) and Mennell, unlike the other authors, used the plural "frictions," although they did not agree on pressure. Kleen prescribed that the pressure be quite hard, and Mennell said it should be light, slowly progressing to deep, depending on the conditions present. Hoffa asserted that the pressure seeks to penetrate deep; Mitchell and Kellogg said that it is moderate.

Grosvenor (1825) and Graham stated that friction is given with long strokes, whereas most of the other authors wanted it done with small circular motions. Graham said friction may be circular or rectilinear (the latter parallel or horizontal to the long axis of the limb). According to Kellogg, the direction is from "below upward," following the large veins, and the motion is centripetal, centrifugal, circular, or spiral rotary. Kellogg also stated that the hands should slip over the skin and that the entire surface of the palms should be used. This view was also shared by Grosvenor and Graham. Hoffa, Bucholz, Despard, and Mennell prescribed that the movement be done with the ball of the thumb or fingers, which remain in contact with the skin and move it over the underlying tissues. Influenced by Ling, several authors used the French term *"massage à friction,"* which movement is no doubt similar to the contemporary friction or frictions.

The modern proponents of friction techniques are Cyriax (1959, 1977, 1978) and Dicke (1978). Cryiax speaks of deep transverse frictions of muscles, tendons, and ligaments; the pulling strokes of Dicke and associates use dry, forceful friction between the fingertips and the skin.

With regard to the tissues to which friction should be applied, Kleen, Mitchell, and Mennell used it on small areas, whereas Graham extended each stroke from joint to joint. There seem to be two very distinct ideas about this movement. One holds that the friction occurs between the hand and the skin surface (e.g., Dicke uses a distinct pattern of short pulling strokes in specific areas). The other (which seems currently to be more acceptable) prescribes that the part of the hand being used be kept in contact with the skin and that the superficial tissues be moved over the deeper (underlying) ones.

Stroking and Effleurage

These movements are so similar that they can be discussed together. Like kneading and petrissage, these French and English terms are almost interchangeable. Mennell did not include the term "effleurage" in his classification of massage movements. It is generally agreed that the direction of the movement is centripetal; however, Mennell and Kellogg differ. They both used the term "stroking," and Kellogg stated that the direction is "with the blood current in the arteries," though he did not mention the amount of pressure. Mennell divided stroking into superficial and deep manipulations. Superficial stroking may be either centripetal or centrifugal, but the pressure, while firm, must be only the lightest touch possible to maintain contact. Deep stroking moves in the direction of the venous and lymphatic flow.

Despard used both stroking and effleurage: the direction of both is centripetal, but the pressure in stroking is vigorous and in effleurage "should vary according to the condition of the patient." Other factors in the movements were very similar, and she described the motion of effleurage as stroking, as did Ling, Mezger, Kleen, and Mitchell.

Ling said the pressure of effleurage varies from the lightest touch to "one of considerable force." Murrell and Kleen said that it varies, whereas Hoffa and Bucholz used light pressure at the beginning of the stroke, increased it over the fleshy part of the muscle, and decreased it again at the end. Mitchell varied the pressure according to the region being treated and used heavy pressure on the upward stroke, keeping the hand in contact to return but with much less pressure. Bucholz also kept the hand in contact for a return stroke, touching the skin very lightly.

Most authors agreed that stroking and effleurage are to be given over large areas. Mennell emphasized that the muscles must be relaxed, and Hoffa and Bucholz said that the movement should follow the anatomic outlines of the muscles. Nearly all authors advocated using the palm of the hand for effleurage and stroking. In addition to the palm, some used the heel of the hand, its edge, the tips of the fingers, the ball of the thumb, and the knuckles for effleurage and stroking. Hoffa, Bucholz, Despard, and Mennell recommended that the palm be in good contact and conform to the contour of the area being treated.

COMPONENTS OF MASSAGE

The factors that must be considered in the application of therapeutic massage techniques are direction of the movement, amount of pressure, rate and rhythm of the movements, media used (including instruments other than the hand), position of patient and the therapist, and duration and frequency of the treatment. Each of these is considered from a historical perspective.

Direction

The literature shows that until the time of Hippocrates the direction of massage was centrifugal (Johnson, 1866). The contributions of Hippocrates to medicine are outstanding, and he demonstrated his genius in the use of massage as well as in many other medical treatments. He favored the centripetal direction for massage movements. He was unusual in his emphasis on clinical observation, and we can assume that he based his choice of direction on clinical observations of the effects of treatment. (The circulation of the blood was not described until nearly two thousand years later.) Asclepiades (125–56 B.C.), a Roman who lived a few centuries after Hippocrates, believed that the body was composed of regularly distributed canals in which nutritive juices moved. Sickness was thought to be a disturbance of the normal movement of these juices. He attempted to restore free flow of the nutritive juices by rubbing but gave no direction for the movement (Johnson, 1866).

Galen, five centuries after Hippocrates, varied the direction of massage movements depending on the purpose of the massage and its relation to exercise. At the beginning of the nineteenth century Ling advocated light stroking in a centrifugal direction and deeper pressure with centripetal movements. This concept has held to the present day. In the superficial stroking technique of Lucas-Championnière, as described by Mennell, the direction may be either centrifugal or centripetal but without deviation once the direction is established (Mennell, 1945). These later writers expressed very clearly what effects were expected from movements in the centripetal direction as compared with those in the centrifugal direction. Murrell (1886) asserted that the direction be "from below upwards" and in the direction of the muscle fibers. Hoffa and Bucholz were among the first to mention that the direction should be congruent with the venous and lymphatic circulation. Mennell said all deep movements of massage should be performed centripetally to aid venous and lymphatic flow. Many authors advocated beginning the movement at the proximal (rather than the distal) portion of a segment, but with the direction of the pressure in each movement being in the direction of venous flow (centripetal) even though the succession of the movements is in the opposite (centrifugal) direction.

Some massage techniques, such as deep friction and connective tissue massage (CTM), are specific about direction of the movement in the area where they are applied.

Pressure

Consideration of pressure seems to have been important from the earliest description of massage movements, although there was no consensus among early practitioners. The Greek authors Herodikus (ca. 500 B.C.) and Herodotus (484–425 B.C.) varied the pressure during the movement: gentle at first, then greater, and toward the end gentle again (Johnson, 1866). Later, Hippocrates distinguished the types of pressure, mentioning gentle, hard, soft, and moderate. He emphasized the importance of selecting the correct pressure for a given technique, to obtain the desired result, as in the frequently quoted statement, *"Hard rubbing binds; soft rubbing loosens; much rubbing causes parts to waste; moderate rubbing makes them grow."*

Ambroise Pare, the most renowned surgeon of the sixteenth century, recognized a difference in the amount of pressure used (Graham, 1884) and described three kinds of friction—gentle, medium, and vigorous—and the effects of each. From the fifteenth through the beginning of the eighteenth century emphasis on heavy pressure seemed to be growing. The extremist in this regard was Admiral Henry (1731–1823) of the British Navy, who believed that "great violence" was important (Johnson, 1866). He described some of the manipulations as painful, "but they cease to be so if persevered in, and become even pleasant." (Rolfing seems to some to be a modern-day application of Henry's beliefs.) Eventually massage became a well-accepted part of medical treatment in the British Royal Navy, where it has a proud tradition (Stockton, 1994).

Beveridge emphasized the importance of touch with varying pressure and the differences in the effects produced depending on the amount of pressure. In the early part of the nineteenth century he wrote, "The finger of a good rubber will descend upon an excited and painful nerve as gently as the dew on the grass, but upon a torpid callosity as heavily as the hoof of an elephant."

Mezger varied the pressure with the type of movement. That for effleurage was gentle, and that for *massage à friction* was "with considerable force" (Berghman & Helleday, 1873). This force must have been considerable, as Colombo, one of his contemporaries, stated that Mezger's patients frequently had blue spots on their bodies. Zabludowski, who was known as the king of German masseurs, criticized the gentle massage advocated by Lucas-Championnière for the treatment of fractures. Zabludowski said that when massage became painless it ceased to be massage and was merely treatment by suggestion; though in a book written later (1903) Zabludowski wrote that massage is not in most cases painful and that when it necessarily becomes painful the pain should subside. Bucholz, writing in 1917, did not agree with Zabludowski's early concepts. He believed all needed effects could be obtained without such abuse of force.

About the same time Kleen and Hoffa showed they appreciated the finesse of technique, together with knowledge, and they regulated the pressure according to the bulk of the tissues, increasing it when working on the belly of a muscle and lessening it at the ends of the muscle. (In this we see recognition of the early concepts of Herodikus and

Herodotus.) They also observed that the proper amount can be judged only by practice.

Throughout the late nineteenth and early twentieth centuries many authors gave the impression that the greater the pressure, the more effective is the massage. They began the treatment or series of treatments with gentle pressure and "worked up" to the pressure tolerance level of the patient. Kellogg stated that the patient's tolerance is established during prolonged treatment, beginning gently and increasing pressure gradually until almost the "whole strength of the operator might be employed without injuring the patient." Despard stated that the "vigour" and amount of pressure should vary according to the condition of the patient, being always gentle at the beginning of the course of treatment and gradually increasing as the patient improves.

Mennell was outstanding in his rationale for the use of massage. He stated that the amount of pressure depends solely on the relaxation of the muscles. When the muscles are relaxed throughout the treatment, even a light pressure must influence every structure throughout the part being treated. He believed that movement can be deep without in any sense being forcible. He reasoned that if the muscles are relaxed they offer no more resistance to the movement than does so much fluid, and any pressure applied on the surface will be transmitted freely to all structures under the hand. He said that practice with a skill that is born only of a delicate sense of touch will show how very light may be the pressure that suffices to compress any structure to its fullest extent and, therefore, incidentally to empty the veins and lymphatic spaces. He also said, "The delusion is deep rooted—and will die hard—that 'stimulation' in massage is impossible without the expenditure of muscle energy and vigour. A delusion, nevertheless, it is." Connective tissue massage techniques use firm pressure but avoid pain.

Rate and Rhythm

Some authors mentioned briefly the rate of massage movements, but few addressed rhythm. Others combined the two. Of the early writers, Herodikus and Herodotus both considered pressure and rate. They advocated gentle and slow movements in the beginning, rapid and heavy ones next, and slow and gentle movements to end (Kellogg, 1919). Hippocrates, describing the treatment of a dislocated shoulder, stated, "It is necessary to rub the shoulder gently and smoothly." None of the users of massage after Hippocrates made mention of rate or rhythm until the eighteenth century. Beveridge evidently considered great speed an advantage: he believed that flexibility of the fingers is important as it permits rapid motion. Ling varied rate according to the type of movement: effleurage should be given slowly; rolling, shaking, and tapotement rapidly. Mezger agreed that effleurage should be given slowly.

Graham, Kellogg, and Bucholz were specific about the

rate (number of strokes per minute) but not about the distance covered in each stroke; thus, the number of strokes had no specific relationship to rhythm. These authors specified different numbers of strokes. For friction Graham specified 90 to 180 strokes per minute. Bucholz prescribed that the speed should depend on the desired effect. ("In irritable cases a slow gentle stroke may produce a marked effect, while in treating an atrophic limb of an otherwise healthy person, considerable speed, up to 50 to 60 times a minute or more, with a good deal of pressure may be applied.") Kellogg adjusted the speed depending on the type of movement and stated the distance to be covered with each stroke. Stroking, he thought, should not cover more than 1 or 2 inches per second; friction, 30 to 80 strokes per minute, depending on the length of the stroke; and petrissage, "not too rapid," 30 to 90 strokes per minute ("more rapid in small parts").

Kleen varied the rate according to the area treated: he thought effleurage on the shoulder and back should be rapid. Lucas-Championnière emphasized that massage should be slow and uniform, with rhythmic repetitions. Zabludowski stated that the area covered to some extent determines the speed. He compared the rhythm to that of music and suggested that a metronome be used in practice, but not as a regular guide. Despard varied the rate and rhythm according to the effect desired. For a soothing effect she recommended effleurage be given slowly and rhythmically, and for a stimulating effect the strokes should be "quick and strong." She varied the rate and vigor according to the condition of the patient and performed all movements rhythmically.

In describing stroking movements some authors distinguished between the rate of the primary stroke and that of the return stroke, making the return stroke more rapid, which creates an uneven rhythm. Mitchell advised this and asserted that a common fault of massage is making the movements too fast. Mennell identified these essentials of superficial stroking: (1) the movements must be slow, gentle, and rhythmic, and there must be no hesitancy or irregularity about it; (2) the time between the end of the stroke and the beginning of the next should be identical with the time of stroking throughout the movement. He believed the rhythm must be even to produce an even stimulus. For the stroke from shoulder to hand, he prescribed 15 movements per minute. For deep stroking, he said, there is no need for great speed, as the flow of venous blood is slow and that of the lymph even slower. He thought that kneading too rapidly is inimical to success, and that for frictions the rhythm should be slow and steady. The movements in connective tissue massage are unhurried, but not of any precise rate or rhythm.

Media

The stories of Homer imply that as early as 1000 B.C. an oily medium was used for massage. According to Homer's Odyssey, beautiful women rubbed and anointed the war-worn heroes to rest and refresh them. Herodotus advised that a "greasy mixture" should be poured over the body before rubbing, and Plato (427–347 B.C.) and Socrates (470–399 B.C.) refer to the benefit received from anointing with oils and rubbing as an "assuager of pain" (Graham, 1913). Olive oil was the preferred medium, and it was believed that the oil itself had some therapeutic value. Roman history records that Cicero's health was much improved by his anointer's ministrations.

Celsus made a distinction between rubbing and unction, or anointing. The rubbing in of greasy substances he called "unction." Other authors later contended that unction could not be performed without friction of some sort. In the days of Galen, the massage following exercise used more oil than the one given before exercise. He recommended rubbing with a towel to produce redness, followed by rubbing with oil for the purpose of "warming up" and softening the body in preparation for exercise.

Henry used unique media. He also devised various instruments and tools that he said "would prevent the nerves and tendons from falling asleep or getting fixed." If these structures were kept in constant motion, "the blood would pass quickly through the blood vessels, leaving no fur behind it, so that ossification which so frequently terminates the human existence is prevented." The instruments were made of wood and bone. Cattle ribs were used principally, as it was very useful to have bent instruments. He also used a hammer with a piece of cork covered with leather as well as the rounded end of a glass vial (Johnson, 1866). Graham followed a similar method to a certain extent for percussion. He suggested that the back of a brush or the sole of a slipper could be used, but even better were India rubber balls attached to steel or whalebone handles (Graham, 1913).

In exceptional circumstances, Murrell said, a bundle of swan feathers, lightly tied together, could be used for tapotement. For reflex stroking Kellogg used the fingernail, the end of a lead pencil, a wooden toothpick, or the head of a pin. On the island of Tonga in the early nineteenth century it is reported that "three or four little children tread under their feet the whole body of the patient" (Graham, 1913). At about this time, the Russians and the Finns used bundles of birch twigs for flagellation before steam baths, and the Hawaiians gave massage while patients were submerged in water.

The more recent users of massage have different opinions about using media for massage. Some object to any sort of medium, and those who use a medium choose either an oily lubricant or a powder. Those who use no medium, or dry massage, assert that it is cleaner; gives a more certain feeling to the hands and steadier movements; is more stimulating; and makes it unnecessary to expose the patient's body. It seems incredible, but frequently massage has been administered with the patient clothed. Galen records that when a gymnast inquired of Quintas what was the value of anointing (rubbing with oil), he replied, "It makes you take off your tunic." Some types of massage do require a dry technique for effective treatment (e.g., deep friction and connective tissue massage).

A variety of compounds, both liquid and solid, have been suggested by those who use oil as a lubricant. The more commonly mentioned ones are olive oil, glycerine, coconut oil, oil of sweet almonds, and neat's–foot oil. Some users prefer solid lubricants because the liquid oils are hard to handle. The solid lubricants suggested are wool fat, petroleum jelly, lanolin, hog's lard, cold cream, and cocoa butter.

Zabludowski was quite specific in his preference for white Virginia petroleum jelly because it was "odorless and tasteless and quite neutral." He said that the chief basis for the use of any lubricant was personal preference. Those who recommend oily lubricants say that they make the skin soft, smooth, and slippery; prevent the pain of pulling hair; and prevent acne. Some of those who are opposed to the use of oily lubricants claim that they promote the growth of hair.

Others who use a medium recommend powder, as they believe it is more pleasant for general massage, makes possible deep kneading, and improves the sense of touch. Several users recommend it particularly to prevent the moisture of the masseur's hands from abrading the patient's skin. Grosvenor recommended the use of "fine hair powder," and writers of more recent date suggest talcum or boric acid powder. A few writers suggest soapsuds as a medium, especially to help remove dead skin from a limb that was casted in plaster.

Mennell said the selection of a medium is a personal preference and believed the best one is the simplest, namely, French chalk, which might be improved by adding oil. He, as well as other users, recommended an oily medium, especially when the skin is dry and scaly. Some suggested that it be used on children and the aged. Of the later users in this group, the reason, though it was not stated, undoubtedly was to avoid abrading sensitive skin; earlier writers believed that the medium itself had curative power.

Position of Therapist and Patient

The early writers gave very little indication of the position of the patient or of the masseur while giving massage. Nothing was written of this until about the seventeenth century. However, a bas-relief of the return of soldiers from war, as described in Homer's *Odyssey*, depicts massage being given to Ulysses. He is seated, and the masseuse is crouching in a most uncomfortable position in front of him giving massage to his leg.

Alpinus said the patient should be "extended horizontally." Many of the later writers described the patient's position in detail and emphasized that the patient should be relaxed—this after the patient had been placed in such a position that relaxation would seem to be utterly impossible. Very few of them gave a rationale for the positions they prescribed, and they seemed to disregard entirely any effect that gravity might have on venous or lymphatic flow. Ling emphasized that the muscles must be relaxed for many movements and yet described rolling and shaking the arm while the seated patient held the arm horizontal with the hand on a table or the back of a chair (Kellgren, 1890).

Grosvenor's position for massage of the lower extremity was described by Cleoburey: "The female rubber [Grosvenor always employed females] is seated on a low stool, and taking the patient's limb in her lap (which position gave her command over it) so as to enable her to rub with extended hands." The position of the patient is not described. One would assume that he or she was seated in a position similar to the one shown in the Greek bas-relief of Ulysses.

Graham said the patient should be in a comfortable position, with joints midway between flexion and extension and warned that if the "manipulator" was too close to the patient his movements would be cramped and that if he was too far away the movements would be indefinite, superficial, and lacking in energy (Graham, 1913).

Kleen described a bench on which the patient was to lie and which was approachable from all sides. The masseur stood or sat beside it. He gave much detail of patient positions for the treatment of various areas. For massage of the neck and throat he had the patient sit on the bench (Kleen, 1921).

Hoffa recommended support to the entire length of the part of the body that is being treated, so that the muscles are relaxed, yet he had the patient sit on a stool for massage of the head, neck, shoulders, and upper arms. For massage of the elbow, forearm, hand, and fingers, an illustration shows the patient sitting with these parts resting on a table. To treat the leg and foot, the patient sits on the table with the foot supported in the lap of the masseur. He said that the masseur's position should be "comfortable and not strained," always beside the patient's bed, and avoiding as much as possible frequent and unnecessary changes of position. For the thigh, the masseur sits beside the reclining patient (Hoffa, 1897).

Zabludowski recommended a comfortable and relaxed position for the patient. The exact position depended on the part to be treated. The patient's glasses were to be removed and the lighting and room temperature adjusted to ensure comfort. Some work might even be done with the patient standing, and small children might be held in the masseur's lap if a table was not available. He emphasized the posture of the masseur and said the standing position was preferred. The masseur should have a sure footing and coordinated movements, to ease his work and avoid too much flexing and extending in many joints. Zabludowski added some quaint rules for the masseur: he should watch his watch chain so it does not bother the patient; he should wear glasses instead of *"pince-nez"* which might slide off the nose if he perspired; he should wear a jersey (knit) undershirt, heavy or light according to the season; he should not work in street clothes, should remove his rings, wear short sleeves, and even remove things from pockets that are in the way when he is sitting (Zabludowski, 1903).

Mitchell (1904) recommended that the patient be reclining, and for some areas that the operator sit on the edge of the bed with the patient's foot in his lap. Bucholz said the patient should be in a comfortable position that would also allow the operator to work with sufficient comfort. Bucholz also did not favor the sitting position for massaging the legs, though he thought it might be used for the foot and calf if the patient was sitting on a table and the "operator" was in front of the patient on a chair (Bucholz, 1917).

Despard recommended that the patient should be in a comfortable position with the muscles relaxed; yet for back stroking she said the patient might stand with the hands resting against a wall or other support (Despard, 1932).

Mennell said the most important factors in performing all stroking movements are the position of the patient and of the masseur, and the relative position of one to the other. He gave no set rules for either's position but said there should be a reason for every position of the masseur and for the position in which the part under treatment is placed. Some of the illustrations in his text show the masseur standing and in others he is sitting. Stroking of the lower extremity was illustrated to point out some common faults of positioning of the patient and of the masseur (Mennell, 1945).

In discussing the effect of massage on venous flow, Mennell considered the effect of gravity to be very important. He recommended that the patient lie recumbent on the table, in a position that allows relaxation of abdominal muscles, with the thighs supported to enhance venous and lymphatic flow from the distal part of the lower extremity. To treat edema of an extremity, he recommended elevating the part while giving the massage. For patients with respiratory problems there are specific positions for postural drainage (see Chapter 9), and the therapist accommodates his or her position and stance accordingly.

In the basic position for connective tissue massage, the patient sits with the back toward the therapist. Lighting is important when the therapist is assessing the patient's problems. In addition to the basic back section, other parts of the body can be treated, and the patient is positioned accordingly (see Chapter 10).

Duration

Galen was one of the first users of massage to address the duration of a treatment, though he advocated a trial-and-error approach. He wrote, "What shall be the duration of the rubbing it is impossible to declare in words; but the director, being experienced in these matters, on the first day must form a conjecture, which shall not be very accurate, but the next day, having already acquired some experience in the constitution of this subject, he will reduce his conjecture continually to greater accuracy."

Grosvenor gave very specific directions for the duration of treatment. He said that friction should at first be continued for an hour, "observing always to rub by the watch" (Cleoburey, 1825; Johnson, 1866). Murrell said the entire duration of a local massage should not exceed 8 to 10 minutes and that other authorities thought 4 minutes was enough. Kleen believed the duration of a treatment was important but that no hard and fast rule could be given. Local massage, he thought, usually should last 15 minutes and general massage at least half an hour and sometimes longer. Hoffa suggested 10 to 20 minutes for local and 30 to 45 minutes for general massage.

Zabludowski said the duration may be 5 to 30 minutes, depending on the size of the affected area, the patient's age, duration of illness, and constitution and habits of the patient. With regard to the time frame over which treatments should continue, he said it depends on the condition to be treated, the prognosis, and so forth, but is usually 2 to 3 weeks. According to Graham, the condition of the patient and the effect of the massage should determine the duration of the treatment. Bucholz said the duration of the treatment should depend on the desired effect. For a fresh injury he stated that 5 to 10 minutes may be adequate, whereas a general massage should last 40 to 50 minutes. Despard prescribed a definite period of time for massaging each area of the body and said the duration of the treatment should increase as the patient's condition improves.

Mennell believed it necessary to consider the age of the patient when administering massage. If the sole aim is to secure a reflex effect, in very young and aged persons, Mennell believed that the duration of treatment should be lessened. For treatment of neurasthenia Mennell said the maximum duration is 75 minutes, which may be attained in comparatively few cases (and never during the earlier stages of treatment). At first, 20 minutes is often sufficient and the treatments may be gradually increased in duration and, toward the end, should be decreased in a similar manner. In cases of injury, however, he emphasized the danger of prolonging the series of the massage treatments in lieu of active exercise as the patient improves.

Frequency

Celsus, a noted medical author though not a physician, wrote merely as an encyclopedist in his *De Medicina* (1665), presenting ideas that appealed to him and were drawn from the available literature. We may assume, therefore, that his writings express some of the ideas that were popular at that time. He gave some details of massage technique and appreciated the value of correct "dosage." He stated, "We should pay no attention to those who define numerically how often anyone is to be rubbed; for this must be gathered from the individual; and if he is very feeble, 50 times may be enough; if more robust, it may be requisite to rub 200 times, and between both limits according to the strength." He also believed treatments should be done less frequently for women, children, and elders than for men (Celsus, 1665; Johnson, 1866).

Grosvenor advised daily treatment (more or less as the case would permit), gradually increased to three times daily. Murrell also believed in frequent treatment (three or four times daily), but each treatment was much briefer than Grosvenor's. Kleen believed massage should be given at least once daily—and in some cases, for injury, several times daily. Hoffa recommended daily massage. Zabludowski advocated daily massage in most cases but believed that the physical and psychological reactions of the patient should determine the frequency. If quick results were desired, he believed treatments should be given twice daily, but in cases that necessitated "weaning from massage" the frequency of treatments should be lessened gradually to two or three per week.

Graham recognized the frequency of treatment as part of the "dosage" of massage, which should be regulated according to the patient's condition. He associated force with the frequency and duration of treatment, local massage being done frequently and general massage at least once daily. In contrast to Zabludowski's weaning from massage, Graham said the frequency could be increased after four or five treatments. Bucholz said that the frequency of treatment depends largely on the patient's social condition but advised twice daily massage in many surgical cases. He believed it wise to begin with short sessions and to increase according to the patient's reaction.

SUMMARY

Historically, many pioneers of massage technique seemed to have no physiologic basis for their techniques, particularly in relation to pressure, rate of movements, and positioning of the patient. The heavy pressure advocated in the fifteenth through the early eighteenth centuries was supplanted by more gentle massage, as introduced by Lucas-Championnière and Mennell in the early twentieth century. It is amazing that this same conclusion was appreciated by Hippocrates, who certainly did not have the scientific and physiologic information available today. At the beginning of the twentieth century Bucholz and Hoffa began to show some rational application of massage technique based upon knowledge of physiology, but in this respect Mennell is outstanding.

Clearly, then, opinions differ widely on most aspects of the various techniques known as "medical massage." Over the centuries some aspects of the techniques have received considerable attention at the expense of others. As a result, it is difficult to identify well-reasoned rationales for most of the techniques used in massage. In this respect, of course, massage treatments were no different from other so-called medical treatments of the same time era. Medical

treatments were often based on anecdotal information. Except for the fact that they appeared to help many patients and seemed worth continuing, medical understanding of massage owed little to "science." Certainly the focus was on the "art" of massage, rather than its "scientific" basis in medical practice. The present text is mindful of the rich tradition of massage treatments and seeks to bring a more reasoned approach to the practice of this ancient art. To this end, each of the various massage strokes is carefully described, and, where appropriate, the clinical and scientific rationale for their use is considered.

References and Bibliography

Beard G. (1952) History of massage technique. Phys Ther Rev 32:613–624.
Berghman G, Helleday U. (1873) Anteckningar om massage. Nord Med Arkin 5(7).
Blundell JWF. (1864) The muscles and their story from the earliest times. London: Chapman and Hall.
Bohm M. (1918) Massage—its principles and technic. Philadelphia: Chas F Saunders.
Broca P. (1876) Sur l'age des sujets à la trépanation chirurgicale néolithique. Bull Soc Anthrop de Paris xi:572.
Bucholz CH. (1917) Therapeutic exercise and massage. Philadelphia: Lea & Febiger.
Celsus AC. (1665) De medicina., Leiden, Nederlands:
Cleoburey W. (1825) System of friction, 3rd ed. London: Munday & Slatter.
Cole J, Stovell E. (1991) Exercise and massage in health care through the ages. In Winterton P, Gurry D (eds): The impact of the past upon the present: Second National Conference of the Australian Society of the History of Medicine, Perth, July 1991. Perth: Hawthorn Press, pp 42–48.
Cyriax J. (1959) Treatment by massage and manipulation. New York: Paul Hoeber.
Cyriax J. (1978) Textbook of orthopedic medicine, vol 1, 7th ed. New York: Macmillan.
Cyriax J, Russell G. (1977) Textbook of orthopedic medicine, vol II, 9th ed. Baltimore: Williams & Wilkins.
Despard L. (1932) Textbook of massage and remedial gymnastics, 3rd ed. New York: Oxford University Press.
de Watteville A. (1885a) The cure of writer's cramp. Br Med J 1:323–324.
de Watteville A. (1885b) Further observations on the cure of writer's cramp. Lancet i: 790–792.
Dicke E, Schliach H, Wolff A, Sidney S. (1978) A manual of reflexive therapy of the connective tissue: "Bindegewebsmassage" (connective tissue massage). Scarsdale, NY: Simon.
Estradere J. (1863) Du massage. Pans, France: Ecole de Medecine.
Feltham E. (1991) Therapeutic touch and massage. Nurs Standard 5(45):26–28.
Green RM. (1951) De sanitate tuenda (A translation of Galen's *Hygiene*). Springfield, IL: Charles C Thomas.
Graham D. (1884) Practical treatise on massage. New York: Wm. Wood.
Graham D. (1913) Massage—manual treatment and remedial movements. Philadelphia: JB Lippincott.

Graham D. (1917) Writer's cramp and allied affections: Their treatment by massage and kinesitherapy. Edin Med J 19:231–239.

Grosvenor J. (1825) A full account of the system of friction adopted and pursued with the greatest success in cases of contracted joints and lameness from various causes. Oxford.

Henry L. (1884) Massage. Aust Med J 6:337–347.

Hoffa A. (1897) Tecknik der Massage. Stuttgart: Ferdinand Ernke.

Jabre J. (1994) "Nerve rubbing" in the symptomatic treatment of ulnar nerve paresthesiae. Nerve Muscle October:1237.

Johnson W. (1866) The anatriptic art. London: Simkin Marshall.

Kamenetz HL. (1960) History of massage. In Licht S. (ed): Massage, manipulation and traction. New Haven: Elizabeth Licht, pp 3–37.

Kamenetz HL. (1985) History of massage. In Basmajian JV (ed): Manipulation, traction and massage, 3rd ed. Baltimore: Williams & Wilkins.

Kellgren A. (1890) The technic of Ling's system of manual treatment. Edinburgh and London: Young J. Pentland.

Kellogg JH. (1919) The art of massage, 12th ed revised. Battle Creek, MI: Modern Medical Publ.

Kleen EAG. (1906) Handbook i massage och sjukgymnastik, Stockholm: Nordin and Josephson.

Kleen EAG. (1921) Massage and medical gymnastics, 2nd ed. New York: Wm. Wood.

Krieger D. (1979) Therapeutic touch: How to use your hands to help or to heal. Englewood Cliffs: Prentice Hall.

Krieger D. (1981) Foundations of holistic health nursing practices: The renaissance nurse. Philadelphia: JB Lippincott.

Lace MV. (1946) Massage and medical gymnastics. London: J&A Churchill, pp 33–35.

Mason A. (1992). Rub, rub, rubbish: Massage in the nineteenth century, Physiotherapy. JCSP 78(9):666.

McMillan M. (1925) Massage and therapeutic exercise. Philadelphia: WB Saunders.

Mennell JB. (1945) Physical treatment, 5th ed. Philadelphia: Blakiston.

Mitchell JK. (1904) Massage and exercise in system of physiologic therapeutics. Philadelphia: Blakiston.

Murrell W. (1886a) Massage as a therapeutic agent. Br Med J i:926–927.

Murrell W. (1886b) Massage as a mode of treatment. London: HK Lewis.

Prunieres A. (1874) Sur les crânes artificiellement perforés et les rondelles crâniennes à l'époque des dolmens. Bull Soc Anthrop de Paris ix:185.

Quintner J. (1993) Apropos rub, rub, rubbish: Massage in the nineteenth century. Physiotherapy, JCSP 79(1):32.

Quintner J. (1994) Aye, there's the rub, down under. Physiotherapy, JCSP 80(8):519–520.

Robins RP. (1885) On writer's cramp. In Braithwaite J (ed): The retrospect of medicine, Vol xcii. London: Simpkin, Marshall, pp 152–155.

Stockton J. (1994) The history of massage and physiotherapy in the Royal Navy. Physiotherapy, JCSP 80(1): 40–42.

Tappan F. (1978) Healing massage techniques—a study of eastern and western methods, Reston, VA: Reston Publishing.

Tappan F. (1988) Healing massage techniques—holistic, classic and emerging methods, 2nd ed. Norwalk, CT: Appleton & Lange.

Thomas's medical dictionary (1886) Philadelphia: JB Lippincott.

Veith I. (1949) Huang Ti. The yellow emperor's classic of internal medicine. Baltimore: Williams & Wilkins.

Zabludowski JB. (1903) Technique of massage. Leipzig: Thieme.

Chapter 2

Basic Requirements for Therapeutic Massage

This chapter deals with the basic requirements for the effective and professional practice of therapeutic massage. Important ethical considerations are clearly relevant to the practice of this medical art, and the basic issues are discussed in some detail. The technical requirements for the administration of massage treatments include the type of equipment to be used, methods of positioning the patient, and the various lubricants, to mention just a few. All of these issues are covered in this chapter, so as to separate them from the descriptions of the basic massage strokes in the next chapter. Each of the issues discussed in this chapter is relevant to the material discussed in most of the remainder of the text.

ETHICAL ISSUES

As a health professional, any therapist should present him- or herself for massage treatments in the same manner as they would to deliver any other treatment modality. Observing the usual high standards of personal hygiene and cleanliness leaves the patient feeling confident of an effective and "professional" treatment. Since massage treatment involves the exposure of the body part to be treated and direct touching of the patient by the therapist, a high standard of ethical practice is essential. Inappropriate touching and unnecessary exposure are to be avoided at all times. Several ethical issues will be mentioned in some of the sections that follow in this chapter.

Therapists should be relaxed in their manner and movements, allowing them to concentrate on their treatment. As in all treatments, an adequate explanation to the patient is an essential prerequisite. There is considerable risk of scratching the patient if jewelry is worn on the wrists or fingers. In this respect, it is advisable for the therapist to work without such jewelry. Effective massage can be

strenuous work, so care and precision of performance are required to reduce the occupational risks of back injury.

KNOWLEDGE OF SURFACE ANATOMY

The effective use of soft tissue massage techniques requires a thorough knowledge and practical application of surface anatomy. Since the therapist's hands are moving the patient's tissues, it is essential that the therapist be familiar with the anatomic structures involved, especially when performing techniques that are designed to affect specific structures, for example, a tendon or part of a muscle. Obviously, if a technique is performed on the wrong structure treatment is unlikely to be successful. Clearly, there can be no substitute for thorough preparation in surface and gross anatomy. Though it is not the intention of this text to review surface anatomy, numerous references will be made to anatomic structures. It will always be assumed that the reader is familiar with the terminology used here.

HAND PREPARATION

The condition of the hands is extremely important to both therapist and patient. They must be clean and well-groomed. The nails should be kept reasonably short and the tips rounded, and they should not injure the patient through any of the strokes. Ideal hands for massage are probably well-padded, warm, supple, and dry. They should express sensitivity and gentleness, firmness and strength. For those learning massage techniques for the first time, suppleness may be increased with various hand exercises. Certain persons seem to have a natural ability to relax the hands and to move them rhythmically, and they will learn the techniques of massage more readily than others; however, anyone who conscientiously spends sufficient time in practice will learn contact and rhythm and acquire good technique.

Hands that have cuts, open sores, warts, or other skin lesions obviously are not suitable for massage treatments. It is obviously very important for therapists to take exceptional care of their hands if they are to be effective in the use of massage. Simple household, automotive, or garden work can be very damaging to the hands. Adequate protection with a suitable hand covering is therefore essential. The use of a high-quality hand or skin conditioner helps keep hands in good condition.

The hands should be washed before and after treatment and in general should always be scrupulously clean. Areas of hard, dry skin can be removed by gently rubbing a very mild abrasive, such as granulated sugar, into the hands. A very small amount of olive oil should be combined with the sugar to produce a paste that is then rubbed into rough areas of the skin. This technique can be repeated several times each day until the areas of hard skin soften. Granulated sugar does not dissolve in olive oil and, therefore, retains its mildly abrasive texture when it is rubbed into the skin. The olive oil also helps to soften the skin.

In massage treatments the hands fulfill two roles: they give movement to the skin, subcutaneous tissues, muscles, and other structures, and they acquire information about the condition of those tissues. In this respect, the hands may be viewed as mobile sensors, relaying information to the therapist on the condition of the tissues they are massaging. Moist, perspiring hands are a great disadvantage to the therapist and may be uncomfortable for the patient. This may be minimized by frequent washing of the hands and drying, possibly with some evaporating spirits.

It is important for the therapist to be relaxed during the application of massage, as most of the strokes are performed, not with the hands alone, but by using body weight and moving the body to different positions. Effective massage can be physically demanding, and the therapist who has strong, flexible hands and good upper body strength will likely find massage treatments much less tiring than those who are not so fit. Various exercises that strengthen and mobilize the hands and upper limbs in general will be

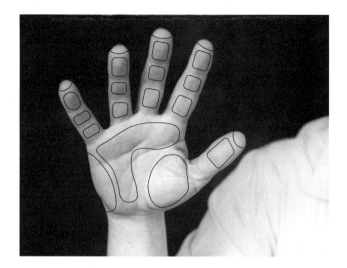

Figure 2–1. Areas of the hand used in massage.
Several areas in the hand can be used for massage. The circumscribed areas include the fingertips and pads, the thumb pad, and the entire palmar surface. The ulnar border of the hypothenar eminence can also be used.

of considerable benefit and should be seen as good "preventive maintenance" for the therapist. Figure 2–1 illustrates several areas of the hand that can be used in massage.

LUBRICANTS: POWDERS, OILS, AND CREAMS

If the therapist has warm, soft, dry hands, use of a lubricant may be unnecessary; however, most massage situations require the use of a lubricant to facilitate movement of the hands over body tissues. Several types of lubricant are available.

Powder

The most common type of lubricant is traditionally a finely powdered French chalk mixture or a mixture of starch, boracic, and chalk. These days, an unscented baby powder is probably the most suitable powder for massage. Heavily scented powders should be avoided, since many people find them offensive and a few are actually allergic to them. Powder has a great advantage over various oils and lotions as it allows the therapist to manipulate deep muscle tissue without risk of the hands' slipping on an oily surface. Powder facilitates the movement of the hand over the skin surface, but when pressure is applied, the hand and skin move together on the deep structures. This effect may be much harder to achieve when oils are used as lubricants.

Soap and Hot Water

Soap and hot water may be used for the dirty or dry, scaly skin that is commonly encountered when a body part has

---

Areas of the Hands That Can Be Used to Administer Massage

- The whole palmar surface of either or both hands
- The ulnar border of the hypothenar eminence
- One or more fingertips
- One or more finger pads
- Either or both thumb pads

been encased in plaster. It is particularly suitable for removing dead, dry skin where the tissues are somewhat undernourished.

Oils and Creams

Many types of oils and creams can be used for massage. They are particularly useful for treating the skin and subcutaneous tissues, especially scars, dry skin, and poorly nourished areas. High-quality olive oil is a commonly used natural oil; baby oil is also suitable.

Various kinds of creams may be used as a substitute for oil (e.g., lanolin, vitamin E, or cold cream). For general use, cold cream may be preferable to liquid oils because of the convenience of application. The cream should be a type that is absorbed slightly by the skin but is not so oily that a large amount remains on the skin after the massage is completed. Only an amount sufficient to allow the hands to glide smoothly over the skin should be used, as too much lubricant prevents a firm grasp of the tissues and leaves an excessive amount on the patient's skin. The right amount depends on the dryness of the patient's skin and of the therapist's hands. Experience will enable the therapist to choose the correct amount. The proper amount of lubricant for one area should be put on both palms and applied to the area with the first stroking movement.

Following treatment, any lubricant left on the skin surface should be removed, unless it is supposed to remain on the skin (e.g., lanolin or some other emollient). The lubricant should be applied sparingly to the hands of the therapist rather then directly to the patient. If the patient is powdered or "flooded" with lubricants, the skin pores may become clogged, an effect that tends to defeat some of the aims of massage.

EQUIPMENT

The most important equipment for successful massage treatment is a pair of well-trained hands directed by an intelligent mind. Other equipment is important however, and massage treatments are practiced with the patient well-supported in all positions. In most cases the patient lies on a proper treatment table (e.g., plinth, couch, bed). Ideally, the table's height should be adjustable to a position that is comfortable for the therapist.

Adequate support for the patient's head, shoulders, and other body parts is extremely important, especially when lying face down. These days, a wide variety of adjustable tables are available that greatly facilitate the practice of massage (Fig. 2–2).

These features help to ensure optimal positioning of the patient and therapist and significantly enhance the efficiency and overall comfort of the treatment for both patient and therapist. Other treatment table designs are available; one example is shown in Figure 2–3. These types of tables are usually made of metal and are operated hydraulically.

Massage can also be given while the patient sits. Small, wooden massage tables traditionally have been used for this purpose, though in recent times a variety of seating devices have been designed for treatment. Figure 2–4 illustrates such a device.

In addition to the equipment already described, two other devices are useful in massage treatments and are worthy of mention. The first is the so-called prone pillow. This device is laid flat on the treatment table and is designed to support the patient's head and shoulders. It is usually quite comfortable and has the greatest advantage of allowing a patient to be reasonably comfortable on a table that has no built-in face hole. Facial tissues should be used on the edges of the face hole to make the treatment more comfortable and hygienic for the patient. Some patients may find these pillows a little uncomfortable if their upper cervical joints are held in an extended position. Minor adjustments to the head position using small folded towels can usually fix any such problems (Fig. 2–5).

Another useful device is a wedge or bolster, a support usually placed so that the patient can lean against it. For this reason, the devices must be placed against a wall or a similar supporting surface. These devices can convert a nonadjustable flat treatment table into a very effective plinth. The wedge can also be used to support the patient's lower limbs. Figure 2–6 illustrates these uses.

The "Ideal" Treatment Table (i.e., One That Provides the Greatest Flexibility of Characteristics)

- Adjustable in height
- Equipped with a face/nose hole
- Made in at least three sections, of which the two end portions can be lifted
- Adjustable forearm rests
- Casters and a lift/lock mechanism

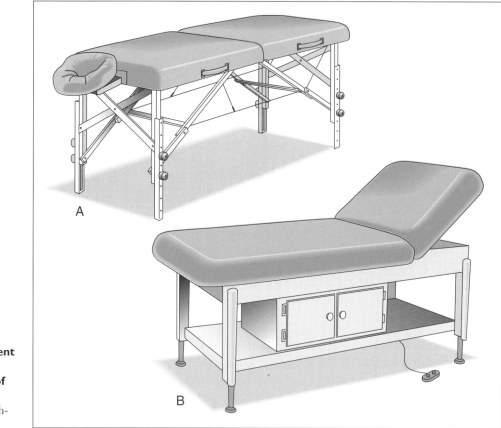

Figure 2–2. Several different types of treatment table suitable for the practice of massage.
Some are of fixed height; others are adjustable.

Figure 2–3. Example of an electrically operated hydraulic treatment table.
Note that the table is of metal construction and operated hydraulically by an electric motor. It has adjustable forearm supports and a face/nose hole in one end, and the other end can also be adjusted. Such a table is usually made of metal, but similar features can be found on wooden plinths, though the height of those is not usually adjustable. The table should not be too wide, because having to lean over the patient places undue stress on the therapist.

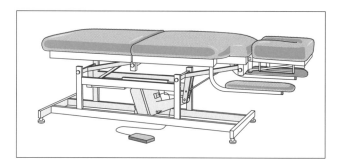

Figure 2–4. Characteristics of a seating device for massage.
The heights of the seat, headrest, and forearm rest are adjustable, making it easy to ensure the patient's comfort. These chairs are very useful in the treatment of the head and posterior neck region.

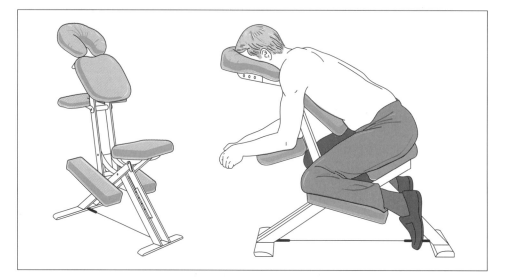

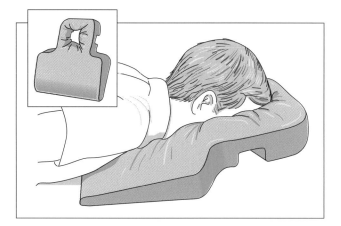

Figure 2–5. A prone pillow supports the head and shoulders.
The pillow is placed under the head and shoulders of the patient, allowing for the face to be supported in the face hole. Most people find these pillows quite comfortable when lying face down.

Other simple devices can also help support the body. For example, sandbags, sheets, towels, and small pillows can all be used to support specific areas of the patient's body when massage is part of a treatment plan. Certainly, it is important for patients to be supported comfortably during treatment; otherwise they may not be able to relax, and treatment may be less effective than it otherwise would be.

DRAPING AND POSITIONING THE PATIENT

The patient's position is crucial for effective massage. An uncomfortable patient will not be able to relax, and this will seriously interfere with the effect of the massage. Enough pillows are required to support all parts of the patient's body, to maximize relaxation. The patient should be kept warm throughout the treatment, and any parts not being massaged should be covered, when possible, with blankets, sheeting, or some similar drape. To induce relaxation in the patient the room should be warm and preferably quiet, and when possible the patient should be treated in private. It is very important at all times to preserve the patient's modesty, and to that end the patient should be adequately covered. At the same time the body parts being massaged must be accessible. The patient's actual position for massage will vary for each patient and each condition. The main criterion is that the patient be well supported and the part to be massaged readily available. The therapist should

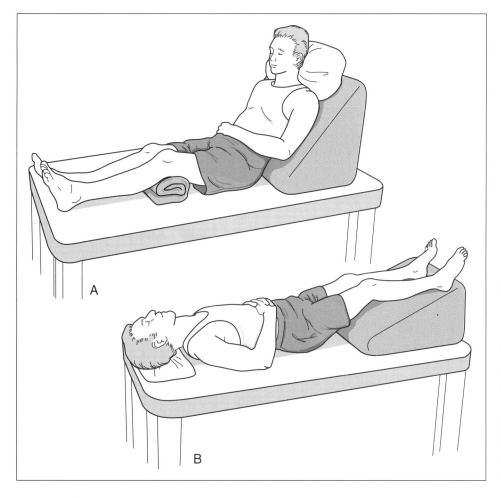

Figure 2–6. A movable "wedge" or "bolster" to support the patient while sitting or lying.
(A) The wedge is used as a support for a patient sitting on the treatment table. Note that for the wedge to be effective some sort of support must be placed behind it. (B) The wedge is used under the patient's lower limbs to elevate them (e.g., in cases of chronic edema in the legs).

stand so that he or she can reach the patient comfortably without having to stoop. Most massage strokes consist of a combination of total body movements plus hand movements in contact with the patient's body. As much as possible therapists should avoid flamboyant gestures, and the massage should be performed slowly and comfortably for the patient.

The patient may be draped with any of a number of different materials. The most versatile one is probably plain sheeting. A single folded sheet can be effective in draping a patient for treatment to any desired body part(s). If possible, the patient's own clothing should not be used for draping, since it is very likely that some massage lubricant will end up on the clothing. In therapeutic massage, the patient is always draped so that only the part(s) to be treated are exposed. There is no situation that requires the patient to be completely naked and exposed. Indeed, sound ethical practice demands that the patient be adequately draped and not unnecessarily exposed.

Many techniques can be used to drape the patient.

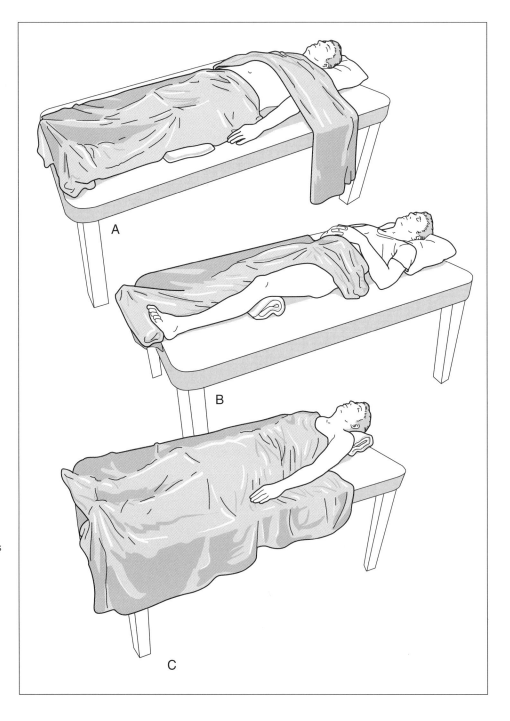

Figure 2–7. **Lying supine (facing the ceiling).**
(A) The patient is draped for treatment to the abdomen. A rolled towel or small pillow can be used to support the neck, and a pillow should also be placed under both knees.
(B) The patient is draped for treatment to the lower limb. A rolled towel or small pillow is useful to support the knee of the limb to be treated. A larger pillow tends to get in the way of the treatment and is best avoided. (C) The patient is draped for treatment to the upper limb. A small rolled towel placed under the neck affords easy access to the shoulder and neck region and is preferable to a large pillow. Note that the upper limb can be treated with the patient in several different positions.

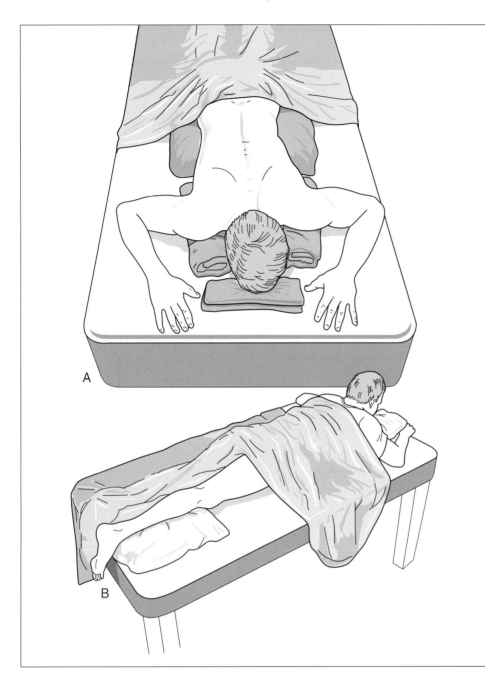

Figure 2–8. Lying prone (facing the floor).
(*A*) The patient is draped and positioned for massage to the back. Several methods can be used to support the patient in this position, but in all cases a pillow should be placed under the shin region of both legs. This will allow some knee flexion, and this takes the stress off of the sciatic nerve and its branches. In addition, a pillow should be placed under the abdomen, so that the lower edge of the pillow is in line with the anterior superior iliac spines. In this position it causes the lumbar spine to remain flat and supported. If the pillow is placed underneath the patient's hips, it causes too much hip flexion and related lumbar extension. The shoulders can be supported by a pillow or by two rolled towels placed at right angles to each clavicle. The patient can rest the head in a face hole in the treatment table or on a folded towel.
(*B*) The patient is draped and positioned for treatment of the posterior aspect of the lower limb. The method of supporting the patient is similar to that shown in *A*, but the draping allows the lower limb to be fully exposed.

Consideration needs to be given ahead of time to the final position of the patient and what draping will be required. For example, wrapping a folded sheet around a patient so that the loose end is in front is not a good idea if the patient will be lying face down because the patient and the therapist will have to struggle to expose the back. A much more effective technique is to place a folded sheet around the front of the patient so that both of the "loose ends" are at the back of the patient. When the patient then lies face down on the treatment table, it will be a simple matter to open the sheets to expose the back. The basic patient positions and typical draping techniques are illustrated in Figures 2–7 through 2–11.

The Most Common Positions for Massage Treatments

- Lying supine (facing the ceiling)
- Lying prone (facing the floor)
- Sitting upright on a plinth with both legs supported ("long sitting")
- Sitting upright on a stool or chair with the upper limb supported on a small table, the end of a plinth, or a pillow on the patient's lap
- Sitting upright on a stool facing a plinth, with the upper limbs and head supported on pillows

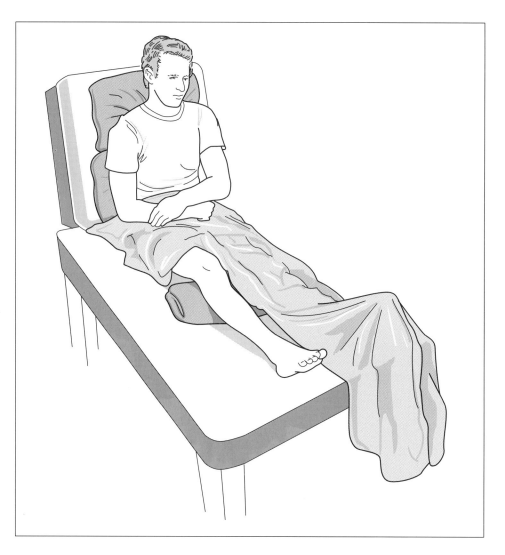

Figure 2–9. Sitting upright on a plinth with both legs supported (long sitting). This position is particularly suitable for treatment to the anterior aspect of the lower limb. The treated limb is best supported at the knee with a small rolled towel, as this allows the therapist's hands to work easily around the knee and calf region. Since the lower limb is the part to be treated, it is quite proper for the patient to wear his or her own clothing on the upper part of the body. If necessary, however, full draping is a simple procedure.

POSITION OF THE THERAPIST

Controlled relaxation of the hands can be achieved only if the therapist's posture permits controlled relaxation and free movement of the arms. When the patient is lying on a bed or treatment table, the so-called standing fall-out (walk standing) position is usually the most efficient stance. Backward and forward swaying with the knees and ankles bent then permits the therapist's arms and hands to be used over a large area with comparatively little movement at the hips and spine. Both feet should remain in contact with the floor at all times, to maintain balance. This swaying motion makes it possible to perform long, stroking movements rhythmically and smoothly, allows proper relaxation of arms and hands, and avoids the unnecessary fatigue associated with performing massage when standing in a strained, stooped position. It also utilizes the weight of the body to regulate the amount of pressure applied. This allows the therapist's body weight to be evenly distributed and makes it possible for him or her to move over a large area without bending the back. This is an important issue, especially since massage can be very strenuous work. Figure 2–12 illustrates the basic concept of good body mechanics in moving along the lower limb of a patient, without the need for much bending.

The height of the treatment table is very important in reducing the risk of back strain for the therapist. Adjustable-height treatment tables are a significant improvement in this regard. The height of the table should be such that the therapist can reach the body part in question while keeping his or her back upright. Fixed-height tables are a real problem for very tall therapists, since they have no option but to bend over the patient. Shorter therapists can remedy the situation by standing on a small platform. In any event, an effort should be made to arrange the plinth at a height suitable for the individual therapist. When the patient is seated on a chair, the best position for the therapist may well be seated and facing the patient.

Since therapeutic massage is performed with the hands, the posture of the upper limbs is also very important. If joint strain is to be minimized, excessive wrist flexion and hyperextension of the fingers must be avoided.

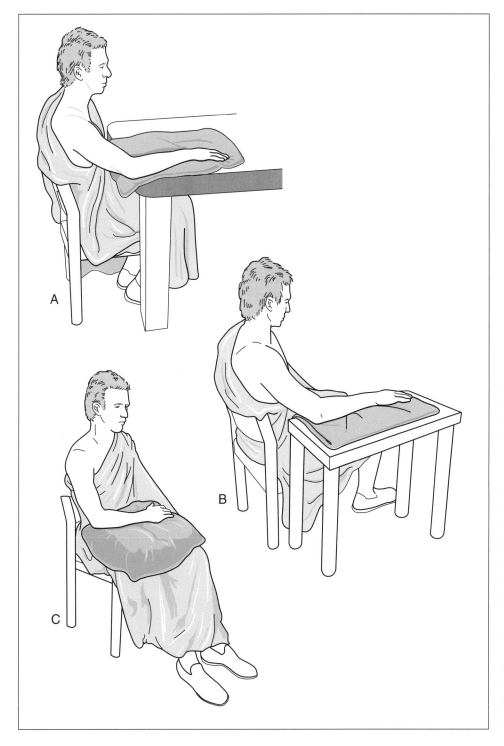

Figure 2–10. Sitting upright on a stool or chair with the upper limb supported on a small table, the end of a plinth, or a pillow on the patient's lap.
These positions are suitable for treatment of the upper limb or a part thereof. (*A*) The patient sits at the end of a plinth with the arm supported on a pillow resting on the table. The draping allows easy access to the shoulder region while maintaining the patient's modesty. (*B*) The patient is in a similar position, but the upper limb is supported on a small table. (*C*) The patient's arm is supported on a pillow resting on the lap. This is particularly useful for the patient who has a very stiff and/or painful shoulder. In all three positions, the therapist may stand or sit to perform the massage.

Good body mechanics is an essential method of preventing injury to the therapist.

COMPONENTS OF MASSAGE

Each massage stroke has its unique characteristics; however, a number of important components of massage are common to all techniques. Each of these is considered briefly here and elaborated upon in the relevant description in Chapter 3. Thoughtful concentration is necessary for the intelligent application of massage.

Comfort and Support

It is obvious that the patient must be positioned comfortably with adequate support so that he or she can relax in the required position. Pillows are usually used to provide

Essential Components of Good Technique in All Massage Treatments

- Comfortable support and positioning of patients so they can be as relaxed as possible during treatment
- Keeping the hands flexible so they fit the contour of the body part being massaged
- Establishing the correct rate of movement
- Maintaining an even rhythm
- Regulating pressure according to the stroke being performed, the kind of tissues being treated, and the purpose of the treatment
- Maintaining proper postural stance and good body mechanics

support, but they can get in the way of effective massage. A suitable alternative is rolled-up toweling placed under the body part, perhaps the neck, shoulder, or knee. A patient who is in significant pain may not be able to keep still for long, and this makes a comfortable and well-supported position all the more important. Folded sheets and/or blankets can be used to drape the patient and also to keep the patient warm.

Relaxation

Relaxation is an important component of massage since the treatment is likely to be much more effective if the patient is as relaxed as possible, especially when techniques to treat muscle tissue are concerned. Relaxation may be thought of on two levels—general and local relaxation. General relaxation describes the state of the entire person; local relaxation refers to a specific body part. In each instance, the therapist tries to facilitate relaxation of the patient by eliminating as many of the factors that inhibit relaxation as possible. At the same time, the therapist promotes

Factors That Tend to Inhibit Relaxation

- Pain or fear of pain
- Fear of unknown treatments
- Strange or new surroundings
- Excessive noise
- Bright lights or total darkness
- Cold, drafty rooms
- Breathing difficulty
- Fear of undressing
- Inadequate support, draping, or positioning
- Psychological factors such as a fear of hospitals or treatment clinics and domestic or personal problems

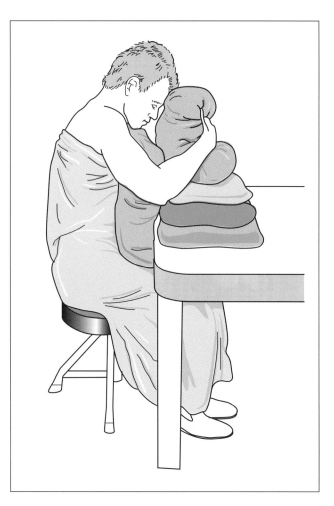

Figure 2–11. Sitting upright on a stool, facing a plinth, with the upper limbs and head supported on pillows. This position is used during treatment of the posterior neck and shoulder region. The patient holds a large pillow close to the chest, so that the patient's chin rests on the upper edge of the pillow. The patient then leans into the edge of the plinth and places the forearms on the pillows stacked in front of him or her. Note that the top pillow is folded in half and the patient rests the forehead on it. This allows plenty of room for the patient to breathe, while the head and face are supported by the pillow. Sufficient pillows should be used so that the patient sits upright and the head leans forward only slightly. This leaves the neck in a comfortable, well-supported position. In addition, the chin is supported by the pillow wedged between the table and the patient. This pillow also serves to keep the draping sheet in its proper position when the arms are lifted up onto the plinth. A similar position can be achieved by the use of a specially designed massage chair (see Fig. 2–4).

relaxation by paying special attention to the comfort and position of the patient.

Specific relaxation techniques may be used to help a tense patient to relax. Two common methods are the *contrast* and the *induction* techniques. In each case, the patient must be supported comfortably (i.e., with enough pillows to fully support the whole body or a part of it).

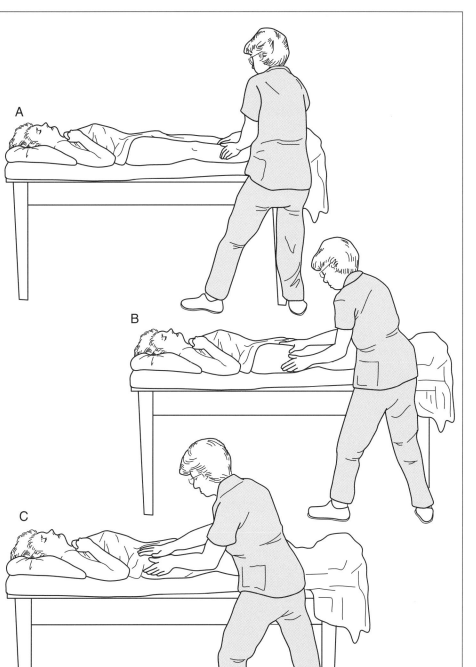

Figure 2–12. An illustration of good body mechanics for a therapist treating the lower limbs.
(A) The therapist's back is held reasonably straight. Progress along the limb is achieved primarily by shifting the body weight forward *(B, C)*. Such positions help to minimize the risk of back injury among therapists.

Environmental Factors That Facilitate Relaxation

- Quiet environment
- Soft lighting
- Moderate temperature
- Draft-free environment
- Clean and tidy treatment area

Contrast Method of Relaxation

The principle of this technique is to facilitate relaxation by teaching the patient to become aware of the difference (the contrast) between tight muscle contraction and relaxation. The technique calls for the patient to contract groups of muscles as intensely as he or she can for about 3 to 5 seconds. The patient is then instructed to relax and "feel" the difference between the two states. As each part of the body is tensed and then relaxed in this manner, the patient gradually achieves general relaxation. Although the contrast technique is often used to promote general relaxation, the principle can also be applied to facilitate local relaxation. The physiologic rationale for the technique is that a muscle relaxes easily immediately after a strong contraction.

Induction Method of Relaxation

As its name implies, a relaxed state is *induced* directly in the patient, usually by talking to him or her. Careful attention to the patient's comfort and support is necessary, and suitable background music is often very helpful. The patient closes his or her eyes and tries to imagine scenes described by the therapist or suggested by music (perhaps the sound of a flowing stream or falling rain). Mental imagery, an important part of this concept, serves to distract the patient's attention from his or her physical body. Muscle contraction is thus greatly reduced and relaxation promoted.

Direction

Massage strokes can be performed in many different directions. Which one is chosen depends largely on the

---

A Typical Sequence of Contractions

- Tense left foot and calf muscles (with toes pointing down and calf muscles contracting), then immediately relax the same muscles.
- Tense left quadriceps, then immediately relax the same muscles.
- Tense right foot and calf muscles (with toes pointing down and calf muscles contracting), then immediately relax the same muscles.
- Tense right quadriceps, then immediately relax the same muscles.
- Contract muscles of both buttocks, then immediately relax the same muscles.
- Contract back extensors, pressing the head and shoulders into the plinth, then immediately relax the same muscles.
- Contract abdominal muscles, tensing the anterior abdominal wall, then immediately relax the same muscles.
- Contract pectoral muscles to roll the upper arms in toward the midline, then immediately relax the same muscles.
- Clench left hand and tense elbow muscles, then immediately relax the same muscles.
- Clench right hand and tense the elbow muscles, then immediately relax the same muscles.
- Contract facial muscles (eyes shut tightly and teeth clenched), then immediately relax the same muscles.

---

purpose of the individual stroke. The directions include centripetal (toward the heart, in the direction of venous and lymphatic flow); centrifugal (away from the heart, in the direction of the arterial flow); and in other specific anatomic directions.

In most cases, the direction of a massage stroke is related to some anatomic structure. For example, effleurage is given in a centripedal direction, since it is designed to promote venous and lymphatic flow. In contrast, deep frictions are performed at right angles to the target fibers (muscle, tendon, or ligament) in order to mobilize them. The specific direction for each stroke is described in Chapter 3.

Pressure

Like the direction of massage strokes, the pressure exerted with each individual stroke varies, depending on the specific purpose of the stroke and the patient's physical problem. The pressure is sometimes constant but in other strokes variable. The choice of pressure depends largely on the function of the stroke. Effleurage is a good example. In this technique the pressure exerted gradually increases throughout each individual stroke to the maximum at the end of the stroke. It always finishes in a group of superficial lymph nodes. The therapist might imagine "pushing" the venous blood and lymph in the superficial vessels. Gradually increasing pressure would be needed, and a definite pause is required at the end of the stroke, to allow the valves in the vessels to close. In contrast, other strokes are extremely light, involving just the weight of the hand moving across the skin.

It is difficult to evaluate accurately the amount of pressure that is actually used, but the effect obtained depends to a great extent on the regulation of the pressure and the stimulation that it produces. Deep pressure may produce a strong stimulation and increase tension and pain, whereas lighter pressure may produce mild stimulation, induce relaxation, and diminish pain. The reaction to external stimulation varies among individuals and with the nature of the lesions under treatment. Specific descriptions of the pressure required for each stroke are given in Chapter 3.

Rate and Rhythm

The rate at which each massage stroke is performed again depends on the particular function of the stroke. In most cases, massage movements are performed relatively slowly, though some, such as hacking and clapping, are performed quite quickly. Mennell stressed that massage movements (except percussion) should be slow, gentle, and rhythmic. He prescribed about 15 strokes per minute for stroking from hand to shoulder. Beard and Wood determined that when the hand or hands move over the tissues at approximately 7 inches per second the desired effects, both mechanical and reflex, can be obtained. This rate, which is the equivalent of Mennell's rate as stated above, should be applied not only to stroking movements but also to the gliding and circular movements of kneading.

Generally speaking, strokes that are performed slowly tend to be more relaxing, whereas rapid strokes are more stimulating. In all cases, it is very important to perform the stroke with the correct rhythm, usually one that is as constant as possible. Continuity of treatment is important and this is achieved by ensuring an appropriate rhythm to the particular massage technique. Chapter 3 indicates the appropriate rhythm and rate at which each stroke is to be performed.

Duration and Frequency of Treatment

Massage treatment can be performed for many different purposes. It can be a general treatment for the whole body, using any number of combinations of strokes; alternatively, techniques can be chosen to achieve a particular effect in a specific structure. For example, one might well use several massage techniques to treat an adherent scar on the hand. The *purpose* of the massage, therefore, determines how long the treatment is to be given and for how many sessions.

Therapeutic massage is performed as part of a total treatment plan. Thus, specific techniques might be integrated with other methods of treatment such as exercise therapy or electrophysical modalities. When performed in these circumstances, each massage technique is practiced several minutes at a time. Numerous repetitions of each stroke are given, depending on the result to be achieved. For example, if the goal of treatment was to mobilize chronic swelling around the ankle region, appropriate massage strokes might be performed until a significant reduction in the swelling is observed. This might take 10 to 15 minutes or longer. In contrast, a full body massage takes much longer to perform and would be somewhere around 45 minutes or longer in duration. Such techniques are rarely used in modern rehabilitation but are popular as recreational massage.

Massage treatments can be given daily, if necessary, or even several times a day. This schedule may be impractical, however, and in practice many different treatment regimens are in common use. Massage, like many other rehabilitation procedures, should not be performed in a prescriptive manner. Unlike medications that require specific dose levels to be effective, massage treatment can be given in many different ways. It is not possible, or indeed desirable, to specify a particular number of treatments because in rehabilitation massage should always be given as part of a total treatment program. It should not generally be used in isolation. The particular goals of a treatment plan determine the type and number of treatments needed to reach a successful outcome, and this may not be known at the beginning of treatment. It is

important to remember that each patient is different and responds differently to treatment.

The duration of the treatment obviously varies according to the size of the area to be treated and the specific pathology. Although the existing problem may be localized to a small area, there will undoubtedly be physiologic disturbances in adjacent areas. Therefore, the treatment may not be limited to the diseased or injured area.

The size and age of the patient also affect the duration of treatment. At any given rate of massage, it takes less time to treat a comparatively small person because the amount of tissue being manipulated is less than that of a large person.

Mennell believed that for very young or aged persons the duration of massage should be curtailed because the reflex arc is more sensitive and the fullest effect is achieved rapidly; this is particularly true if the sole aim of the massage is to secure a reflex effect. To this end, the number of movements should be reduced rather than the rate increased (the latter practice, sometimes thoughtlessly followed, defeats the purpose of the massage).

In discussing the "dosage" of massage, various medical authorities recognize the variability of application and the difficulty of specifying doses. It would seem impossible to avoid either too little treatment or too much if the duration of each treatment is specified. Mennell emphasized the importance of intelligent observation of the patient by the therapist during treatment and the danger of over- or undertreating. He believed, however, that unless at some time there is evidence of an overdose it is quite possible that too little treatment has been given. This emphasizes the need for constant and intelligent observation of the patient and the response to the treatment.

Changes in Signs and Symptoms

As the condition of the treated tissue changes, it may be necessary to alter the duration of treatment. Keeping in mind that massage is a means to an end, the duration of the treatment may be shortened gradually as it accomplishes the desired results. If massage has not accomplished the desired results, it may be that the duration has been too brief or too long. The therapist should observe the patient closely if he or she is to appreciate the need for the change and adapt the duration of treatment accordingly. The duration of any massage treatment should therefore vary according to the lesion being treated and the size of the area, the rate of the movements, the age of the patient, and any change in signs and symptoms. To obtain the maximum benefit from any massage treatment and to avoid inadequate treatment or an overdose, it is essential that therapists have good scientific knowledge of massage and of its physiologic effects and that they apply the massage thoughtfully and intelligently, observing carefully its effects.

Chapter 3

A Classification and Description of Massage Strokes

The brief review of the history of massage in Chapter 1 clearly shows that there have been, and still are, many different ways of defining the various massage techniques. This chapter provides specific information about each of the traditional massage strokes that make up the system known as Swedish remedial massage. The definitions and descriptions represent a current view of the various techniques. Of course, some of these descriptions of the strokes are at variance with earlier ones. This is not surprising, given the considerable disagreement over terminology. Indeed, it is hoped that the classification and descriptions detailed in this chapter are logical, accurate, and worthy of adoption. In most cases, examples are given of each of the strokes to several body parts, and many of these strokes are also featured in Chapters 5 and 6, which address general and local massage techniques.

The specific effects of each stroke and the common contraindications are also given in this chapter, to bring together all of the information on each stroke. Contraindications to massage are discussed in more detail in Chapter 4. Since massage sequences are formed by combining different strokes, it was felt that the information about each stroke would be more useful if it were presented in a single chapter.

CLASSIFICATION

Individual massage strokes can be classified in a number of ways. Here, they are grouped on the basis of the way in which each one is performed (e.g., a pressure stroke or percussion). Individual strokes are classified as described in Table 3–1.

DESCRIPTION

Stroking Manipulations

Definition
A stroking movement is performed with the entire palmar surface of one or both hands moving in any direction on the surface of the body.

Purpose
Stroking is useful to begin a massage sequence. It allows the patient to become accustomed to the feel of the therapist's hands and, likewise, gives the therapist an opportunity to get the feel of the patient's tissues. When

Table 3.1. A Classification of Massage Strokes	
MANIPULATION (STROKE)	VARIATIONS
Stroking	Superficial
	Deep
Effleurage	
Petrissage (pressure)	Kneading
	Picking up
	Wringing
	Skin rolling
Tapotement (percussion)	Hacking
	Clapping
	Beating
	Pounding
Vibration	
Shaking	
Deep frictions	Transverse
	Circular

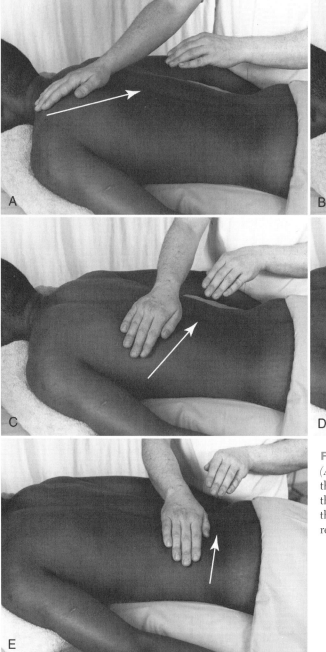
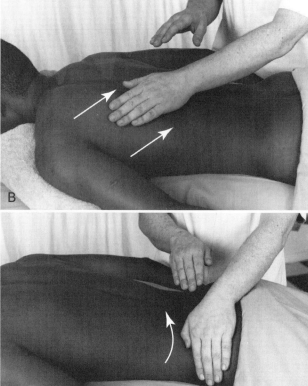

Figure 3–1. Stroking to the back.
(*A–C*) Stroking is performed in a diagonal pattern to cover the patient's back region. Hands are used alternately and the direction of the movement can be changed to cover the area in a different direction (e.g., across the low back region [*D,E*]).

performed slowly it helps a patient to relax. It is also useful for joining sequences of other strokes.

Basic Technique and Direction of Movement

Stroking can be given in any direction; however, the direction should be one that is convenient for the operator and comfortable to the patient. It usually moves in one direction at a time. Typically, the strokes move along a line parallel to the long axis of the body (lengthwise) and/or across the long axis. It can also be given at an angle to the long axis (diagonally). Figures 3–1 to 3–3 show the direction of the stroking.

The movement should be continuous while the hand is in contact with the skin. It must be rhythmic; otherwise, the stimulus will be uneven. The beginning of each stroke must be definite, but smooth. The manipulation may be performed with one or both hands. Both hands may be used, either alternately or simultaneously. When both hands are used alternately, one hand is lifted off the patient

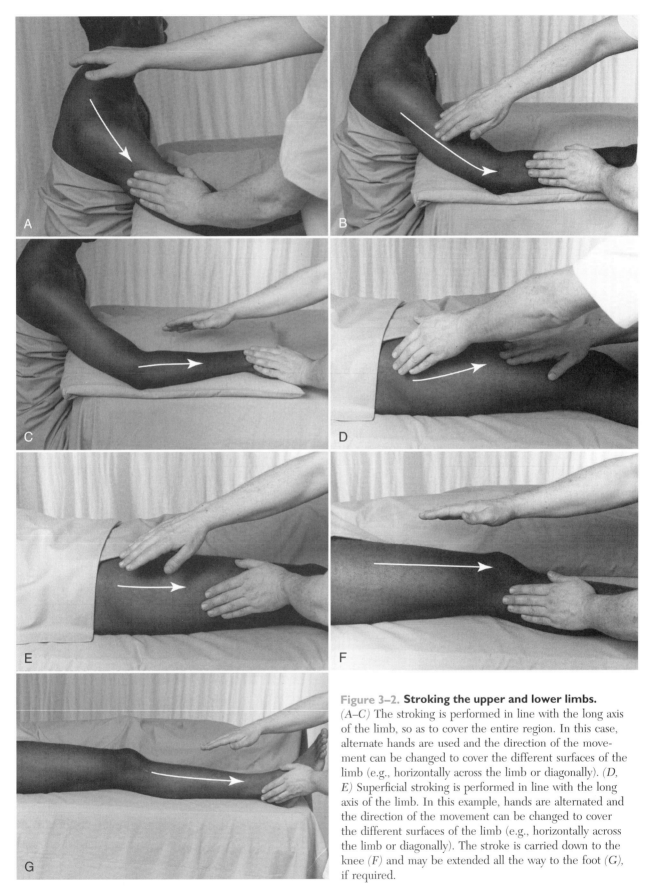

Figure 3–2. Stroking the upper and lower limbs.
(A–C) The stroking is performed in line with the long axis of the limb, so as to cover the entire region. In this case, alternate hands are used and the direction of the movement can be changed to cover the different surfaces of the limb (e.g., horizontally across the limb or diagonally). *(D, E)* Superficial stroking is performed in line with the long axis of the limb. In this example, hands are alternated and the direction of the movement can be changed to cover the different surfaces of the limb (e.g., horizontally across the limb or diagonally). The stroke is carried down to the knee *(F)* and may be extended all the way to the foot *(G)*, if required.

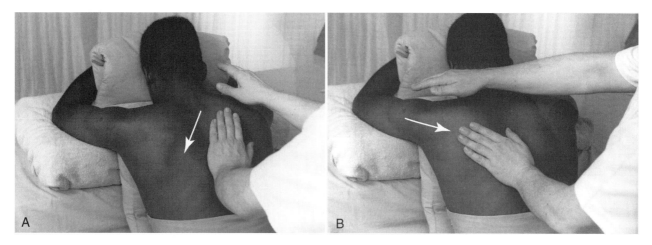

Figure 3–3. Stroking the posterior neck and shoulder region.
(A) The stroking is performed in a vertical pattern to cover the patient's posterior neck and shoulder region. Hands are alternated, and the direction of the movement can be changed to cover the area in a different direction (e.g., horizontally across the region or [B] diagonally.)

while the other makes contact. For stroking small areas such as the face the finger tips may be used instead of the whole hand.

Rate of Movement

Stroking may be slow or fast. Performed slowly, it tends to be relaxing. Performed quickly, it has a more stimulating effect on the tissues.

Depth and Pressure

The depth and pressure used for stroking techniques depend largely on the type of stroking being used. In general, "superficial" stroking tends to use lighter pressure, whereas deep stroking uses much greater pressure and, therefore, affects deeper structures.

Variations

Superficial Stroking

Superficial stroking is usually slow and gentle but firm enough for the patient to be conscious of the passage of the hand throughout the movement. When given in this manner, the stroke is extremely relaxing for the patient.

Deep Stroking

Deep stroking is given with much greater pressure and is usually performed rather slowly. Given in this manner, it tends to stimulate the circulation to the deeper muscle tissue. For this reason, it is generally given in the direction of the venous and lymphatic flow. In many ways, it is very similar to effleurage.

Figures 3–1 through 3–3 illustrate stroking to various parts of the body.

Effects of Stroking

Therapeutic effects are produced mainly through direct mechanical impact on the tissues and reflexly through the sensory nervous system.

- Significant relaxation, producing a sedative effect, may be obtained and may help relieve pain and muscle spasm (pain-gate mechanism).
- When performed rapidly and lightly stroking has a stimulating effect on sensory nerve endings, resulting in a generalized, invigorating effect.
- Deep stroking may cause dilation of arterioles in the deeper tissues and in superficial structures.

Therapeutic Uses of Stroking

- As a means of helping the patient to become accustomed to the touch of the therapist's hands. Aids general or local relaxation.
- As a way of providing information about the patient's tissues to the therapist.
- To help relieve muscle spasm and, therefore, indirectly to relieve associated pain.
- To help relieve flatulence or other intestinal movement disorders, by mechanical effects on the intestinal contents.
- To promote relaxation and induce sleep in persons who have insomnia.

Contraindications to Stroking

- Large open areas (e.g., burns or wounds).
- *Gross* edema, if there seems to be danger of splitting the skin.

- Marked varicosities if damage to the vein wall might result. (Very light stroking may be possible.)
- Areas of hyperesthesia (i.e., those very sensitive to touch).
- Extremely hairy areas (if stroking causes pain).

Effleurage Manipulations

Definition

Effleurage (from the French, *effleurer:* to skim over) is a slow, stroking movement performed with increasing pressure in the direction of flow in the veins and lymph vessels (i.e., centripetal direction). Whenever possible, the stroke finishes, with a definite pause, in a group of superficial lymph glands.

Purpose

Effleurage is a stroke designed to move the contents of the superficial veins and lymph vessels. It is particularly useful as a means of facilitating circulation and as a stroke that can be used between manipulations that tend to mobilize tissue fluids. For example, after a series of deep kneading strokes to a muscle, effleurage given to the area will help to move the fluids that have been mobilized by the kneading. It is also a very useful stroke to finish off a massage sequence.

Basic Technique and Direction of Movement

Effleurage is always given in the direction of the venous and lymphatic flow (i.e., toward the heart, in a centripetal direction). The manipulation is performed with the palmar surface of one or both hands, working either alternately or simultaneously. Small areas such as the face or foot can be treated with the fingers or the thumb of one or both hands.

The hand or hands must be relaxed and molded accurately to the shape of the part being treated. The stroke should be smooth and rhythmic and is directed toward a group of lymph glands, following the course of superficial veins and lymphatics always working from distal to proximal areas. At the end of each stroke the hands may be allowed to gently stroke back to their starting position, or they may be lifted from the surface of the body and returned through the air to the starting position for the next stroke. Each method has advantages and disadvantages; so, in practice, either is suitable.

Rate of Movement

Effleurage is performed quite slowly (about 6 or 7 inches per second). This is because the pressure exerted on the tissues is much greater than just the weight of the therapist's hands. Rhythm is extremely important with this stroke: as usual, it should be even and relatively constant.

Depth and Pressure

To affect the contents of the superficial veins and lymphatics, effleurage must be performed with significant pressure. Pressure should gradually increase so that the venous blood and lymph are pushed through the veins and lymph channels. There should be a definite pause at the end of each stroke, at or near the lymph glands. This allows the valves in the vessels to close, thus minimizing back flow. These changes in pressure during the stroke make it important to maintain firm but comfortable pressure on the tissues. Effleurage to a variety of body areas is depicted in Figures 3–4 through 3–6.

Effects of Effleurage

- By mechanical pressure, the flow of blood in the superficial veins is moved toward the heart. When pressure is relaxed the valves in the veins prevent backward flow.
- Lymph flow is accelerated in a similar way, and this results in more rapid elimination of waste products, which promotes healing.
- Owing to the increased flow in the veins and lymphatics, congestion in the capillaries is relieved and the blood flows more readily into the capillary bed, thus stimulating the circulation and facilitating healing.
- Mobility of the superficial soft tissues is increased, which in turn increases range of motion in joints and limb segments.
- If the effleurage is performed deeply it may cause dilation of the superficial arterioles through the axon reflex, thus stimulating circulation.

Therapeutic Uses of Effleurage

- As a technique to accustom patient and therapist to the feel of the treatment.
- To join various massage manipulations and so give continuity to the massage.
- To follow up deeper strokes (e.g., kneading, friction) and enhance absorption of waste products.
- For circulation disturbances (e.g., chronic edema, some heart conditions, lower motor neuron disturbances).
- In the subacute and chronic stages of soft tissue injuries, to promote absorption of inflammatory exudate.
- To relive pain and promote relaxation.

Contraindications to Effleurage

- Large open areas (e.g., burns, ulcers, open wounds).
- *Gross* edema if there seems danger of splitting the skin.
- Marked varicosities if damage to the vein wall may result (very light effleurage may be possible).
- Areas of hyperesthesia (i.e., those very sensitive to touch).
- Extremely hairy areas (if this causes pain).

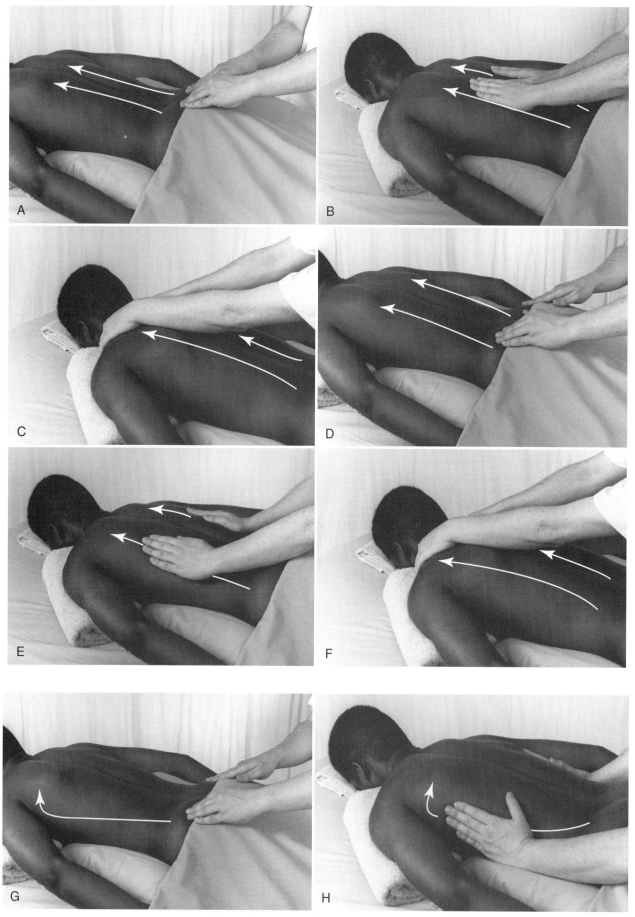

Figure 3–4. Legend on opposite page.

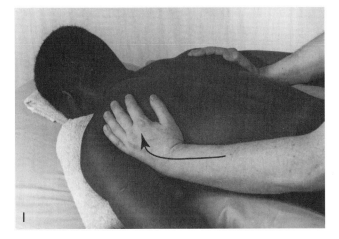

Figure 3–4. Effleurage to the back.
Effleurage is performed on the back moving from the sacrum toward the head. Both hands are used, the movements being mirror images of each other. The first stroke begins with the fingertips on the sacrum (A) and passes toward the head in a straight line (B). At the upper fibers of the trapezius muscle, the hands turn outward to pass over the muscle belly to finish in the supraclavicular fossae, the fingertips being allowed simply to fold over (C). The second stroke begins just lateral to the first one on the sacrum (D) but passes more laterally up the back (E) in a similar fashion, once again to finish in the supraclavicular region (F). Finally, the third stroke begins with the fingertips in a position similar to that for the previous stroke (G). This time, however, the fingertips point outward and the hands pass up the sides of the chest wall (H) to finish with the ulnar border of each hand in the respective axillary region of the patient (I).

- Chronic swelling in the lower limb associated with congestive cardiac failure or any other heart condition with which lower limb edema is associated.

Petrissage (Pressure) Manipulations

Petrissage (from the French, *pétrir:* to knead), or pressure manipulations, covers several different massage strokes that are characterized by firm pressure applied to the tissues. In the majority of cases, these strokes aim to mobilize deep muscle tissue or the skin and subcutaneous tissues. Four distinct types of stroke are discussed in this section: kneading, picking up, wringing, and skin rolling.

Kneading

Definition
Kneading is a manipulation in which the muscles and subcutaneous tissues are alternately compressed and released. The movement takes place in a *circular* motion. During the pressure phase of each stroke, the hand(s) and the skin move together on the deeper structures. During the release (relaxation) phase, the hand(s) glide smoothly to an adjacent area and the movement is repeated.

Purpose
Kneading strokes have a strong mechanical action and are designed to affect deep tissue. In particular, kneading aims to mobilize muscle fibers and other deep tissues, thus promoting the normal function of muscles, which is not only to contract to produce movements but also to lengthen and allow movement in the opposite direction. To allow this, muscle fibers and other structures must be mobile.

Kneading is also useful for mobilizing chronic swell-ing, especially where such swelling has become organized and is preventing normal joint and limb motion.

Basic Technique and Direction of Movement
Kneading is a stroke in which the hand(s) and the skin move together on the deeper structures, during all times in which pressure is applied to the tissues. It can be performed with several parts of one or both hands, including the entire palmar surface and the pads/tips of the fingers or thumbs. In each case, the basic direction of the movement is circular. Pressure is applied during half of the circular motion and released during the other half, to provide relaxation of pressure. The technique can be performed in a stationary manner (stationary kneading), but it is more usual for the hands to move across the body surface. Movement of the hands is achieved during the relaxation phase of each circular motion; the hands usually move in parallel lanes. Figure 3–7 illustrates this concept. It is common to all types of kneading.

Rate of Movement
Kneading is performed rather slowly because of the pressure exerted on the tissues. If it is performed too quickly, it is likely to be ineffective and/or uncomfortable for the patient. The rate of movement is similar for both stationary kneading and the more common "mobile" version. When using the whole hand(s), each circular movement should take about 3 to 4 seconds to complete. Obviously this is much less if one is using the finger or thumb pads/tips to perform the massage, as they are so much smaller.

Depth and Pressure
As its name implies, kneading requires significant pressure on the tissues if it is to be effective; however, the pressure

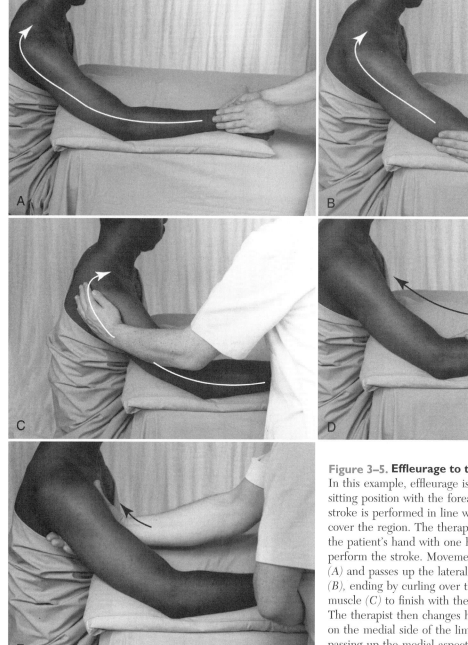

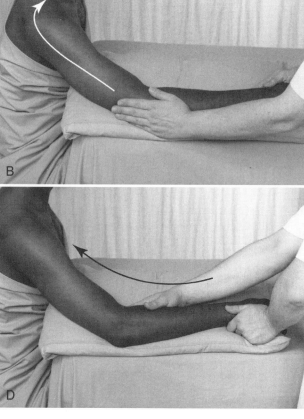

Figure 3–5. Effleurage to the upper limb.
In this example, effleurage is performed with the patient in a sitting position with the forearm supported on a pillow. The stroke is performed in line with the long axis of the limb to cover the region. The therapist faces the patient and supports the patient's hand with one hand while using the other to perform the stroke. Movement begins at the hand or wrist (A) and passes up the lateral aspect of the forearm and arm (B), ending by curling over the posterior fibers of the deltoid muscle (C) to finish with the palm in the supraclavicular fossa. The therapist then changes hands and performs the stroke on the medial side of the limb, beginning at the wrist and passing up the medial aspect of the forearm (D), to finish in the axillary lymph glands (E).

must be adapted to the tissues being treated and it can be performed rather lightly, especially on more delicate structures such as the backs of the hands or face. It is important for the pressure to be applied during only half of each circle. At such times, the hand(s) are *not* moving on the skin; rather, the hand(s) *and* the skin move over the deeper structures. It is not easy to quantify the actual pressure needed during kneading, but the experienced therapist will be able to apply the correct amount of pressure to produce effective treatment of the deep tissues without harming the patient.

Variations

Several variations of the basic kneading stroke are used and these are explained in the following sections.

Compression Kneading

This basic kneading stroke is also called "palmar kneading," "circular kneading," "flat-handed," and "whole-hand kneading." As its name implies, it involves the entire palmar surface of either or both hands. In this manipulation the tissues are compressed upwards and inwards, in a circular motion against the underlying tissues, and then

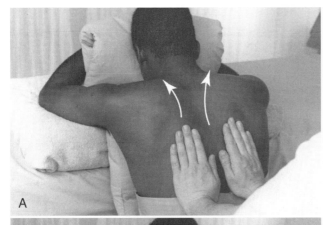

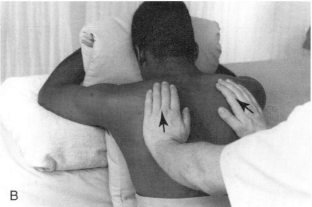

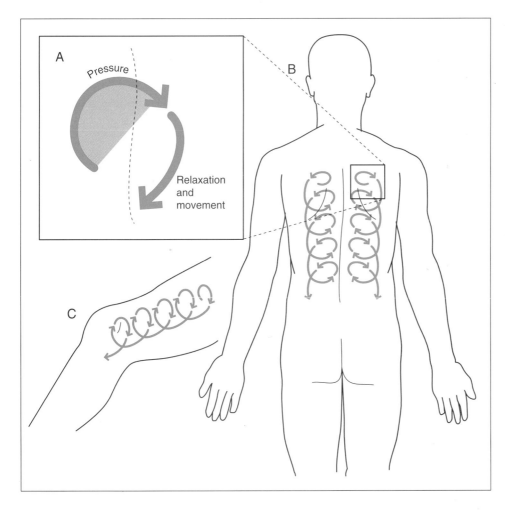

Figure 3–6. Effleurage to the posterior neck and shoulder region.
The therapist stands behind the seated patient. The stroke begins with the fingertips together in the midline approximately at the middle to the lower border of the scapulae (A). The stroke is performed in an upward direction (B), moving toward the base of the neck, finishing by allowing the hands to pass over the top of each trapezius muscle (C), to end with the palms in the supraclavicular lymph nodes.

Figure 3–7. Basic technique and direction of movement during kneading strokes.
The basic movement is circular. Pressure is applied during one half of the circle, and relaxation and movement are allowed during the other half (A). Progress of the hands along the body surface is usually achieved by moving them in a series of parallel lanes, as on the back (B). The same concept is applied to the thigh (C), except that the hands now work on either side of the limb, usually beginning proximally.

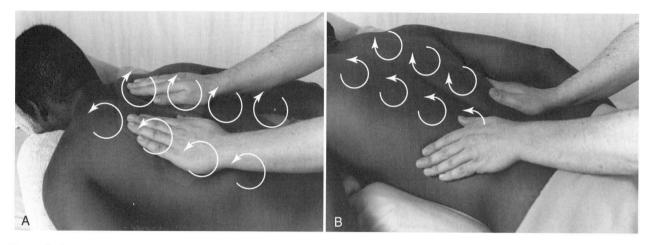

Figure 3–8. Compression kneading to the back muscles.
The stroke usually starts at the upper fibers of the trapezius muscle and progresses along the back *(A)* toward the sacrum. If required, the fingers may turn outward slightly as the hands reach the lumbar region *(B)*. This helps to avoid too much extension of the wrists at the sacral region. To avoid pinching the tissues, it is better to perform the technique with the two hands working "out of phase" (i.e., one hand compresses moving upward and inward, while the other relaxes moving downward and outward).

released. A large area of the body can be covered by overlapping lanes of the individual circular strokes. If the tissues are flat, such as the back region, both hands can be used on the same plane of motion (side by side). In the limbs, however, the hands may work opposite to each other. This usually produces more movement of the whole muscle masses involved. Figure 3–8 illustrates the basic technique and Figure 3–9 demonstrates hand positions for kneading (squeeze kneading in this case) muscles in the thigh when the hands work opposite each other.

Squeeze Kneading

Squeeze kneading is similar to the basic kneading technique: this time, however, the tissues are pressed upward and lifted away from the underlying tissues, squeezed gently, and then allowed to relax. The squeezing is produced by a "lumbrical" action of the fingers, the tissues being squeezed between the palm and the fingers. It is usually performed on relatively large muscle masses, such as those in the thigh; however, it can be performed on small muscles by squeezing the tissues between the thumb and

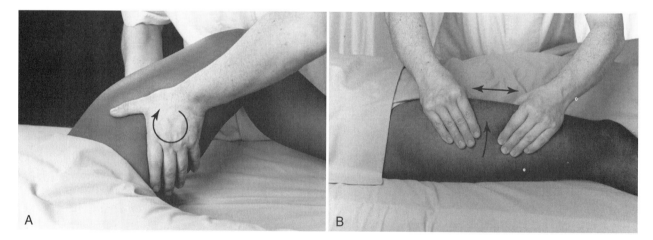

Figure 3–9. Kneading to the thigh muscles.
Two different techniques are illustrated. In *(A)* the therapist's hands work opposite to each other. Compression is applied to the tissues between the hands, but, again, the hands work out of phase with one another. This technique works very well when it is possible to get both hands on either side of a muscle mass. It is easiest to start at the proximal part of the limb (hip) and work toward the distal part (knee). *(B)* Kneading is performed by lifting the muscle mass away from the bone and "passing" it from one hand to the other in a circular motion. It is also possible to introduce an element of the wringing technique (see Fig. 3–16) at the same time, producing a deep kneading motion in the muscle.

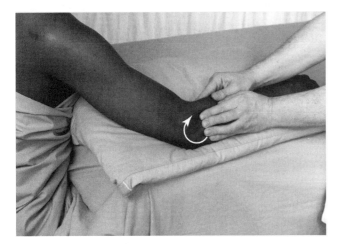

Figure 3–10. Finger pad kneading to the elbow region.
In this example, the therapist's hands work in opposition to each other. The fingers may work either in phase or out of phase with each other, depending on the therapist's preference. The technique works very well around irregular-shaped surfaces such as the face, elbow, knee, and ankle.

the finger pads. Figure 3–9 illustrates squeeze kneading to the thigh muscles. This is also a good example of the therapist's hands working opposite each other and out of phase.

Finger Pad Kneading

The basic circular kneading stroke is performed with the pads of one or more finger tips, using either hand or both. If the hands are placed opposite each other, for example, around the elbow region, then the fingers usually work in phase with each other. It is quite possible, however, for the fingers to work out of phase, and this is simply a matter of

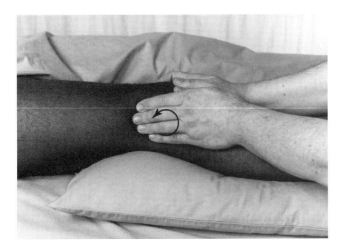

Figure 3–11. Finger pad kneading around the patella.
In this example, the therapist's hands are again working opposite to each other, and the fingers may work either in phase or out of phase.

preference. The technique is very useful for treating small to medium-sized areas and areas of irregular shape (e.g., around the ankle). When both hands are used, they may work side by side in some situations, or opposite each other, as in Figures 3–10 and 3–11, which illustrate finger pad kneading around the elbow and knee regions, respectively.

Thumb Pad Kneading

Basic circular kneading strokes are performed with the pads of one or both thumbs, usually working side by side. This technique is especially useful along fusiform muscles (e.g., the flexors and extensors of the wrists and fingers or the anterior tibial muscles). It is also very useful for the treatment of very small areas in the hand, foot, and face. Figure 3–12 illustrates the stroke.

Reinforced Kneading

The basic kneading technique is performed with one hand on top of the other, to reinforce the stroke. It is useful for treating very large patients, when extra effort is required for effective treatment. This is especially true if the therapist is of relatively small stature and the patient very large. The technique is illustrated in Figure 3–13.

Knuckle Kneading

For small areas where greater depth is required (e.g., the sole of the foot) the dorsal surface of the middle or proximal

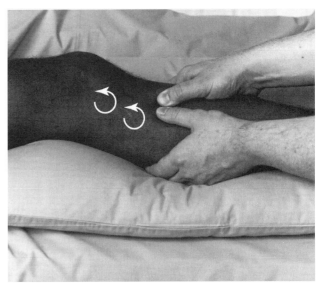

Figure 3–12. Thumb pad kneading to the anterior tibial muscles.
In this example, the therapist's hands work side by side. The thumb pads may work either in phase or out of phase with each other, depending on the therapist's preference. The technique works very well around small irregular-shaped surfaces such as the face, elbow, knee and ankle. It is also very useful on long fusiform muscles such as those in the forearms and legs.

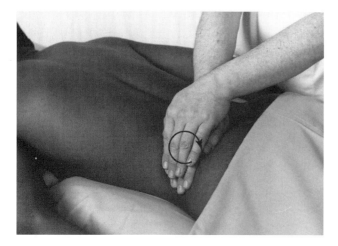

Figure 3–13. Reinforced kneading to the lumbar muscles.
One hand reinforces the other in this technique. The basic circular kneading technique is followed, simply using one hand reinforced by the other. This technique provides extra pressure that is useful for very large muscle masses or large patients.

phalanges may be used. Significant pressure can be generated with the closed fist, applying the same basic circular motion (Fig. 3–14).

Picking Up

Definition
In picking up, one or more muscles are grasped, lifted away from the underlying tissues, squeezed, and released. The grasping and releasing is performed in a circular motion, usually in the same direction as the muscle fibers.

Purpose
Picking up is a technique performed largely on muscle tissue for the purpose of mobilizing individual or groups of muscles. It has a significant mechanical action on the muscle fibers and is designed to increase muscle mobility, thus facilitating normal joint and limb function.

Basic Technique and Direction of Movement
The usual technique is a single-handed manipulation of a muscle or muscle group. The tissue to be treated is grasped with the whole hand, the thumb being well abducted. On very wide muscle groups the hands may be used together to give a wider grasp. The initial pressure is upward and inward in a circular motion toward the tissues. The tissues are then grasped by the palm of the hand, the fingers and thumb being controlled by the intrinsic muscles (a lumbrical action). The tissues are lifted away from the underlying structures by a movement of wrist extension. The tissues are released, and the hand glides along the muscle belly to repeat the stroke.

A variation of this basic technique is a two-handed technique in which the tissues are grasped and lifted away

from underlying tissues by one hand and then "passed" to the other while still lifted away from deeper structures. The muscle is then released by the second hand. Progress is made along a muscle by passing the tissues from one hand to the other.

Rate of Movement
The movement should be slow, continuous, and rhythmic, and the whole muscle belly should be treated, generally from origin to insertion. Care should be taken to keep the grasp soft and supple and avoid pinching the tissues.

Depth and Pressure
Picking up is a type of petrissage and is therefore a pressure manipulation. Sufficient pressure must be exerted to grasp and lift the muscle tissue away from the underlying structures. The tissues are then squeezed before being released. All this requires considerable pressure. In general, picking up is not as "deep" a technique as compression kneading. Figure 3–15 illustrates picking up to the deltoid, biceps, triceps, thigh, and calf, respectively.

Wringing

Definition
Wringing is a manipulation in which the tissues are lifted with both hands and compressed alternately between the fingers and thumb of opposite hands.

Purpose
Wringing is rather similar to picking up in its purpose. It is also a technique performed largely on muscle tissue, for the purpose of mobilizing individual muscles or groups of

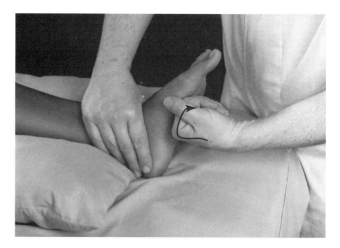

Figure 3–14. Knuckle kneading to the muscles on the sole of the foot.
This is a modified kneading technique that is useful for applying extra pressure to the deep muscle layers on the sole of the foot. It could be used on other large muscle masses where extra pressure is required.

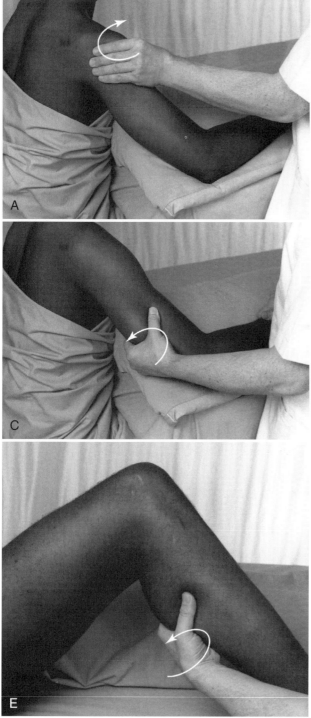

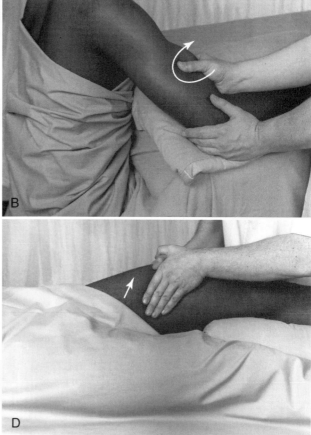

Figure 3–15. Picking up to muscles in the upper and lower limbs.
(A) The deltoid muscle is picked up using a single-handed technique. The biceps (B) and triceps (C) muscles are treated similarly. In all three examples, the patient is seated comfortably at the end of a treatment table with the upper limb supported on a pillow. (B) Note that the therapist's left hand provides counterpressure to support the arm when the biceps muscle is treated. Similar counterpressure is often needed when performing this technique with one hand. (D) The quadriceps muscle is picked up using a two-handed technique. The thumbs are crossed, and the muscle is lifted away from the underlying bone. A single-handed technique is used to pick up the calf muscles (E).

them. It has significant mechanical action on the muscle fibers because of the twisting motion that is imparted to the tissues. Like picking up, it is designed to increase muscle mobility, thus facilitating normal joint and limb function.

Basic Technique and Direction of Movement
The hands are placed along the axis of the muscle with the thumbs well abducted from the fingers. The tissues are grasped with both hands; lifted, using a lubricant action; and then compressed between the fingers and thumb of opposite hands. The movement of the tissues is gained by alternately flexing and extending the wrists, producing a motion similar to that of wringing a wet cloth.

The hands move alternately down the long axis of the muscle, working across the muscle fibers and stretching the tissues. Wringing is used chiefly on large and loose groups of muscles. The techniques can be modified, however, to accommodate smaller muscles. In this case, wringing may

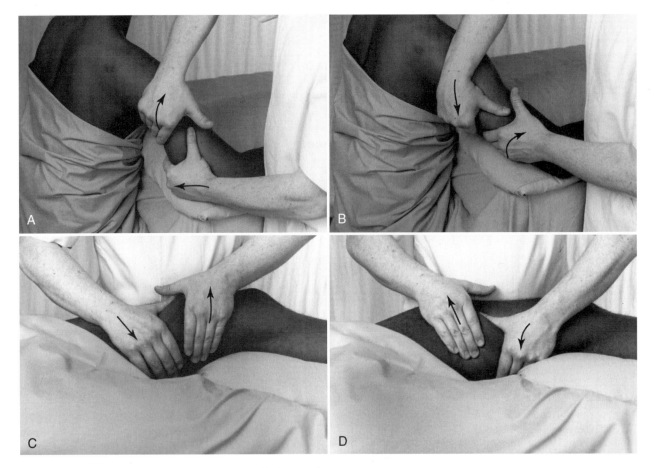

Figure 3-16. Wringing to the upper and lower limb muscles.
With the patient seated and supported comfortably, wringing to the triceps can be performed. *(A, B)* The twisting motion of the hands as they move across the long axis of the muscle group is illustrated. Pressure is applied, alternating between the fingers of one hand and the thumb of the other. *(C, D)* In a similar approach wringing to the medial thigh muscles is depicted.

need to be performed with the tips of the fingers and thumbs instead of the whole hands.

Rate of Movement
The stroke is performed at slow to medium speed—about 4 to 6 inches per second on a large muscle—and somewhat more slowly on smaller muscles. This stroke requires a particularly even rhythm if it is to feel comfortable to the patient. If the rhythm and pressure are erratic, it will be difficult for the patient to relax and for the technique to be effective.

Depth and Pressure
Since the tissues are grasped and lifted from the deeper structures during wringing, it is obviously a stroke that demands reasonable pressure. It is a deep stroke designed to mobilize deep muscle tissue. As always, pressure must be regulated so that it does not pinch the patient and cause pain. Figure 3–16 illustrates wringing to the triceps and thigh muscles, respectively.

Skin Rolling

Definition
In skin rolling the skin and subcutaneous tissues are rolled over the deeper structures.

Purpose
Skin rolling is designed to mobilize the skin and subcutaneous structures. Since the skin is folded over on itself it is also likely to move the contents of the superficial vessels and thus to improve circulation to the area. Normal joint and limb movements require a normal degree of extensibility in the skin and subcutaneous tissues. Skin rolling is designed to mobilize the skin, and therefore improve joint and limb function that has been compromised by excessive immobility of the skin.

Basic Technique and Direction of Movement
The hands lie flat, side by side on the skin surface with the thumbs stretched apart as far as possible. The extended

fingers draw the tissues toward the thumbs, with a lumbrical action. This produces a fold of skin between the fingers and thumbs. The thumbs then compress the tissues toward the fingers; rolling them around the body part in a wavelike motion, away from the therapist. The motion is repeated on the adjacent portion of skin.

Rate of Movement

Skin rolling is usually performed quite slowly (about 4 to 6 inches per second) and taking care not to pinch the tissues and cause pain.

Depth and Pressure

This stroke is performed to the skin and subcutaneous tissues and does not require significant pressure to be effective; however, if the skin and deeper structures are tight and/or the patient has a significant layer of body fat, it may be difficult to lift up a roll of skin without pinching the patient and causing pain. If the skinfold thickness is more than 1 inch, the pressure may need to be reduced a little to prevent pinching.

The skin and deeper structures are much more mobile in some parts of the body than in others. This means that it may be difficult if not impossible to perform the technique properly on some body parts. In any area that is naturally tight and relatively immobile (e.g., around the lower lumbar and sacral region) this technique cannot be performed very well. In addition, it may not be possible to perform this technique on patients whose skinfold thickness is greater than 2 to 3 inches, since it may be impossible to effectively produce a comfortable fold in the skin while lifting the tissues away from deeper structures. It is much easier to perform effective skin rolling if the skin is loose. (*Note:* This technique is easy to practice on an animal that has very mobile skin, such as a cat or a dog.) Figure 3–17 illustrates skin rolling over the posterior thoracic region.

Effects of Petrissage

On the Circulation

- By alternately compressing and then relaxing the muscles, the veins, both superficial and deep, alternately empty and refill. Congestion in the capillary beds is thus relieved, and the flow into them from the arterioles is improved.
- The flow of lymph is stimulated by the same mechanical means.
- Given vigorously petrissage causes vasodilation in the skin. The skin temperature of the part may also rise slightly. This effect produced by the axon reflex and perhaps by the liberation of substances that produce vasodilation.

On Muscles

- Increases the blood supply.
- Metabolic waste products are more readily eliminated owing to increased venous and lymphatic flow.
- Slow, rhythmic petrissage relaxes muscles and reduces pain.
- Posttraumatic scar tissue in a muscle may be stretched by slow, deep petrissage, particularly wringing. This promotes normal joint and limb function.

On the Skin and Subcutaneous Tissues

- Increased blood supply is important for promoting the resolution of inflammatory processes of the skin and subcutaneous tissues.

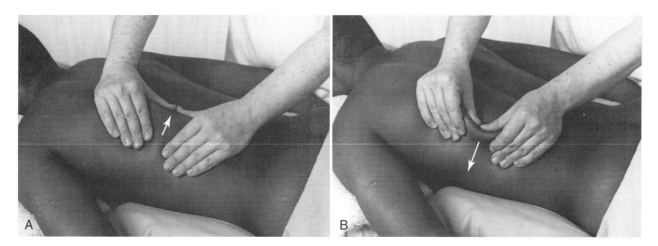

Figure 3–17. Skin rolling to the posterior thoracic region.
(*A*) The hands are placed side by side, with the fingers and thumbs stretched apart. A large fold of skin is lifted up from the underlying tissues using a "lumbrical action." (*B*) This fold of skin is pushed away from the therapist by moving the thumbs toward the fingers. In this fashion, the skin is rolled around the chest wall. The movement is then repeated on the adjacent tissues, with the hands moving down the back from the shoulder to the sacrum.

- The skin is mobilized by the manipulations, and that promotes its elasticity.

Therapeutic Uses of Petrissage

- To facilitate deep and superficial circulation to an affected body area.
- To mobilize muscle contractures.
- To mobilize the skin and subcutaneous tissues.
- To help resolve chronic edema.
- To help relieve pain and muscle fatigue.
- To promote relaxation.

It is important to remember that petrissage usually is not given in cases of acute trauma to large areas of muscle, particularly if there has been significant bleeding into the tissues. Once the initial acute phase is over, very gentle petrissage can help to remove the inflammatory exudate and help facilitate healing. To obtain the correct effect it is necessary to choose the appropriate manipulation. It will be necessary to adapt the manipulation to the area and the condition under treatment.

Contraindications to Petrissage

- Deep kneading to acute muscle tears (especially intramuscular hematomas).
- Kneading around acutely inflamed joints.
- Skin diseases (especially acute dermatitis, psoriasis, or any communicable skin infection).
- Damage or disease of blood vessels (especially thrombophlebitis and deep vein thrombosis).
- Hyper- or hypotonic limbs (very gentle massage only).
- Malignant disease (cancer or tuberculosis) in or near the area being treated.
- Bacterial infections in or near the area being treated, especially infections in joints.

Tapotement (Percussion) Manipulations

Classification

Tapotement (from the French, *tapôter:* to tap), or percussion manipulations as they are also known, cover several different massage strokes that are characterized by various parts of the hand striking the tissues at a fairly rapid rate. The hands usually work alternately, and the wrists are kept flexible so that the movements are light, springy, and stimulating. In the majority of cases these strokes aim to stimulate the tissues, either by direct mechanical means or by reflex action. Four distinct types of stroke are discussed in this section: clapping, beating, hacking, and pounding.

Clapping

Definition

Clapping is a single- or two-handed stroke in which the cupped hands strike the skin surface rapidly, compressing the air and causing a vibration wave to penetrate the tissues.

Purpose

Clapping is designed to stimulate the tissues by direct mechanical action. When performed over the lungs, the mechanical waves help to loosen secretions. Brisk, light clapping performed over muscle tissue stimulates muscle activity by direct mechanical activation of muscle spindle afferents.

Basic Technique and Direction of Movement

Clapping is usually performed with alternate movements of the palmar surfaces of the loosely cupped hands. The stroke is carried out by alternate flexion and extension of the wrists, the rest of the arm being as relaxed as possible. Figure 3–18 shows the position of the cupped hand.

Rate of Movement

Clapping is performed quite rapidly since it aims to stimulate the tissues. The actual rate is determined by the therapist's ability to coordinate the wrist movements, but it should be as fast as is comfortable for patient and therapist.

Depth and Pressure

Clapping is a stroke that is performed rapidly but lightly. This is why it is performed with wrist movement rather than elbow flexion and extension. The elbows should be held in a comfortable position somewhere near full

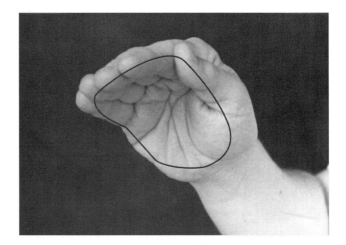

Figure 3–18. The cupped hand position used to perform clapping.
The hand is cupped by flexing the metacarpophalangeal joints and extending all the other joints in the fingers. The thumb is held close to the side to form part of the edge of the cup. As the hand strikes the tissues, the air trapped in the cup is compressed slightly, setting up a vibrating wave that travels into the tissues (i.e., the mechanical stimulus is transferred into the tissues). On no account should the fingers be held stiffly, as this produces a stinging or slapping effect.

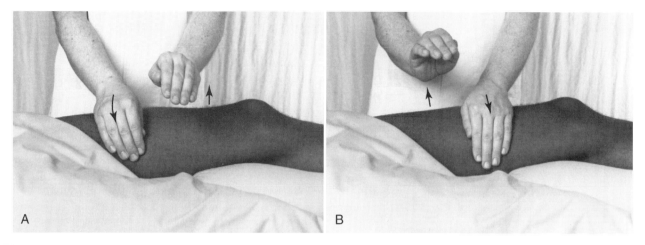

Figure 3–19. Clapping to the inner thigh muscles.
(A, B) The therapist stands at right angles to the long axis of the muscles to be treated. With the elbows held almost straight, the cupped hands alternately strike the skin surface and move up and down the length of the muscle. Note the flexion and extension at the therapist's wrists rather than the elbow joints.

extension, but the actual stroke is performed by alternate wrist flexion and extension and not by elbow movement. In this way, the stroke can be performed lightly and rapidly, with the hands moving over the entire area to be treated. Figures 3–19 and 3–20 illustrate clapping to the inner thigh muscles and the lungs, respectively.

Beating

Definition
Beating is a single- or two-handed stroke in which the loosely clenched fist strikes the part so that the dorsal aspect of the middle and distal phalanges of the fingers and the heel of the hand make contact with the tissues.

Purpose
Beating is similar to clapping and is designed to stimulate the tissues by direct mechanical action. Though it is similar to clapping, beating is more stimulating. On certain areas (e.g., the sacrum) the manipulation may be done with one hand only, at a slow rhythm. The relaxed hand drops on the part with the terminal phalanges extended. This is known as sacral beating.

Basic Technique and Direction of Movement
Beating is usually performed with alternate movements of the dorsal aspect of the middle and distal phalanges of the loosely clenched hands, together with an area of the palm near the wrist joint. The stroke is carried out by alternately

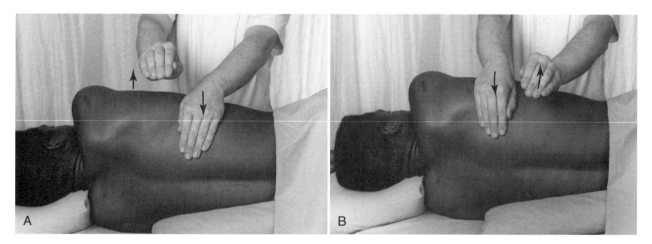

Figure 3–20. Clapping over the lungs to loosen secretions.
The therapist stands at right angles to the long axis of the thorax. With the elbows held almost straight, the cupped hands alternately strike the skin surface (A, B) and move up and down the thorax, over the lungs. Again, movement is produced by flexion and extension at the wrists rather than the elbow joints. This technique may also be performed over a folded towel. This damps the effect of the stroke, allowing the therapist to exert greater pressure without causing a slapping sensation on the skin surface.

flexing and extending the wrists; the rest of the arm is as relaxed as possible. The hands move along the body part being treated so as to cover the entire area involved.

Rate of Movement
Beating is performed quite rapidly, since it aims to stimulate. The actual rate is determined by the therapist.

Depth and Pressure
Beating is a stroke that is performed rapidly and with rather more pressure than clapping, since it is a more stimulating stroke. As in clapping, the elbows should be held in a comfortable position somewhere near full extension. The actual stroke is performed by alternate wrist flexion and extension, not by elbow movement. The hands move across the area in a manner similar to that of clapping. Figure 3–21 illustrates beating to the inner thigh muscles.

Hacking

Definition
Hacking is a single- or double-handed stroke in which the lateral edges and dorsal surfaces of the fingers strike the skin surface in rapid succession to create a strong, stimulating effect.

Purpose
Hacking is used to stimulate the skin and subcutaneous and muscle tissue.

Basic Technique and Direction of Movement
The therapist, standing at right angles to the long axis of the muscles to be treated, flexes the elbows and abducts the shoulders so that the forearms are nearly horizontal, with the wrists near full extension (a praying position). The movement is a rapid alternation between pronation and supination of the forearms with the hands working "out of phase" with each other. It is the ulnar borders and dorsal

surfaces of the third, fourth, and fifth fingers that actually strike the skin surface. The hands move back and forth along the muscles to be treated.

The movement is one of rapidly alternating pronation and supination with slight radial and ulnar deviation. During the movement, the palmar surfaces almost touch each other. It is important for the fingers and hand to be relaxed during the stroke; otherwise the fingers strike the skin surface and cause an uncomfortable sensation for the patient. The manipulation is performed across the muscle fibers, and bony areas are carefully avoided.

Hacking is usually performed with two hands, but it can be done with only one. This variation might be useful in the treatment of small muscles, when it is difficult to fit two hands into the area.

Rate of Movement
This is a difficult stroke to master because it has to be performed as rapidly as possible. It requires considerable coordination of effort, and it is better to perform it correctly at slower speeds than faster but incorrectly. The most common mistake in the performance of hacking is to flex and extend the elbows rather than to rotate the forearms. This can easily produce too much pressure, and the stroke ceases to be light and stimulating.

Depth and Pressure
Hacking must be performed rapidly but lightly. There is no pressure other than the weight of the relaxed fingers striking the skin surface in rapid succession. This produces a characteristic sound, as each finger is clearly audible as it strikes the surface. Figure 3–22 illustrates hacking to the inner thigh muscles.

Variations
In *ulnar border hacking* the movement is performed in a similar way but uses the ulnar border of the hand and fingers on large fleshy areas for a deeper effect. *Point*

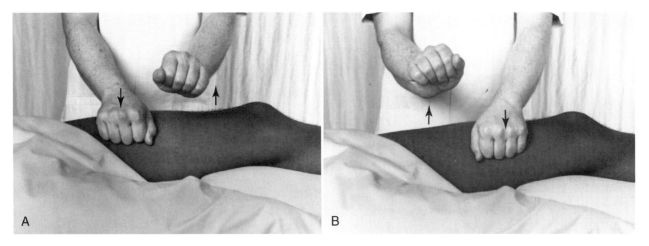

Figure 3–21. Beating to the inner thigh muscles.
(A,B) The basic alternating wrist action in beating is illustrated. The stroke is performed quite rapidly and with a little more pressure than that used with clapping.

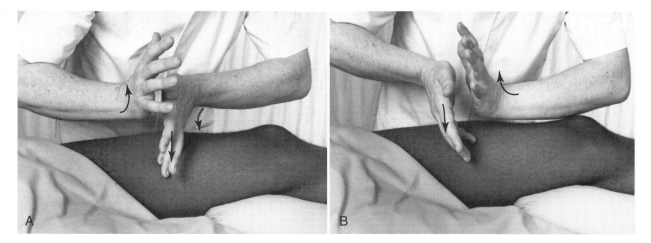

Figure 3–22. Hacking to the inner thigh muscles.
The therapist stands at right angles to the long axis of the muscles to be treated. The forearms are nearly horizontal, and the wrists are almost fully extended. The movement is a rapid alternation between pronation and supination of the forearms (*A, B*) with the hands working out of phase with each other. The lateral and dorsal surfaces of the third, fourth, and fifth fingers strike the surface one after the other, producing a characteristic sound. The hands move back and forth along the muscles to be treated.

hacking is carried out by the finger tips only, when the wrist is alternately flexed and extended. It is used only on the face.

Pounding

Definition
Pounding is a movement in which the ulnar borders of the loosely clenched fists alternately and in rapid succession strike the part to be treated.

Purpose
Pounding is another of the stimulating strokes. It is somewhat deeper than hacking, as the hands are lightly clenched and the ulnar borders are used to strike the tissues. This allows greater depth to the stroke.

Basic Technique and Direction of Movement
Pounding is a stroke that looks very similar to hacking. The therapist stands at right angles to the long axis of the muscles to be treated with elbows flexed and shoulders abducted so that the forearms are nearly horizontal. The wrists are near full extension. The movement consists of rapid alternation of pronation and supination of the forearms, with the hands working out of phase with each other. The fists are loosely clenched, and it is the ulnar borders of the hands and fifth digits that actually strike the skin surface. The hands move back and forth along the muscles to be treated.

Rate of Movement
The movement should be as rapid as the coordination of the therapist allows; however, good technique should not be sacrificed for speed.

Depth and Pressure
Since the ulnar borders of the hands are used to strike the surface, this is a much deeper stroke than hacking. It is therefore suitable for the stimulation of large, deep muscle masses.

Effects of Tapotement

Mechanical Effect. If percussion is given over the thorax with the patient in a suitable postural drainage position, adherent mucus may be loosened and moved along the respiratory tract so it can be coughed up.

Reflex Effects. Owing to the axon reflex there is reddening of the skin. At first there is vasoconstriction secondary to stimulation of vasomotor nerves, but this is followed by vasodilatation. Hacking over the spinal muscles may induce a general sense of warmth and invigoration, owing to the stimulation of the sensory branch of posterior primary rami. Tapotement over muscle fibers produces a stretching effect that reflexly facilitates muscle contraction (via the stretch reflex). Sensory nerve endings (especially the mechanoreceptors) are stimulated, and this may give rise to pain relief via a spinal gating mechanism.

Therapeutic Uses of Tapotement

- Treatment of chronic chest conditions such as cystic fibrosis and bronchiectasis.

- To provide a general stimulating effect in a massage sequence to any part of the body.

- To relieve neuralgia after amputation, trauma, or another pathologic process.
  (*Note:* Tapotement should not be performed over bony areas or over muscles that are either hypertonic or hypotonic.)

Contraindications to Tapotement

- Vigorous clapping may cause obvious damage to the underlying lung tissue, if given over *severe rib fractures* (flail chest). Only very fine, gentle vibrations may be used in the presence of a rib fracture.
- Clapping to the thorax in cases of *acute heart failure,* especially if associated with coronary thrombosis, due to the obvious possibility of an embolism.
- Clapping to the thorax in cases of *acute pulmonary embolism,* as it may cause blockage of pulmonary vessels.
- In cases of *severe hypertension,* vigorous shaking and vibration may increase blood pressure to dangerously high levels, especially if the patient is "tipped" during treatment.
- Tapotement can be painful or uncomfortable for a patient with *hyperesthesia.*
- *Flaccidity* places the patient at risk for overstretching a muscle.
- *Spasticity* may be significantly increased.
- On *newly formed scar tissue* it may interfere with healing or stimulate overproduction of such tissue.
- It may increase damage to tissue involved with *acute traumatic edema.*
- If the area to be treated is involved with *cancer or tuberculosis,* it risks spreading the disease.

Vibration

Definition
Vibration is a single- or double-handed technique in which a fine shaking movement or tremor is conveyed to the tissues by the hand or finger tips.

Purpose
Vibration is a stroke designed primarily to help loosen secretions in the lungs. It may also be used as a stimulating technique over muscle tissue, since it can stimulate a stretch reflex.

Basic Technique and Direction of Movement
The hand or finger tips are placed lightly on the part. The elbow should be nearly straight, but the arm must remain relaxed. When given over the thorax to loosen and remove lung secretions, the hands may be placed successively over each of the various lung segments. The movement may be in and out, up and down, or made by moving the hand to cover a larger area.

Rate of Movement
If vibrations are given to help loosen lung secretions they should be delivered during the *expiratory* phase of breathing. During the actual vibratory movement, the shaking may be quite rapid, but it is performed only as the patient breathes out.

Depth and Pressure
Vibrations are usually rather fine in quality. Little pressure is applied during the actual shaking of the chest. Figure 3–23 illustrates the technique of vibrations applied to the thorax.

Shaking

Definition
Shaking is a single- or double-handed technique in which a significant rhythmic shaking movement or tremor is conveyed to the tissues by the hand or finger tips.

Purpose
Shaking is a stroke designed primarily to assist in the loosening of secretions from the lungs. It is similar to vibration but is usually performed rather more "coarsely" than vibrations. It may also be used as a stimulating technique over muscle tissue, since it can stimulate a stretch reflex.

Basic Technique and Direction of Movement
The part is held with one or both hands, which move from side to side, in and out, or up and down. When given to the thorax, the manipulation is timed to coincide with the expiratory phase of respiration. The therapist's hands may remain stationary or may move over the skin to cover a larger area.

Rate of Movement
When shaking is given to help loosen lung secretions, it should be timed with the patient's respirations and given

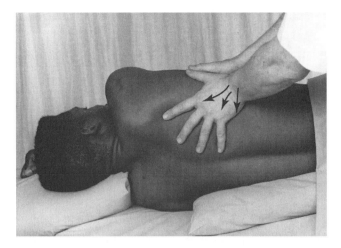

Figure 3–23. Vibrations to the thorax to help loosen lung secretions.
In this example, the patient is in the side-lying position with the end of the plinth tipped up. The therapist's hands are placed on the chest wall with the fingers spread wide so that the palms of the hands are about level with the eighth rib in the midaxillary line. Slight resistance may be given as the patient breathes in, and the fine vibratory movement is imparted only as the patient breathes out.

during the expiratory phase of breathing. Since the movement is rather coarse, as compared with vibrations, it is usually a little slower.

Depth and Pressure

Shaking is a more vigorous stroke than vibrations, and, therefore, rather more pressure is applied during the actual shaking of the chest. Otherwise the two strokes are very similar.

Effects of Vibrations and Shaking

Mechanical Effects. When given over the thorax, they loosen adherent mucus.

When applied over the stomach and intestine the manipulations cause movement of gases.

Vibrations may help resolve edema.

Reflex Effects. Vibrations applied over nerves may relieve pain (spinal gating mechanism). The technique may also be used to facilitate a muscle contraction (stretch reflex).

Therapeutic Uses of Shaking and Vibrations

- For chronic chest conditions and after chest surgery to loosen mucus and aid expectoration.
- To relieve flatulence.
- To help resolve chronic edema. (A mechanical vibrator may be more useful in the relief of chronic edema.)
- For the relief of some cases of neuralgia.

Contraindications to Shaking and Vibrations

- Shaking or vibrations may cause obvious damage to the underlying lung tissue, if given over *severe rib fractures* (flail chest). Only very fine, gentle vibrations may be used in the presence of a rib fracture.
- To the thorax in cases of *acute heart failure,* especially if associated with coronary thrombosis, due to the obvious possibility of an embolism.
- To the thorax in cases of *acute pulmonary embolism,* as it may cause blockage of pulmonary vessels.
- In cases of *severe hypertension,* vigorous shaking and vibration may increase blood pressure to dangerously high levels, especially if the patient is "tipped" during treatment.
- In cases of *hyperesthesia,* vibration and shaking may be too uncomfortable/painful.
- *Spasticity* will probably increase if vibration or shaking is used on a spastic muscle group.

Deep Frictions (Cyriax Frictions)

Deep friction massage is a rather different technique than the massage strokes described previously. In effect, it is a massage system in itself, though it is designed principally to affect the connective tissues of tendons, ligaments, and muscles. The most famous modern exponent of deep friction massage was James Cyriax, and his writings on the subject have become the established standards for the techniques (Cyriax, 1966; Cyriax & Coldham, 1984).

Definition

Deep frictions consist of small, accurately localized, deeply penetrating movements performed in a circular or transverse direction. These deep strokes are usually carried out by the finger tips, though the thumb pad or palm can also be used.

Classification

Transverse movements are a series of short, deep strokes performed transversely across the fibers of the target tissue. A series or three or four *circular* movements are performed on the same spot, gradually getting deeper and deeper into the tissues.

Purpose

Deep frictions are designed to mobilize tendons, ligaments, joint capsules, and muscle tissue, particularly if chronic adhesions or inflammation is present.

Basic Technique and Direction of Movement

To obtain the firm contact with the skin that is necessary to apply friction movements, it is important that no lubricant be used. Friction movements over dry, scaly scar tissue should be applied without a lubricant, and when the treatment is completed, a small amount of lubricant should be applied to the area with stroking movements. The two types of friction strokes are quite different and will be described separately.

Transverse Frictions

Transverse frictions are performed at right angles to the long axis of the fibers in the structures involved (i.e., across the fibers). These following important points of technique must be emphasized:

Massage must be given on exactly the correct spot.

Accurate localization of the lesion is essential if the technique is to be successful. A thorough knowledge of anatomy and excellent palpation skills are essential for the therapist.

The structure to be treated must be placed on full stretch.

The structure to be treated is usually a tendon, ligament, joint capsule, or muscle. Placing it on maximum stretch requires accurate anatomical knowledge and applied understanding of the biomechanics of the involved tissues.

The fingers must move with the skin and subcutaneous tissues on the deeper ones.

The finger tips and the skin surface must move together on the deeper tissues; otherwise the strokes are ineffective and

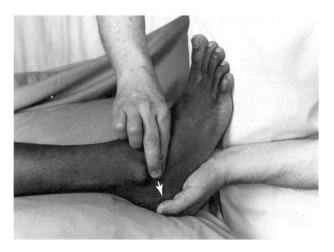

Figure 3–24. Transverse frictions to the lateral ligament of the ankle.
The lateral ligament is first put on maximum stretch by inverting the forefoot and calcaneum. In this position, the exact point of tenderness is first determined and the friction stroke delivered at right angles to the fibers of the ligament. Pressure gradually increases during each pass across the ligament, until significant pressure has been achieved. This gives the stroke its deep effects. In this case, the friction stroke is applied by the index finger reinforced by the middle one.

it is easy to blister the skin. In hot weather the skin should be washed and dried, and if necessary evaporating spirits may be given to the part afterward to dry the skin surface.

The movement is delivered with a transverse motion across the fibers.

It is essential that the movement be performed at right angles to the direction of the fibers. This has been found to be the most effective method of mobilizing striated muscles. In addition, a slight arc of motion across the fibers is desirable, since most of the structures treated are not flat in cross section but curved. As the fingers move across the structure, pressure is usually applied *in one direction only,* either forward or backward. This produces a series of pulling or pushing strokes.

The movements must have sufficient depth and sweep to reach the lesion.

This may require reinforcement by using two fingers or thumbs when treating a large muscle like the quadriceps. The strokes should begin lightly and the pressure should gradually be increased until sufficient depth is reached. If the massage stroke is too localized the mobilization will be ineffective, and often painful. To be effective it must cover a sufficient area.

Transverse frictions, properly administered, can be very demanding on the terminal joints of the therapist's fingers. To help prevent problems and to maintain effective treatment, a custom-made finger splint may be helpful

(Steward, Woodman, & Hurlburt, 1996). A variety of applications of transverse frictions are depicted in Figures 3–24 through 3–26.

Circular Frictions

These may be performed with the tips of the second, third, and fourth digits or with the thumb. The fingers may be

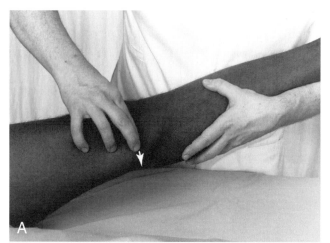
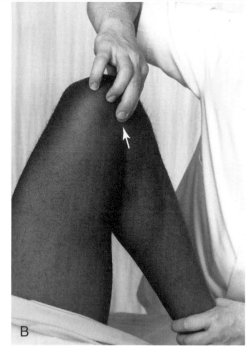

Figure 3–25. Transverse frictions to the medial ligament of the knee.
The ligament to be treated is first put on maximum stretch. In the case of the medial (tibial collateral) ligament of the knee this can be achieved with the knee in either full extension *(A)* or full flexion *(B).* In this position, the exact point of tenderness is first determined and the friction stroke delivered across the fibers of the ligament. Pressure gradually increases during each pass across the ligament, until a significant pressure has been achieved. The stroke is delivered with the index finger reinforced by the middle one.

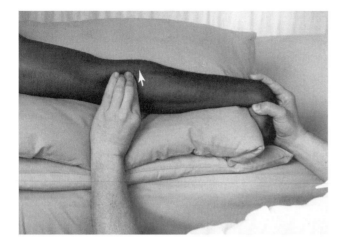

Figure 3–26. Transverse frictions to the common extensor origin of the forearm muscles.
The common extensor origin is first put on maximum stretch by fully flexing the wrist and fingers with the elbow in extension and pronation. In this position, the exact point of tenderness is first determined and the friction stroke delivered on a curve that follows the contours of the arm and at right angles to the fibers of the tendon. Pressure gradually increases during each pass across the ligament until a significant pressure has been achieved. This gives the stroke its deep effects. In this case, the friction stroke is applied by the index finger reinforced by the middle one.

reinforced by the corresponding digits of the other hand if greater depth is required. When the finger tips are used, a small "tripod-like" arrangement is made with the tips of the index, middle, and ring fingers, respectively. The index and ring finger tips touch each other and the middle finger sits on top of them. An alternative technique is for the therapist to use the tip of the index finger reinforced by the middle one.

The fingers should be pressed obliquely into the tissues before beginning the movement and then should move in very small circles, going slightly deeper with each successive one. In this way the superficial tissues are moved over the deeper ones. When the required depth has been obtained (usually after three or four circles) the pressure is released gradually and the fingers are lifted to an adjacent area so that the manipulation can be repeated. Figure 3–27 illustrates circular frictions to an interspinal region.

Rate of Movement
Both transverse and circular frictions are performed slowly with a steady rhythm.

Depth and Pressure
Both transverse and circular frictions are very deep strokes. Significant pressure is applied to a very small area of tissue, and it is important that the fingers do not move across the skin, lest a blister result because of the pressure. In both cases, pressure is gradually increased with the first few

passes over the tissue being treated. This helps the patient to become accustomed to the sensation. It will be somewhat uncomfortable or painful but should not be unbearable.

Duration of Treatment
Treatment may last 5 to 20 minutes at each session; this may be repeated two or three times a week, as long as is necessary.

Effects of Deep Frictions
The deep sustained pressure on the tissues causes local damage and liberates a histamine-like substance (H substance) and other metabolites that act directly on the capillaries and arterioles in the local area, causing vasodilation. The magnitude of the response depends on the depth of the manipulation and on how long it was performed.

The local vasodilatation produces an increase in the amount of tissue fluid in the area, which distends the area. In effect, the stroke produces controlled inflammation of the target area and at the same time mobilizes the structures that were not moving correctly. If the manipulation is sustained for some time very little sensory effect is felt by the patient, but initially the manipulation can be painful. Producing pain in the patient is in fact a very useful therapeutic strategy. Painful stimulation is a well-known

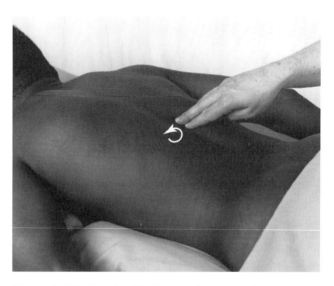

Figure 3–27. Circular frictions to the interspinous region.
With the patient comfortably positioned lying prone, the exact location of the problem area is first determined. The tips of the first three digits are used to form a small tripod-like arrangement. Pressure is applied through the fingertips in a small circular movement, gradually getting deeper. Three or four circles on each tender area usually is sufficient before a pause is given. The technique can then be repeated several times. The sensation for the patient is expected to be uncomfortable or painful, but not unbearable, during the actual application.

technique for the treatment of chronic pain, particularly that associated with myofascial pain syndromes. It can be achieved using electrical stimulation or manual techniques. In fact, deep friction is an excellent example of a manual treatment that produces a very effective, if painful, response.

Therapeutic Uses of Deep Frictions

Scar tissue secondary to fibrositis or trauma is often painful and immobile. Tissues of the body all have their own natural mobility and elasticity, and this may be impaired by any local organization of fibrous tissue. Production and organization of fibrous tissue is the inevitable result of trauma or a rheumatic inflammatory process that does not heal properly. The result will likely be a painful loss of joint and limb function. Deep frictions, along with other interventions in a planned treatment program, are useful for the management of muscle tears, musculotendinous lesions, tendinitis and partial tendon ruptures (tenoperiosteal tears), tenosynovitis, ligament sprains, induration of subcutaneous areas, and scar tissue.

Contraindications to Deep Frictions

The major contraindications to deep frictions are similar to those for other strokes, particularly those involving significant pressure on the tissues.

- Acute muscle tears (especially intramuscular hematomas)
- Acutely inflamed joints
- Skin diseases (especially acute dermatitis, psoriasis, or any communicable skin infection) in the area to be treated
- Damaged or diseased blood vessels (especially thrombophlebitis and deep vein thrombosis) in the area to be treated
- Neoplasm or tuberculosis in or near the area being treated
- Bacterial infections in or near the area being treated, especially infections in joints

References

Cyriax J. (1960) Clinical applications of massage. In: Licht S (ed): Massage, manipulation and traction. Baltimore: Waverley Press, pp 122–139.

Cyriax J, Coldham M. (1984) Textbook of orthopaedic medicine, Vol 2. London: Bailliere Tindall, pp 9–21.

Steward B, Woodman R, Hurlburt D. (1995) Fabricating a splint for deep friction massage. JOSPT 221(3):172–175.

Chapter 4

Mechanical, Physiological, Psychological, and Therapeutic Effects of Massage

According to the great Arabic philosopher and scientist Avicenna (980–1037), "The object of massage is to disperse the effete matters [metabolites] formed in the muscles and not expelled by exercise. It causes the effete matter to disperse and so remove fatigue" (Gruner, 1930). This statement from Avicenna clearly shows that classical scholars were very interested in understanding the mechanisms by which massage might have its beneficial effects.

Although soft tissue massage has been perfected over many thousands of years, there are relatively few scientific studies into its effects and efficacy. The great majority of writings on the subject of massage have concentrated more on a description of the techniques and the observed effects of the treatment than on efforts to investigate these effects scientifically. Only comparatively recently has much interest been seen in the objective measurement of the effects of massage. In this chapter we discuss both the traditional descriptions of the effects of massage and some recent laboratory data.

Soft tissue massage has three basic effects on the patient: mechanical, physiological, and psychological. Each of these broad areas is considered separately here, although they are, of course, closely related. In fact, the primary effects of massage are mechanical, but they produce physiological and psychological effects in the person. An understanding of these effects leads to a reasoned description of the therapeutic indications and probable contraindications for massage.

> ## Mechanical Effects of Massage
>
> - Movement of:
>   Lymph
>   Venous blood
>   Lung secretions
>   Edema
>   Intestinal contents
>   Hematoma contents
> - Mobilization of:
>   Muscle fibers
>   Muscle masses
>   Tendons
>   Tendons in sheaths
>   Skin and subcutaneous tissue
>   Scar tissue
>   Adhesions

MECHANICAL EFFECTS

Squeezing, pulling, stretching, pressing, and rubbing strokes have obvious mechanical effects on tissues. The mechanical forces associated with each technique affect the tissues in a variety of ways. For example, the various techniques of kneading and wringing would be expected to have a considerable mobilizing effect (loosening or stretching) on the skin and subcutaneous and muscle tissue, owing to the alternate squeezing and stretching of the strokes. In contrast, the gradually increasing pressure of effleurage would be expected to push the venous blood and lymph in the superficial vessels toward the heart, thus promoting good circulation and resolution of chronic edema and hematoma. In a similar manner, the pressure and direction of stroking and effleurage techniques promote movement of the intestinal contents.

The principal effects of each of the basic massage techniques were outlined in Chapter 3. While the mechanical effects of massage are important to identify, it is the physiological effects that need to be considered in some detail, since these give rise to the therapeutic potential of massage. The primary effect of massage, then, is to produce mechanical stimulation of the tissues by means of rhythmically applied pressure and stretching. Pressure compresses soft tissues and distorts the networks of nerve ending receptors. Stretching applies tension on soft tissues and distorts the nerve ending plexuses of receptors. By enlarging the lumens of blood vessels and lymph vessel spaces these two forces affect capillary, venous, arterial, and lymphatic circulation. We can demonstrate axon reflex. We can stimulate a variety of receptors, both superficial and deep, in the skin, muscles, and tendons; in ligaments and joint capsules; and in many of the deeper organs of the body. Massage can also loosen mucus and promote drainage of excess fluids from the lungs.

How these mechanical forces are applied is determined largely by the therapist's choice of massage techniques (stroking, friction, kneading, percussion, vibration) and his or her skill in adjusting the duration, quality, intensity, and rhythm of the stimulus (see Chapter 3). What effects massage may have is not as well understood or as well defined. Many claims have been made for the use of massage, many of which are based largely on clinical experience, both objective reports and anecdotal testimonials. Some are rationalizations of hypotheses based on knowledge of anatomy and physiology. Some are based on controlled laboratory studies, and some can definitely be described as wishful thinking. Comparatively little has been written on massage, and relatively few studies have been made.

The effects of massage have been described and classified in several ways. Mennell referred to mechanical (pressure and tension), chemical, reflex, and psychological effects. Other authors discussed general and local effects. These effects might also be classified as mechanical, physiological (including reflex), and psychological. A purely mechanical effect can be demonstrated by stroking superficial veins and, with direct pressure, removing the blood from the portion of the vein being stroked.

Lucas-Championnière's technique of obtaining relaxation of muscles in spasm following a fracture by superficial stroking can be explained only as a reflex (physiological)

effect. Mennell's (1945) caution against "rubbing a disability into a patient's mind" when massaging a part that has sustained a minor injury stresses a purely psychological effect. It is probable, however, that most massage treatments produce their effects as the result of a combination of mechanical, physiological, and psychological factors.

PHYSIOLOGICAL EFFECTS

The mechanical effects of massage give rise to a number of important physiological effects.

Effects on Blood and Lymph Flow

Since all massage techniques involve some degree of manipulation of the skin and underlying tissues, it is reasonable to expect that they would have a considerable effect on the flow of blood and lymph in these tissues. In addition, swelling that had accumulated in such tissues would be expected to be similarly affected; however, Mennell believed that it is impossible to affect arterial circulation directly via the mechanical effects of massage. He theorized that applying massage pressure in the direction of the venous flow is comparable to the effect of squeezing any soft tube to empty it of fluid. If the muscles are relaxed they constitute a soft mass containing tubes filled with fluid. Any pressure applied to the mass should push the fluid in these tubes in the direction in which the

---

Physiological Effects of Massage

- Increased blood and lymph flow
- Increased flow of nutrients
- Removal of waste products and metabolites
- Stimulation of the healing process
- Resolution of chronic edema and hematoma
- Increased extensibility of connective tissue
- Pain relief
- Increased joint movement
- Facilitation of muscle activity
- Stimulation of autonomic functions
- Stimulation of visceral functions
- Removal of lung secretions
- Sexual arousal
- Promotion of local and general relaxation

---

pressure is applied; therefore, if sufficient pressure is applied to the entire mass the deeper veins will also be emptied. Such pressure might at the same time retard arterial blood flow if it is forceful enough to compress the arteries and the veins. Theoretically, if the amount of

venous blood brought to the heart can be increased by massage the heart rate or the stroke volume might be increased and a greater amount of arterial blood would thus be carried to the periphery. In fact, there is little evidence of such a simple mechanical reaction of the arterial and arteriolar system to massage. Wakim (1949, 1955) found that following deep stroking and kneading massage the average increase in total blood flow in normal, rheumatoid arthritic joints was inconsistent. Moderate, consistent, and definite increases in circulation were observed after such massage to flaccid, paralyzed extremities. Vigorous, stimulating massage resulted in consistent and significant increases in average blood flow of the massaged extremity but produced no change in blood flow in the contralateral unmassaged extremity.

According to Pemberton (1932, 1939, 1950) the nervous system, probably through the sympathetic division, contributes to a reflex influence on the blood vessels of the parts concerned. He believed that it is probable, therefore, that vessels in the muscles or elsewhere are emptied during massage not only by virtue of being squeezed but also through a reflex action.

Pemberton stated that microscopic observation thus reveals that massage may cause almost all the smaller vessels to become visible because it promotes blood flow through them. Although there is little information on the type of massage that was used, several convincing experiments have been performed that show that massage increases circulation of the blood.

Wolfson (1931) studied the effect of deep kneading massage on venous blood flow in normal dog limbs and found that massage caused a great increase in flow initially, which was followed by a fairly rapid decrease to a less than normal rate even before the end of stimulation. Immediately after cessation of the procedure he noted that the flow rate slowly increased again to normal. He concluded that the actual volume of blood that passes through the limb during the period of stimulation and recovery is not greater than normal but that there is more complete emptying for a short time, so that a larger volume of fresh blood is brought to the part. He suggested that it would seem logical to use short but frequent massage treatments.

Carrier (1922) has shown that light pressure produces almost instantaneous, though transient, dilatation of the capillary vessels, whereas heavier pressure may produce more enduring dilatation. Microscopic observation of fields in which only a few capillaries are open shows that pressure may cause nearly all the smaller vessels to become visible.

Pemberton (1945) described the work of Clark and Swanson, who made cinematographic studies of the capillary circulation in the ear of a rabbit utilizing a permanent window for observation. These studies demonstrated that following massage more capillaries were opened and the rate of flow was faster. A change in the blood vessel wall was evidenced by the "sticking" and emigration of leukocytes. The increased blood flow as a result of massage was demonstrated as long ago as the mid-1890s (Brunton & Tunnicliffe, 1894–1895).

Many have claimed that the reflex effect of superficial stroking improves cutaneous circulation, especially blood flow in superficial veins and lymphatics; aids in the exchange of tissue fluids; increases tissue nutrition; and assists in the removal of the products of fatigue or inflammation; however, as long ago as 1939, Wright stated that such claims must be examined critically in the light of present-day knowledge of physiology. He maintained that it was difficult to make positive statements about reflex effects produced by massage. More than 50 years later, the situation is in many ways rather similar.

Severini and Venerando (1967) reported that superficial massage produced no significant changes except in skin temperature. Deep massage did however increase blood flow and systolic stroke volume and decreased systolic and diastolic arterial pressure and pulse frequency. Interestingly, deep massage was also associated with increased blood flow in the untreated contralateral limb. This effect was also demonstrated by Bell (1964), who showed that after deep stroking and kneading of the calf of one leg for 10 minutes plethysmographic studies showed blood volume—and thus the rate of blood flow—had doubled, an effect that lasted 40 minutes, as compared with only 10 minutes after exercise. Bell recommended massage to treat edema of fractures because of its effects on venous and lymphatic flow. Severini and Venerando (1969) also combined massage with a hyperemia-producing drug (containing vanillyl and butoxyethyl nicotinate). The combined treatment led to a significant and prolonged rise in skin temperature. When the drug was used alone or with superficial massage there was no change in circulation in muscles, but with deep massage there was an appreciable and effective increase in blood flow in muscles.

On a more central level, Barr and Taslitz (1970) showed that systolic and diastolic blood pressure tended to decrease after a 20-minute back massage. Delayed effects were an increase in systolic pressure and a small additional decrease in diastolic pressure. The heart rate increased.

In the lymphatic capillaries and plexuses of the skin and subcutaneous tissue, lymph can move in any direction. Its movement depends on forces outside the lymphatic system. Its course is determined by factors such as gravity, muscle contraction, passive movement, and massage. If obstruction of the deeper lymphatics occurs in a part it is still possible to keep the superficial lymphatics open, and, if the part is massaged or given opportunity to drain by gravity, lymph moves through these other channels in the direction of the external force.

Animal experiments show that there is very little lymph flow when a muscle is at rest. Von Mesengeil's and Kellgren and Colombo's studies on the effects of massage on lymph flow observed increased lymph flow when the muscles were massaged (Cuthbertson, 1933). Von Mesengeil "repeatedly injected China ink into corresponding articulations of rabbits. One joint was massaged and the corresponding one left as a control. In the legs without massage, the tendency of the colored material to pass toward the heart was very small, but in those legs subjected to massage there was great absorption of the ink above the joint in the intermuscular connective tissues and in the lymphatic glands. The lymphatics passing up to the glands were deeply stained black."

Kellgren and Colombo found, "Massage always had a sure and effective influence in increasing the rapidity of the absorption of substances injected into animals in all the organs which can be subjected to manipulations—subcutaneous tissues, muscles, articulations, and serous cavities. The course which the injected substance followed during its absorption was always that of the nearest lymphatics and the glands into which they pass. Deep effleurage was probably less effective than the squeezing and rolling of muscles and subcutaneous tissue." McMaster (1937) also showed that massage increased lymph flow by experiments in which the limbs of normal healthy subjects were massaged after intradermal dye injections.

Drinker and Yoffey (1941) cannulated the cervical lymph trunks in an anesthetized dog and were able to sustain lymph flow all day long by massaging the head and neck above the cannulas. When the massage was stopped, lymph flow either ceased or was negligible. The investigators state that, in treating chronic inflammatory conditions in which fibrosis is sure to advance if tissue fluid and lymph remain stagnant in the part, massage in the direction of lymph flow is the preeminent artificial measure for moving extravascular fluid into lymphatics and for moving lymph onward toward the bloodstream.

Drinker and Yoffey also found that the effects of posture were very obvious and that lymph flow from a dependent, quiescent part was practically negligible. Therefore, to influence the flow of lymph most efficiently in any area it seemed logical that the part should be elevated during the application of massage.

Ladd and coworkers (1952) compared the effects of massage, passive motion, and electrical stimulation on the rate of lymph flow in the forelegs of 15 dogs and found that massage was "significantly more effective than either passive motion or electrical stimulation in this series of animals." All three procedures were found to increase lymph flow much above that of the control period.

The idea of using mechanical forces to affect the circulation of blood and lymph is not limited to manual massage techniques. In recent years, a variety of pneumatic devices have been developed that deliver a series of controlled (and often graduated) pressure changes along a limb surface. In effect, these devices perform a kind of mechanical massage. They have proved to be of considerable benefit in the treatment of many acute and chronic circulation disorders but especially lymphedema (Yamazaki, Idezuki, Nemoto, & Togawa, 1988). Of course, manual massage techniques also have an important role to play in the management of lymphedema (Mason, 1993).

Massage has been studied for its effect on circulation, as a means of preventing pressure sores (Dyson, 1978; Ek, Gustavsson, & Lewis, 1985; Olson, 1989). Massage for this purpose, however, does not follow traditional massage techniques. In most cases, it takes the form of a short period (30 to 60 seconds) of "skin rubbing," the intention being to stimulate circulation to the areas of skin that are prone to develop pressure sores. Not surprisingly, the results of this kind of massage are difficult to interpret, let alone to use as a basis for making recommendations. In some studies this type of massage seemed to increase local circulation; in others, it appeared to decrease it. It seems unlikely that rapid skin friction massage would produce the kind of genuine increase in circulation that would prevent pressure sores. This is because this type of massage simply produces a small degree of mechanical friction on the skin surface. This would probably show up as a slight and short-lived change in surface temperature. On the other hand, a different kind of massage would be expected to produce a more profound effect on the circulation, especially if it involved deep kneading to muscles around the area, were that possible. A more efficient way of producing a rapid change in skin blood flow is massaging the area with an ice cube. In this case it is the cold stimulus that produces profound vasodilation after the initial vasoconstriction (Michlovitz, 1996). Undoubtedly, a brief massage with an ice cube is likely to be much more effective than a similar period of skin rubbing.

Effects on the Blood

More than 90 years ago Mitchell (1904) stated that in both healthy and anemic persons the red cell count increased after massage. In anemic subjects the increase is greatest 1 hour after treatment. Schneider and Havens (1915) also showed that abdominal massage will increase the hemoglobin and red cell count in blood taken from the finger at ordinary barometric pressures. Pemberton (1950) stated that massage unquestionably increases the hemoglobin and red cell values in the circulating blood and that there is a limited but definite increase in the oxygen capacity of the blood after massage. Lucia and Rickard (1933) found that massage consisting of gentle but firm stroking of a rabbit's ear at the rate of 25 strokes per minute for 5 minutes caused a local increase in the blood platelet count.

Bork, Karling, and Faust (1971), reporting the effects of whole body massage on serum enzyme levels in normal persons, showed a significant rise in serum glutamic oxaloacetic transaminase, creatine phosphokinase, lactic dehydrogenase, and MK. Because of these effects they feel that whole body massage is contraindicated for patients with dermatomyositis, especially serious cases.

More recently, Ernst and colleagues (1987) showed that a 20-minute whole body muscle massage causes a dilution effect and changes blood fluidity. This was observed in both normal subjects and patients with ankylosing spondylitis. When these effects are coupled with the increased blood and lymph flow produced by massage it can clearly be seen that this form of treatment has a significant role to play in maintaining and enhancing the overall nutrition of the tissues.

Effects on Metabolism and the Healing Process

Very little recent experimentation has been reported on the effects of massage on metabolism, although several studies were performed more than 50 years ago. Cuthbertson (1933) reviewed the existing literature on this subject and conducted several experiments of his own. These were his findings:

- Urine output is increased, especially after abdominal massage.
- Excretion of acid is not altered, and there is no change in the acid-base equilibrium.
- Excretion rates for nitrogen, inorganic phosphorus, and sodium chloride are increased.
- In normal persons there is no immediate effect on the basal consumption of oxygen or on pulse rate or blood pressure.

Pemberton (1939) believed, "In general the studies which have been made suggest broad and general influences may be exerted by massage and that it has no immediate or large effect on general metabolism per se." He agreed with the view that its cumulative effect on various metabolic processes lies in its effects on the circulation of the parts concerned.

The resolution of acute trauma or of chronic inflammation (healing process) consists of a cascade of interrelated changes in the affected tissues. These changes depend entirely on the efficiency of local circulation to the part, since all of the materials needed to resolve the inflammatory process must arrive at the scene via the bloodstream. In addition, all of the waste products must be removed from the area via the blood and lymph channels (Evans, 1980). Since massage has such profound effects on the blood and lymph systems, it seems obvious that it has the potential to be useful in stimulating the healing process, in both the acute and the chronic phases of recovery.

It is important to remember the crucial importance of the lymphatic system in removing plasma proteins and other large molecules once they have been deposited in the interstitial fluid. These molecules are too large to reenter the capillaries and must be eliminated via the lymphatics. Facilitation of healing is therefore the by-product of the other (more direct) effects (e.g., increased blood and lymph flow) on the tissues.

Effects on Muscle Tissue

More than 100 years ago Maggiora (1891) described the physiological action of massage on muscle tissue. Many other writers have also described the effects of massage on muscle tissue. Much of the literature on the effects of massage contains a relatively large number of positive statements and implications about the effects of massage on muscles, as compared with its effects on other systems and tissues of the body. Some of these statements cannot be substantiated by clinical observation or by scientific research. The present review considers separately the effects of massage on normal and abnormal muscle tissue.

Normal Muscles

Kellogg (1919) observed, "Massage produces an actual increase in the size of the muscle structures. The muscle is also found to become firmer and more elastic under its influence." McMillan (1925) wrote, "The muscles are strengthened and made to grow by manipulation." According to Despard (1932), "Massage improves the nutrition of the muscles and consequently promotes their development." These observations are not supported by contemporary authorities who generally agree that massage does not increase muscle strength.

Mennell (1945) believed that the theory that advocated kneading a muscle ("working a muscle up") and thereby making it stronger was a complete "delusion." He stated, "By one means alone can muscular strength be developed, and that is by muscular contraction, and no form of massage can do more than aid this means indirectly," and again, "To use massage aright we must consider it entirely as a means to an end, that end being restoration of function." As a means to an end, massage may be useful in making it possible for a muscle to perform more exercise and thus develop its strength. This fact has been proven by experimental work done by Rosenthal, Mosso, and Maggiora (and by others cited in Cuthbertson, 1933), who have shown that a muscle fatigued by work or by electrical stimulation will be restored much more rapidly and thoroughly by massage than by rest alone of the same duration.

Nordschow and Bierman (1962) studied 25 normal, healthy, active subjects to determine whether massage manually applied could cause measurable muscle relaxation in normal human subjects, expressed as increased muscle length. A "finger-to-floor" test was used to measure tension in the posterior muscles of the back, thighs, and legs as each subject, standing with knees straight, bent forward and attempted to touch the floor with the fingertips. Following such an attempt, each subject then assumed a comfortable, well-supported prone position for 30 minutes of rest. The "finger-to-floor" test was then repeated. The subject then reassumed the prone position and was given 30 minutes of massage, 15 to the back and 15 to the posterior aspect of the lower extremity, allowing 7.5 minutes per limb. The authors concluded that manual massage can cause relaxation, which is expressed as increased muscle length. Bell (1964) reported that muscle fatigue was relieved more quickly by massage and rest than by rest alone and suggested alternate "bouts" of exercise and massage in therapy (as is frequently done in some sports).

In a preliminary report, Smith and colleagues (1994) studied the effects of athletic massage on delayed-onset muscle soreness, creatine kinase, and neutrophil count. Their results indicate that massage reduces the negative effects of exercise on normal muscle. Presumably these effects are due to the increased circulation of blood and lymph, effectively "washing out" the by-products of exercise.

The term "muscle tone" is often used to describe the quality of a muscle that is firm and "ready to contract"; however, muscles at rest show no electromyographic activity (Goodgold & Erberstein, 1983), and, therefore, a muscle that exhibits tone cannot be at rest: it must be in a state of minimal contraction. Although some statements in the literature imply that massage increases muscle tone, evidence to support this claim is inconclusive, at best. Theoretically, however, several massage strokes would be expected to increase the fusimotor drive to a muscle. For example, any of the tapotement strokes (hacking, beating, pounding) would be expected to increase muscle spindle firing and, therefore, fusimotor output. Indeed, this is the mechanism by which massage strokes facilitate muscle contraction. It amounts to direct stimulation of stretch reflexes within the stimulated muscle.

Pathologic Conditions of Muscle

Fibrosis tends to occur in immobilized, injured, or denervated muscles. Significant shortening of the parallel and series elastic components (contracture) is often the end result. The muscle as a whole becomes shorter than its normal resting length, mainly because the fibrous tissue lacks elasticity and adhesions form between layers of connective tissue.

With the careful use of various massage techniques it is possible to apply tension on this fibrous tissue, the objective being to prevent adhesions from forming and to break down small adhesions that have already formed. The techniques best suited to this purpose are various forms of petrissage and deep friction. When supplemented by appropriate exercise and stretching regimens massage techniques are an essential component in the restoration of muscle length and of normal function. A number of experimental studies have investigated the effects of massage on both injured muscle and denervated muscle. These are considered separately here, since the issues involved in each case are significantly different.

Injured Muscle

Some of the earliest experimental work in this area was described by Lucas-Championnière (cited in Mennell, 1945), who summarized the results of the work of Castex on the effects of massage on injured muscles. Animal muscles were subjected to crushing injury; then massage was given to one group and another group was used as controls. The muscle tissue of both groups was later examined microscopically. The untreated parts showed the following characteristics: (1) dissociation into fibrils of the muscle fibers, as shown by well-marked longitudinal striation; (2) hyperplasia (often simple thickening) of the connective tissue; (3) an increased number of nuclei in the connective tissue; (4) interstitial hemorrhages; (5) an enlargement of blood vessels, with hyperplasia of their adventitious coats; and (6) usually intact sarcolemma (but, in one section, multiplication of nuclei gave an appearance that somewhat resembled interstitial myositis).

In contrast, the massaged limbs had the following features: (1) normal-looking muscle; (2) no secondary fibrous bands separating the muscle fibers; (3) no fibrous thickening around the vessels; (4) greater general muscle bulk; and (5) no signs of hemorrhage.

Denervated Muscle

Although massage has been used quite extensively for treatment of denervated muscle, there is little information in the literature on its effectiveness. Some studies have been performed, however, mainly in an effort to determine its effect on the histopathologic changes in the muscle itself, on atrophy, and on the strength of the muscle. At present no firm conclusions can be drawn from these results.

Chor and associates (1939) conducted an experiment to study the effects of massage on atrophy and the histopathologic changes that occur in denervated muscle in primates. Two groups of rhesus monkeys were subjected to unilateral section of the sciatic nerve; the nerves were then immediately sutured, and the extremity was immobilized in a plaster cast. After 4 weeks, massage (stroking and kneading) and passive motion were applied for 7 minutes daily to one group, while the control group was kept at complete rest. After intervals from 2 months for some animals to 6 months for others, the muscles were examined microscopically to determine the histopathologic changes. The muscles kept at rest were pale and surrounded by thickened septa of fibrous tissue with whitish and yellowish streaks throughout. Microscopically, this fibrosis was clearly demonstrable, both surrounding muscle fibers and replacing atrophic ones. The massaged muscles were supple and elastic and showed considerably less fibrosis and adhesions.

How much muscle function is restored after reinnervation is determined largely by the ratio of functioning muscle fibers to fibrous tissue that has replaced degenerated muscle fibers. To some extent preventing the formation of inelastic fibrous tissue and adhesions, massage helped maintain a favorable ratio for greater recovery of function.

In an earlier study, Chor and Dolkart (1936) studied atrophy of muscle from disuse and atrophy of denervated muscle. They observed that atrophy secondary to disuse of a skeletal muscle develops slowly and is associated with very simple structural changes. The loss of muscle bulk was attributed to a diminished quantity of sarcoplasm in the individual muscle fibers, the atrophic muscle fibers being narrower and packed closer together. The characteristic cross-striations persist; there is no actual degeneration of the muscle fibers. The intramuscular blood vessels remain unaltered.

The muscle atrophy that follows nerve section or lesions of the anterior horn cells (e.g., poliomyelitis) is more than wasting from disuse. Its course is very rapid, and characteristic changes occur. In addition to the shrinkage of the muscle fibers, degeneration of these cells follows. The cross-striations disappear, and breakdown of the muscle cells ensues. In later stages, the disintegrated muscle cells are replaced by fibrous tissue and fat. Changes also occur in the intramuscular blood vessels. The number of capillaries increases, and the small intramuscular blood vessels show hypertrophy of the endothelium and an increase in their fibrous structure.

Chor and coworkers believed that atrophy and degeneration of denervated skeletal muscle are inevitable and then showed that massage did not prevent atrophy up to a period of 6 weeks, but because of its effect on the amount of fibrous tissue formed, it did enable the muscles to return to normal more rapidly upon reinnervation.

In an early study, Langley and Hashimoto (1918) considered the effects of massage in denervated muscles from a single rabbit. Firm massage was begun on the third postoperative day. Treatment was discontinued on the seventh day because open lesions developed on the limb. Treatment was started again on the 11th day with "gentler" massage, which was continued until 23 days after denervation. They concluded that the effect of the treatment on atrophy was slight at best and that an increase in the growth of connective tissue is a possible result of massaging denervated muscle.

Hartman and colleagues (1919) tested both weight and work capacity of denervated muscles in 37 rabbits. One leg of the animals was given kneading and stroking massage. Both legs were given passive exercise. Treatment was continued for periods of 7 to 190 days. No significant differences were noted. The investigators suggested that the weight of the muscle did not necessarily indicate the amount of contractile tissue present, since structural mass and function of the muscles differed considerably in 17 of the muscles tested.

Hartman and Blatz (1920) later tested the power of denervated gastrocnemius muscles of 60 rabbits. The muscles on one side were massaged for periods of 2 to 20 minutes daily, and both legs were given daily passive movement. The muscles were tested at intervals of 10 to 14 days. They concluded (1) that "the treated limb on the whole did not appear to be any better off than the control"; (2) that massage was of no value; and (3) that there was invariably a decrease in power, and no significant difference between treated muscles and controls.

Wright (1939) stated that more rigorous proof was required for the claims that muscle wasting can be prevented or muscle nutrition improved by providing massage but not movement. He believed that some local effects are undoubtedly produced in the muscle and that they may be due to chemical agents liberated into the blood to produce local or general effects. He also believed that some of the metabolites of muscle activity may be liberated by massage. He questioned whether direct mechanical stimulation can produce a direct muscle response in denervated muscle as reflex reactions are excluded.

Suskind and coworkers (1946) studied the denervated gastrocnemius muscles of cats. Two 5-minute periods of effleurage and kneading were given daily to one limb; the other limb served as the control. The strength and weight of the muscles were measured 28 days after sectioning. Results showed that the denervated muscles treated with massage were heavier and stronger than their untreated contralateral controls. The effect on muscle weight was slight but statistically significant. It seemed that massage had lessened the gradual loss of contractile strength observed in skeletal muscle after denervation.

Wood and associates (1948) reported the effects of massage on weights and tensions of the anterior tibial muscles of 14 dogs. Bilateral section of sciatic nerves was done, and one leg was given a 10-minute period of stroking and kneading massage daily. The other leg was used as the control. The muscles were tested at intervals of from 13½ to 36 weeks after denervation. Results showed that all anterior tibial muscles in the treated animals appeared pale and small in bulk as compared with normal anterior tibial muscles. There was also a greater proportion of tendon to total bulk than in normal muscles, and a greater proportion of fatty tissue. It was impossible to distinguish treated tissue from untreated muscle on gross examination. Histologic sections from anterior tibial muscles of treated animals (treated and untreated muscles) showed no significant histologic differences. Wood concluded, "Massage was not effective in delaying denervation atrophy, as indicated by losses in strength and weight and by examination of histological sections in experimentally denervated anterior tibial muscles of the dog."

The primary effects of massage on muscle tissue can be summarized as follows:

• Massage does not directly increase the strength of normal muscle; however, as a means to an end it is more effective than rest in promoting recovery from fatigue produced by excessive exercise. Theoretically, then, massage makes it possible to do more exercise, which, in turn, increases muscular strength and endurance. This is an important factor in treatment. It would seem logical that massage should be given between periods of exercise when exercise is used to develop muscle strength and endurance. This is particularly relevant for sports medicine.

- Generally speaking, massage does not increase muscle tone, but certain strokes can be used to facilitate muscle activity (especially percussion techniques).

- Massage may reduce the amount of fibrosis that inevitably develops in immobilized, injured, or denervated muscle.

- Massage does not prevent atrophy in denervated muscle. Even though a muscle may undergo considerable wasting, if fibrosis is minimal and circulation and nutrition are good, a small muscle may have greater power than a muscle with larger mass if the mass is the result of overgrowth of fibrous tissue that interferes with the function and recovery of the remaining innervated muscle fibers.

- The aims of massage in the treatment of denervated muscle should be to maintain the muscles in the best possible state of nutrition, flexibility, and vitality, so that after recovery (if this is possible) from trauma or disease, the muscle can function at its maximum.

Effects on Bones and Joints

Key and colleagues (1934a and b) conducted an experiment to determine the effects of heat, massage, or active exercise on local atrophy of the bone caused by immobilization of the part. Ten patients with normal lower extremities were used. Both extremities were placed in casts, which were bivalved and removed during treatment. One extremity was used as a control; the other was treated. The massage was given 10 minutes twice daily for 6 weeks. Roentgenograms were made before and at the end of the experiment. No significant differences were observed between the treated and control limbs. The investigators concluded that short periods of heat (five patients), massage (two patients), or active exercise (three patients) had little, if any, effect on local atrophy of bone secondary to immobilization in a plaster of Paris cast. These results are interesting; however, the experiment was performed on very small numbers of subjects and the results are certainly inconclusive.

In the past, massage was used widely in the treatment of fractures, and it was considered beneficial for aiding repair of the associated soft tissue injuries. It has not been established that massage actually helps heal bone. It was the opinion of the Fracture Committee of the American College of Surgeons that, in the process of normal bone repair after fracture, "The effectiveness and rapidity of growth of tissue are dependent upon efficient circulation in the parts. . . . Therefore every effort must be made from the beginning to help the efficiency of the circulation."

Mock (1945) believed that, since recent research had shown the tendency for callus to be formed along the lines of the new blood vessels formed at the site of fractures, any treatment that enhanced circulation in the area of the fracture without producing motion of the fragments should promote deposition of callus. Of course this may be a

difficulty with many of the deeper massage strokes, whose objective is to deliberately squeeze and stretch the deeper muscle tissues. It is hard to see how these techniques can be given effectively without causing movement of the bone fragments at a fracture site; however, if the fracture site is stable, massage techniques might be very useful.

Many of the structures that surround the various joints of the body, such as ligaments, bursas, capsules, and tendons, are often the locus of chronic problems. In many instances of chronic dysfunction treatment is aimed at breaking down scar tissue in these structures and adhesions between them. Traditionally, deep friction massage has been the technique of choice, since its strong mechanical effect on scar tissue is obviously useful in restoring normal, painless range of motion to an affected joint (Cyriax, 1960, 1984; Hammer, 1993).

Effects on the Nervous System

Little direct information is available in the literature on the actual effects of massage on the function of the human nervous system. Nonetheless, it is possible to describe some likely effects based on what is known of the neurobiology of the system. For example, whenever the skin is touched or the underlying tissues are manipulated, sensory receptors in a variety of tissues are activated. Afferent signals pass into the spinal cord, form synapses with various spinal neurons, and eventually find their way to the sensory cortex and other brain centers. At a spinal level, several spinal reflexes could be triggered, depending on the type and depth of massage technique and the part of the body being massaged. Similar reflex activation is likely at a variety of autonomic centers and brain nuclei. Some of these concepts are discussed in the next section on the effects of massage on pain. Clearly, there are many potential pathways by which soft tissue massage might have direct and indirect effects on the nervous system.

A number of recent studies have shown that many direct effects are indeed possible. Very clear evidence from several well-controlled studies shows that massage (kneading) performed directly on a muscle causes significant depression of the amplitude of the H-reflex response, but only during the period of massage (Morelli, Seaborne, & Sullivan, 1991; Sullivan, Williams, Seaborne, & Morelli, 1991). This effect was also recorded in patients with spinal cord injury (Goldberg, Seaborne, Sullivan, & Leduc, 1994).

Goldberg and colleagues (1992) studied the effect of two intensities of massage on H-reflex amplitude and showed that a deeper massage technique produced a more pronounced reduction in H-reflex amplitude than did superficial massage. In all of the studies cited above, the inhibitory effect of the massage on H-reflex amplitude effectively lasted only during the massage phase. Some subjects (especially those with spinal cord injury) did show a tendency for the inhibitory effect to continue when the massage had ceased, but it did not last long enough to be useful therapeutically. These results are also important because they indicate that massage of a muscle tissue and its related structures (e.g., skin, subcutaneous tissues) can change the level of excitability of the spinal motor neurons. The effect is reflex in nature and is likely to be associated with increased firing of the pressure-sensitive receptors in muscle, especially the Golgi tendon organs, which are known to inhibit their relevant alpha motor neurons.

The sedative effect of a general massage can easily be demonstrated, and Mennell (1945) stated, "There is probably an effect on the central nervous system as well as a local effect on the sensory, and possibly the motor, nerves."

Despite promising early experimental studies on reflex control of circulation and neuromuscular responses to massage (Cuthbertson, 1933; McMaster, 1937; Pemberton, 1945) and strong support for hypotheses that massage has definite reflex effects, such effects seem to be hypothesized for want of any other rational explanation. Just what specific reflex mechanisms are responsible has not been made clear, nor has how simple or complex the reflex action(s) may be. Much work still must be done to clarify and verify these concepts by controlled clinical and laboratory studies, correlated with current physiological and neurophysiologic concepts.

The work of Barr and Taslitz (1970) is an example of the kind of studies that need to be done for a variety of massage treatments. In addition to the effects on blood pressure and heart rate of a 20-minute back massage Barr and Taslitz report these: (1) increased skin sweating and, thus, decreased resistance to galvanic current (galvanic skin response); (2) after a slight decrease in body temperature (0° to 0.1°C) in the control period, an increase from 0° to 0.2°C at the end of the massage; and (3) increased pupil diameter, which, in their opinion, may or may not have been a result of massage. Their results indicate an increase in sympathetic activity in most indexes.

The idea of producing specific effects in the nervous system, or indeed in neural control of many organs and systems, is not a new one. Traditional acupressure and many Eastern massage techniques are intended to affect a variety of nervous system functions. Examples of this principle can also be found in theories of reflexology, which hold that direct manual stimulation of various body areas (mainly, but not exclusively, the feet and hands) produces effects elsewhere in the body, and of the Japanese system of massage known as *shiatsu*. These concepts are discussed in more detail in Chapters 11 and 12.

Effects on Pain

Since the very earliest of times, primitive humans probably knew that vigorous rubbing of an injured area relieved pain. Such behavior is clearly instinctive and is displayed by humans and many animals. Rubbing the skin stimulates cutaneous mechanoreceptors, and these afferent signals are able to block the transmission—and possibly the perception—of nociceptive (pain) signals. This effect is easy to demonstrate and is one that most people have experienced. These same cutaneous receptors can also be stimulated by other modalities such as mechanical vibration and electrical stimulation.

In the past three decades, new theories and research on pain and its mechanisms of generation, transmission, perception, and treatment (Wall, 1994) have had a significant bearing on the ancient art of massage. This new understanding has led to a revival of interest in the use of electrical stimulation (Mannheimer & Lampe, 1984; Robinson & Snyder-Mackler, 1995) and many forms of manual mobilizing technique (Grieve, 1994).

A complex picture has developed that provides a rationale for intervention in a variety of soft tissue problems, including various chronic pain syndromes. The specificity of nociceptors and mechanoreceptors and their relationship to the transmission and eventual perception of pain have been elucidated, together with the alteration of tonic levels of muscle activity. Since it is known that manual stimulation of afferent fibers carrying sensory information can have a significant effect on pain, this constitutes strong scientific support for the use of massage as a therapeutic measure to relieve pain.

Beginning with the work of Melzack and Wall (1965) the concept of a neural "gate" in the region of the dorsal horn of the spinal cord gray matter has been central to intervention or research strategies involving pain. Although the original theory has undergone much review and revision, the central concepts remain intact.

All gates are designed to control the movement of something. When a gate is open, passage is permitted (possibly in both directions), and when it is closed a passage is denied. In this regard, the spinal gate is no different. Various cells are able to control the flow of nociceptive information (pain) from distal body parts to central sites in the nervous system. Nociceptive information is transmitted by small-diameter, slowly conducting fibers (A-delta and C fibers). The gate may be "closed" by specific sensory impulses from mechanoreceptors (large-diameter fibers) in a variety of structures, but particularly in the skin. When the gate is closed, nociceptive input is reduced, and this may significantly reduce the level of pain perceived by the patient. Descending impulses are also able to affect the ability of the gate to open or close. It should be remembered that the actual nociceptive signals are not in themselves painful. They are simply nerve impulses traveling in the peripheral and central nervous system. Only when these signals reach the higher brain centers are they interpreted as pain.

The neurophysiological basis for gate control is a complex and developing model. It involves not only the neural pathways of the system but also complex interactions between various brain structures and neurotransmitters and hormones (enkephalins and endorphins). The area has been reviewed extensively in many texts that deal with different aspects of the physiology and management of pain. A detailed description is well beyond the scope of this text, and interested readers are referred to Wall (1994) for an excellent review of the subject.

Clearly, then, massage techniques have the capacity to produce significant afferent input by direct stimulation of large-diameter mechanoreceptors in many structures. Depending on the techniques in question, these structures will be mainly in the skin or in the skin and the deeper tissues. In either case, activation of the spinal gating mechanism, descending pain suppression influences, and release of endogenous opiates are reasonable explanations for pain relief produced by massage techniques.

Interaction of the somatic and the autonomic nervous systems and of the musculoskeletal and the visceral systems has always been assumed. In recent years better understanding has shown that these interrelationships are more direct and predictable than was previously thought. An example of this better understanding can be found in the clinical approach to referred pain. It has long been assumed that referred pain is only the central interpretation of visceral or deep musculoskeletal pain through spinal connections to areas overlying the painful structures or related to them. In this view permanent relief of this type of pain is achieved only by removing the original cause. Temporary relief usually involves a central-acting drug that blocks the transmission or perception of pain. It has been demonstrated, however, that the peripheral pain site may contain reflexes that respond to direct peripheral intervention and that this intervention may even have a positive influence on the central cause of pain. This concept is illustrated particularly well in the trigger points of the myofascial pain syndrome (see Chapter 11). In this case a variety of methods (some manual) can be used to desensitize the painful trigger points (Travell & Simons, 1983, 1992).

The effects of massage on circulation of blood and lymph may also contribute to pain relief. Since certain massage techniques have a significant effect on the circulation they may be expected to enhance removal from an affected area of "pain metabolites" (e.g., kinins). This washing out effect could be a significant contribution to pain relief achieved with soft tissue massage.

Pain relief can also come from the relaxation effect produced by certain massage techniques (Meek, 1993). If muscle spasm is a significant cause of pain, then clearly reducing the muscle spasm will help to relieve the pain. The more generalized relaxation that can be achieved with massage may also contribute to pain relief, especially if such pain is of a central nature.

In recent years, nonpharmacologic methods have become popular among nurses for the relief of pain in terminally ill patients (Degner & Barkwell, 1991; Mobily, Herr, & Nicholson, 1994; Weinrich & Weinrich, 1990). The concept of therapeutic touch holds that pain relief is achieved without actually touching the patient (Heidt, 1991; Krieger, 1979, 1981; Owens & Ehrenreich, 1991). Technically, such techniques are not massage since they do not produce mechanical effects in the tissues. Their effectiveness must therefore be attributed to other (as yet undefined) mechanisms.

Effects on the Viscera

Abdominal Viscera

Until quite recently there was little published information on the effects of massage on the abdominal viscera. Mennell (1945) believed that the forceful abdominal massage that once was used primarily for its mechanical effects derived from a poor understanding of the gut. He pointed out that the slightest tap on the exposed intestine of a frog causes instant spasm of that portion plus cardiac inhibition, and that the effect of manipulation on involuntary muscle of the intestines can be observed during abdominal surgery. Excessive handling may result in over-stimulation and temporary paralysis of the involuntary (smooth) muscle. This might produce the opposite effect—inhibition of normal bowel function rather than stimulation.

Mennell believed that it was impossible to empty the small intestine mechanically. He believed that any action of massage on the intestines is almost, if not entirely, a reflexive response to the pressure of mechanical stimulation. This stimulation can increase peristalsis and thus hasten the emptying of the intestinal contents. He pointed out that some portions of the large intestine are quite constant in their relationship to the abdominal wall, and thus the direction of the passage of the contents in the duodenum, the ascending and descending colon, and the iliac colon can be followed.

Beard and Wood were convinced that massage of the abdomen by kneading and deep stroking (see Local Massage of the Abdomen, Chapter 6) is effective in stimulating peristalsis to promote evacuation of flatus and feces from the large intestine. These procedures may be performed by the patient while seated. The contents of the abdomen, with the exception of the duodenum and fixed portions of the colon, may easily be displaced or glide away from any pressure exerted on the abdominal wall, making it impossible to exert any mechanical effect of massage.

Klauser and coworkers (1992) conducted a well-controlled study of the effects of abdominal wall massage on colon function in both normal subjects and patients with chronic constipation. This important study showed no significant differences in colon function in the two groups. Despite anecdotal reports from earlier writers, the results of this study place in serious doubt the efficacy of such massage for the treatment of chronic constipation. Other authors (Emly, 1993) have drawn similar conclusions about the effects of abdominal wall massage.

Mennell believed that, though it may be possible to produce a mechanical effect with massage to some abdominal organs (e.g., prostate), the effects probably reflect a reflex reaction to mechanical stimulation. He said that it may be possible also to produce reflex contraction of smooth muscle of the spleen, but physiologically it is difficult to explain any beneficial effect. To expect any benefit from "shaking up the liver," as earlier writers had recommended, was quite wrong, according to Mennell, though abdominal massage may stimulate portal circulation and, thus, liver functions.

Massage treatment of the pancreas has been suggested by some writers. Mennell thought it might be affected reflexly, but it seems likely that this is only an indirect effect of improved general vascular tone. Being a hollow organ, the gallbladder is, according to Mennell, amenable to the mechanical effects of massage.

Because knowledge of the effects of massage on the abdominal viscera is quite limited, and until more information is available, it would seem unwise to perform any type of abdominal massage except to affect abdominal muscles—and possibly indirectly to influence the circulation and, through reflex response to pressure, to stimulate activity of the involuntary muscles of the intestines.

Special techniques are required for massage of specific organs, and they should be applied only by persons specially trained in these techniques. (Because of the harm that can result from abdominal massage it should not be included in a general massage unless medical consultation has first been sought.)

Other Visceral Organs

Mennell questioned the use of massage for the kidneys. Although he noted that by kneading the kidneys during cystoscopy it is possible to see urine pass from the ureter into the bladder, he doubted that this is clinically practical.

Direct massage of the heart is used as an emergency treatment in certain circumstances. When an abdominal incision has been made, the surgeon may massage the heart, either by compressing it between the diaphragm and the ribs or by incising the diaphragm and directly grasping the heart. Mennell knew of no direct action on the heart that could be achieved by externally applied massage movements, other than the obvious mechanical compression. Indeed, Kouwenhoven and associates (1960) reported a 70% long-term survival rate for patients with cardiac arrest who were given closed-chest cardiac massage (see Appendix).

Some forms of massage might be expected to affect various organs of the body by virtue of their reflex effects. Connective tissue massage is an obvious example: stimulation of specific areas on the posterior trunk region is expected to produce effects on a variety of organs and structures elsewhere in the body. This concept relies on evoking an autonomic reflex by stimulating cutaneous afferents reflexly related to specific organs and structures (see Chapter 10).

Another example of the potential for massage techniques to reflexly affect the various organs of the body is expressed in the treatment concept of acupressure (see Chapter 12). In this case, finger pressure applied to specific points on the body is designed to produce reflex effects in various organs and systems. This is yet another excellent example of the principle of a remote site effect, in which stimulation at one part of the body produces an effect elsewhere, even in an apparently unrelated area.

Effects on Lung Secretions

Percussive and vibratory massage techniques can be used in combination with other measures of chest physical therapy to prevent or treat acute and chronic lung conditions. The few controlled studies on the effects of chest physical therapy do not separate the effects of the various measures; however, many clinicians stress the importance of these types of massage techniques in the treatment of conditions such as emphysema, cystic fibrosis, bronchiectasis, asthma, atelectasis, and pneumonia.

Cyriax (1960, 1984) stated that percussive techniques, combined with postural drainage, can dislodge mucus and mucopurulent material from the bronchi and that gravity and vibration help to move the secretions from the insensitive periphery of the lungs to the area where the cough reflex is elicited. Such measures have been advocated in standard texts for many years. For example, Bendixen, Egbert, Hedley-White, Laver, and Pontoppidan (1965) recommended vibration and percussion with cupped hands (clapping) to shake loose secretions. Percussion is used in cases of "sticky, thick secretions that defy normal coughing efforts." Likewise, Cherniack, Cherniack, and Naimark (1972) believed that the role of physical therapy in the care of patients with acute respiratory failure could not be overemphasized. They advocated that while postural drainage is being performed to stimulate removal of secretions "the chest should be pummeled with rapid repetitive strokes and vibrated" by the therapist, and that the patient should frequently cough and expectorate the loosened secretions.

Current texts on the topic (Hillegass & Sadowsky, 1994; Irwin & Techlin, 1995; Watchie, 1995) continue to stress the importance of proper airway clearance and the need to teach the patient to use simple but effective home treatment techniques. For a more complete discussion of these issues, see Chapter 9.

Effects on the Skin

Little is known about skin metabolism, so it is difficult to evaluate how it might be affected by massage. Earlier writers proposed that massage had a direct effect on the superficial layers of the epidermis that "freed" the openings of the sebaceous and sweat glands. The mechanism was improved circulation, which directly improved the function of these glands (Krusen, 1941). Other early writers thought that sweating was not significantly increased but that sebaceous secretions might be expressed (Wright, 1939).

According to Rosenthal (cited in Cuthbertson, 1933) massage increases the temperature of the skin by 2° to 3°C. He found that neurasthenic persons showed a greater increase in skin temperature than normal healthy persons in response to massage, and that women showed a greater increase than men. He explained the differences by the fact that the entire nervous system, including the vasomotor nerves, is stimulated more easily in neurasthenic persons than in normal ones and in women more than in men. The increase in skin temperature may be due to direct mechanical effects and to indirect vasomotor action.

Severini and Venerando (1967) found that both superficial and deep massage led to a significant drop in skin temperature at the site of application. Barr and Taslitz (1970) observed increased sweating and decreased skin resistance to galvanic current in response to massage. They found much variation in skin temperature changes in both control and treatment periods and felt they could not infer that massage either increased or decreased skin temperature.

Clinical observation shows that, following massage to a part that has been in a cast for some weeks, definite improvements in the texture and appearance of skin can be noted. If the skin has become adherent to underlying tissues and scar tissue has formed, friction movements and tension are used to loosen the adherent tissues mechanically and to soften the scar.

Bodian (1969) recommended massage to enhance the cosmetic results of eyelid surgery. The mechanism of the method he describes "seems to be stretching and disruption of excess scar tissue." He found this massage useful in treating thick scars of the eyelid, keloids, overcorrected ptosis, overcorrected entropion, postoperative ectropion, and shallow fornices.

Since the skin is the organ that first comes into direct contact with the therapist's hands, it is not unreasonable to expect that massage has at least some effects on skin. These effects can be helpful or harmful. For example, if too much powder or oil is used on the skin, it is likely that the skin surface will become clogged with residue of the lubricant.

Effects on Fatty Tissue

Many have claimed over the years that massage removes deposits of adipose tissue. Krusen (1941) asserted that clinical observations did not support this theory and that attempts to reduce local fat deposits are futile.

Rosenthal (cited in Cuthbertson, 1933) investigated this problem experimentally. Vigorous massage was applied to certain areas of the abdominal wall of animals. Microscopic studies of the massaged and untreated areas showed no change in the fat in treated areas, even when the massage had been forceful enough to cause frequent small hemorrhages. Wright (1939) and Kalb (1944) came to similar conclusions.

> ## Psychological Effects of Massage
> - Physical relaxation
> - Relief of anxiety and tension (stress)
> - Stimulation of physical activity
> - Pain relief
> - General feeling of well-being (wellness)
> - Sexual arousal
> - General faith in the laying on of hands

PSYCHOLOGICAL EFFECTS

Few reports of experimental research on the psychological effects of massage have been published. Most people are familiar with the soothing effect of gentle massage, even when no lesion or physical disability is present (defined earlier as "recreational massage"). In therapeutic massage, the therapist's concentrated attention to the patient, combined with the pleasant physical sensations of the massage, often establishes a close and trusting personal relationship. In these circumstances, patients may reveal to the therapist problems, worries, and facts about their health that they had thought too trivial to report to a physician. In this situation the therapist listens and holds any information in confidence. The therapist is careful to see that the patient does not become too dependent in the relationship and encourages him or her to report relevant information to a physician.

Massage treatment can have negative psychological effects. The time and attention devoted to massage may exaggerate the seriousness of the disability in the patient's mind. Mennell (1945) warned, "It is easier to rub a disability into a patient's mind than it is to rub it out of his limb." Care must therefore be taken to reassure the anxious patient and to correct any misunderstandings about the reasons for treatment.

Many of the physiologic effects of massage described earlier have a significant psychological component. For example, pain relief has a psychological concept, since it is strongly dependent on the patient's perception. In this way, pain relief is a legitimate psychological effect of massage.

Physical Relaxation

Most people find that massage treatments are extremely relaxing. Certain strokes in particular promote physical relaxation; however, the concept of relaxation is not principally a physical one. It is just as much psychological as physiological. For muscles to relax, especially in an entire limb or the whole body, the person must be able to minimize the cortical drive passing to the relevant spinal motor neurons. This requires a conscious effort to "let go." The reason some people find it very difficult to relax their limbs might well be their inability to let everything go at the psychological level. Suitable massage techniques can contribute to this process, as they help the patient let his or her muscles and limbs relax.

Relief of Anxiety and Tension (Stress)

Relief of tension through massage is strongly linked to the promotion of relaxation identified previously. A patient who has significant anxiety and tension (stress) will find it very hard, if not impossible, to relax. As massage promotes relaxation it also helps to reduce anxiety and tension. This is because relaxation requires psychological release from anxiety and tension. This is one of the main reasons why recreational massage is so popular as part of stress reduction programs.

Stimulation of Physical Activity

Certain massage techniques are quite stimulating and produce a strong sense of invigoration. These techniques have proved very useful in the sporting world and have given rise to the concept of sports massage, which simply reflects the notion of using certain massage techniques to promote physical activity and optimal performance. A strong psychological impact often results from the application of suitable massage techniques.

Pain Relief

The physiological processes involved in pain relief through massage were discussed previously; however, the perception of pain is largely a psychological concept. It has important physiological substrates, but it requires the conscious mind for awareness of pain. Thus, pain relief achieved with massage is as much a psychological effect as it is a physiological one. This is one reason why massage treatments can be so helpful for terminally ill patients who suffer significant pain.

Sexual Arousal

Massage techniques have, of course, been used for countless centuries as a means of stimulating sexual arousal. There is, in fact, little difference in the actual massage strokes involved. The major difference, however, lies in what areas of the body are massaged.

Stimulation of the skin of a number of body areas (erogenous zones) can produce sexual arousal. These include all genital areas, buttocks, insides of the upper thighs, breasts, neck, and many areas of the face. Stimulation of any such area has the potential to produce sexual arousal, especially if that is the intention of both parties. Sexual arousal is not a simple reflex matter, requiring only sufficient stimulation of certain body areas. It is as much a psychological process as it is physical: sexual arousal occurs in the mind. Peripheral stimulation certainly helps, but the entire process is not a simple reflex action. Sexual arousal is not a treatment goal of therapeutic massage, and for this reason, many erogenous zones should be carefully avoided.

General Feeling of Well-Being (Wellness)

There is little doubt that massage treatment is, by and large, a very pleasant form of therapy. The general state of relaxation and stress relief, possibly coupled with pain reduction, have the effect of inducing a feeling of well-being in the patient. This feeling might also be linked to the liberation of endogenous opiates or some other substances as yet unidentified. At the very least, massage is a significant way of achieving a sense of wellness, and this may account, in part, for the popularity of recreational massage around the world.

General Faith in the Laying on of Hands

Many people, especially older ones, have great faith in the religious healing technique called the laying on of hands, a procedure in which the hands of a "healer" are placed on or close to the affected area and some kind of "healing force" is transferred to the tissues. This rather old idea has gained renewed interest, especially among nurses (who call it "therapeutic touch" (Heidt, 1991; Krieger, 1979, 1981; Owens & Ehrenreich, 1991). It is used widely for chronic pain management.

The idea that healing might be facilitated by touching the patient is, of course, very old and common to many ancient cultures. Indeed, this may be why it resonates to this day, even in more technologically advanced societies. If the act of touching a person makes that person believe (a psychological construct) that healing will take place, then it is not too difficult to imagine that healing could, in fact, happen. If we adopt the premise that the human mind has the power to control all aspects of body functions it is quite conceivable that the mind could bring about positive physical changes in the body, including healing and pain control. Since these effects can be produced by massage and related activities, it could be classified as a psychological effect of the treatment that brings about real physiological changes.

PRINCIPAL THERAPEUTIC EFFECTS

The therapeutic effects of massage should now be obvious, since they are based on the mechanical, physiological, and psychological effects of massage described earlier: relaxation (local and general), pain relief, increased range of joint and limb motion, stimulation of blood and lymph circulation, and facilitation of healing. Each of the strokes described in Chapter 3 is listed in Table 4–1. This table indicates the effects associated with specific strokes, since,

Table 4.1	THERAPEUTIC EFFECTS OF SOFT TISSUE MASSAGE
STROKE	EFFECTS
Effleurage Stroking Skin rolling	Stimulation of superficial blood and lymph flow; mobilization of skin and subcutaneous tissue; promotion of local and general relaxation; relief of pain
Kneading Wringing Picking up	Mobilization of muscle tissue; stimulation of deeper circulation; promotion of relaxation; relief of pain
Hacking Beating Pounding Clapping	Stimulation of muscle activity and deep circulation
Clapping Vibrations Shakings	Mobilization and removal of lung secretions
Deep friction	Mobilization and pain relief in tendons, muscles, ligaments, and joint capsules

clearly, different strokes produce different effects. Much of this information has also been detailed in Chapter 3, under the headings for individual strokes.

PRINCIPAL USES OF THERAPEUTIC MASSAGE

The mechanical, physiological, and psychological effects of massage give rise to the therapeutic effects. In turn, the therapeutic effects are the basis for the therapeutic uses (also known as the therapeutic indications). These, too, should now be obvious.

Principal Uses of Therapeutic Massage

- To aid general or local relaxation
- To relieve pain
- To treat specific problems:
  Chronic edema
  Scar tissue (superficial or deep)
  Lesions of muscles, tendons, ligaments, or joints
  Hematomas (superficial or deep)
  Chronic constipation (little evidence supports this claim)
  Facilitation of movement
  Prevention of deformity

GENERAL PRECAUTIONS AND CONTRAINDICATIONS

Specific contraindications for each massage stroke are described in Chapter 3. A summary is provided below for readers' convenience. The presence of one of these conditions does not necessarily mean that treatment cannot be given; rather, careful consideration must be given before any treatment is performed.

It is possible to conceive of three types of contraindication:

- **Absolutely contraindicated** (massage must never be given under any circumstances)
- **Usually contraindicated** (usually massage may not be given)
- **Rarely contraindicated** (in rare cases massage may not be given)

In determining whether a patient can safely receive massage, good judgment is always needed, as it is not always easy to identify contraindications. Even when contraindications are present, circumstances may warrant ignoring the usual practice. For example, for a terminally ill patient massage may be very helpful in relieving pain, though it might otherwise be contraindicated. In fact there are very few absolute contraindications to massage. The following examples are provided to explain the basic rationale.

General Contraindications to Massage

- Acute infection
  Bones (e.g., osteomyelitis)
  Joints (e.g., septic arthritis)
  Skin (e.g., dermatitis)
  Muscle (e.g., myositis)
  Subcutaneous tissue (e.g., cellulitis)
- Skin disease (e.g., psoriasis)
- Cancer or tuberculosis in the area to be treated
- Areas of severe hyperesthesia
- Presence of foreign bodies (e.g., grit, glass)
- Diseases of blood vessels (e.g., thrombophlebitis)
- Massage may be given, but with great care, to patients who have marked varicosity of the veins, hemophilia, or gross edema.

Massage should not be given in areas of tumor or infection that could be spread by the treatment (this falls into the category of *usually contraindicated*). Examples of this are skin conditions such as psoriasis, any malignancy, and any kind of joint or bone infection.

Massage should not be given over areas in which foreign bodies such as glass and dirt are embedded, because of the obvious risk of causing more damage. Massage is also contraindicated in the presence of disorders of the blood vessels. It could produce local damage to the vessels or, in rare instances, free an embolus in a limb involved with thrombophlebitis.

It is important to remember that contraindications generally apply to the area being treated. It is quite safe to treat areas that are not affected. For example, it would be safe to massage the neck and shoulders of a patient who had significant arterial disease in the lower limbs.

As always, the causes of the patient's current signs and symptoms are extremely important. For example, a patient may present with chronic, gross swelling around the feet, ankles, and lower legs. On the surface, this seems an ideal indication for massage to mobilize the fluids and remove the swelling; however, if the swelling is the result of underlying congestive heart failure, that might well contraindicate treatment unless the heart condition was well controlled. In this instance, swelling in the legs is probably a mechanism by which the patient's inadequate cardiovascular system has "off-loaded" fluid into the periphery as a means of reducing the pumping load on the heart. Mobilizing this fluid back into the cardiovascular system might overtax the patient's heart. This example highlights the importance of understanding the reasons for the patient's signs and symptoms.

General Precautions

Massage is a relatively safe treatment; however, patients can come to harm if given inappropriate or inadequate treatment. Careful assessment of the patient's total situation is obviously needed. The following list contains many "common sense" precautions that need to be observed before, during, and after massage.

1. Obtain an accurate medical diagnosis.

2. Perform an appropriate physical (clinical) examination to determine how the medical condition is affecting the patient and develop a suitable treatment plan. Remember that massage techniques are best used in combination with other rehabilitation techniques rather than as the sole treatment.

3. Check carefully for possible contraindications to treatment.

4. Drape, position, and support the patient properly.

5. Ensure a high standard of cleanliness, especially for the therapist's hands.

6. Perform the massage properly while monitoring the patient's response.

7. Assess and document the patient's response to treatment so that modifications can be made if necessary.

SUMMARY

Soft tissue massage techniques have predictable mechanical effects on the tissues being manipulated and these effects cause measurable physiological changes in the person being massaged. These effects are therapeutically useful in the treatment of a variety of conditions. Soft tissue massage has been investigated for many decades, but it is evident that the studies on the effects of massage briefly reviewed in this chapter have in many instances omitted any mention of the details of the massage applications. Therefore, conclusions drawn by the experimenters and clinicians had to be stated in quite general terms. Indeed, many references on the clinical use of massage state that "massage does (or does not) . . ."; "massage will (or will not) . . ."; "massage should (or should not) be used for . . ."; or "massage is indicated (or contraindicated) in the treatment of. . . ." Such absolute statements are seldom based upon knowledge or consideration of the effects of specific types, amounts, or sequences of massage techniques applied to specific tissues. There is still a great need to conduct controlled clinical and laboratory studies to evaluate the many possible combinations of the various components of massage.

There can be no doubt that massage has many beneficial mechanical, physiological, and psychological effects to offer, nor can there be any doubt that massage has many useful therapeutic applications. Despite ever more sophisticated medical technology, the ancient art of massage is still likely to reserve an important place in the 21st century and well beyond. It seems most unlikely that any machine will be able to replace the sensitivity and power of trained human hands working in contact with another human being. The current popularity of various concepts of holistic health will also likely ensure that massage will continue to be a popular health care practice for the foreseeable future.

References and Bibliography

Barr JS, Taslitz N. (1970) Influence of back massage on autonomic functions. Phy Ther 50:1679–1691.

Bell AJ. (1964) Massage and the physiotherapist. Physiotherapy, JCSP 50:406–408.

Bendixen H, Egbert L, Hedley-White J, Laver M, Pontoppidan H. (1965) Respiratory care. St. Louis: CV Mosby, pp 99–101.

Bodian M. (1969) Use of massage following lid surgery. Eye, Ear, Nose Throat Monthly 48:542–547.

Bork K, Karling GW, Faust G. (1971) Serum enzyme levels after "whole body massage." Arch Dermatol Forsch 240:342–348.

Brunton TL, Tunnicliffe TW. (1894–1895) On the effects of the kneading of muscles upon the circulation, local and general. J Physiol 17:364.

Carrier EB. (1922) Studies on physiology of capillaries: Reaction of human skin capillaries to drugs and other stimuli. Am J Physiol 61:528–547.

Cherniack RM, Cherniack L, Naimark A. (1972) Respiration in health and disease, 2nd ed. Philadelphia: WB Saunders, p 452.

Chor H, Cleveland D, Davenport HA, Dolkart RE, Beard G. (1939) Atrophy and regeneration of the gastrocnemius-soleus muscles: Effects of physical therapy in monkey following section and suture of sciatic nerve. JAMA 113:1029–1033.

Chor H, Dolkart RE. (1936) A study of simple disuse atrophy in the monkey. Am J Physiol 117:4.

Cuthbertson DP. (1933) Effect of massage on metabolism: A survey. Glasgow Med J (new 7th series) 2:200–213.

Cyriax J. (1960) In Licht S. (ed): Massage, manipulation and traction. New Haven: Elizabeth Licht.

Cryiax J. (1984) Textbook of orthopaedic medicine, Vol 2, 11th ed. Treatment by manipulation, massage and injection. London: Bailliere-Tindall.

Degner L, Barkwell D. (1991) Nonanalgesic approaches to pain control. Cancer Nurs 14(2):105–111.

Despard LL. (1932) Textbook of massage and remedial gymnastics, 3rd ed. New York: Oxford University Press.

Drinker CK, Yoffey JM. (1941) Lymphatics, lymph, and lymphoid tissue: Their physiological and clinical significance. Cambridge: Harvard University Press, p 310.

Dyson R. (1978) Bed sores—the injuries hospital staff inflict on patients. Nurs Mirror 146:30–32.

Ek AC, Gustavsson G, Lewis DH. (1985) The local skin blood flow in areas at risk for pressure sores treated with massage. Scand J Rehab Med 17:81–86.

Emly M. (1993) Abdominal massage. Nurs Times 89(3):34–36.

Ernst E, Matrai A, Magyarosy I, Liebermeister RG, Eck M, Breu MC. (1987) Massage causes changes in blood fluidity. Physiotherapy, JCSP 73(1):43–45.

Evans P. (1980) The healing process at cellular level: A review. Physiotherapy, JCSP 66(8):256–259.

Goldberg J, Seaborne D, Sullivan S. (1992) The effect of two intensities of massage on H-reflex amplitude. Phys Ther 72(6):449–457.

Goldberg J, Seaborne D, Sullivan S, Leduc B. (1994) The effect of therapeutic massage on H-reflex amplitude in persons with a spinal cord injury. Phys Ther 74(8):728–737.

Goodgold J, Erberstein A. (1983) Electrodiagnosis of neuromuscular disease. Baltimore: Williams & Wilkins.

Grieve GP. (1994) Modern manual therapy of the vertebral column. London: Churchill Livingstone.

Gruner OC. (1930) A treatise on the canon of medicine of Avicenna. London: Lazac.

Hammer WI. (1993) The use of transverse friction massage in the management of chronic bursitis of the hip or shoulder. J Manipulative Physiol Ther 16(2): 107–111.

Hartman FA, Blatz WE. (1920) Treatment of denervated muscle. JAMA 74:878.

Hartman FA, Blatz WE, Kelborn LJ. (1919) Studies in regeneration of denervated mammalian muscle. Am J Physiol 53:109.

Heidt P. (1991) Helping patients to rest: Clinical studies in therapeutic touch. Holistic Nurs Pract 5(4):57–66.

Hillegass EA, Sadowsky HS. (1994) Essentials of cardiopulmonary physical therapy. Philadelphia: WB Saunders.

Irwin S, Techlin JS. (1995) Cardiopulmonary physical therapy. St. Louis: CV Mosby.

Kalb SW. (1944) The fallacy of massage in the treatment of obesity. J Med Soc NJ 41:406–407.

Kellogg JH. (1919) The art of massage, 12th ed revised. Battle Creek, MI: Modern Medical Publ.

Key JA, Elzinga E, Fischer F. (1934a) Local atrophy of bone I. Effect of immobilization and of operative procedures. Arch Surg 28:935–942.

Key JA, Elzinga E, Fischer F. (1934b) Local atrophy of bone II. Effects of local heat, massage, and therapeutic exercise. Arch Surg 28:943–947.

Klauser AG, Flaschentrager J, Gehrke A, Muller-Lissner SA. (1992) Abdominal wall massage: Effect on colonic function in healthy volunteers and in patients with chronic constipation. Z Gastroenterol 30:247–251.

Kouwenhoven WD, Jude JR, Knickerbocker GG. (1960) Closed-chest cardiac massage. JAMA 173:1064–1067.

Krieger D. (1979) Therapeutic touch: How to use your hands to help or to heal. Englewood Cliffs, NJ: Prentice Hall.

Krieger D. (1981) Foundations of holistic health nursing practices: The renaissance nurse. Philadelphia: JB Lippincott.

Krusen FH. (1941) Physical medicine. Philadelphia: WB Saunders, p 335.

Ladd MP, Kottke FJ, Blanchard RS. (1952) Studies of the effect of massage on the flow of lymph from the foreleg of the dog. Arch Phys Med 33:611.

Langley JN, Hashimoto M. (1918) Denervated muscle atrophy. Am J Physiol 52:15.

Licht S. (1960) Massage, manipulation and traction. New Haven: Elizabeth Licht.

Lucia SP, Rickard JF. (1933) Effects of massage on blood platelet production. Proc Soc Exper Biol Med 31:87.

Maggiora A. (1891) De l'action physiologique du massage sur les muscles de l'homme. Arch Ital Biol 16:225–246.

Mannheimer J, Lampe G. (1984) Clinical transcutaneous electrical nerve stimulation. Philadelphia: FA Davis.

Mason M. (1993) The treatment of lymphodema by complex physical therapy. Aust J Physiother 39(1):1–5.

McMaster P. (1937) Changes in the cutaneous lymphatics of human beings and in the lymph flow under normal and pathological conditions. J Exp Med 65:347.

McMillan M. (1925) Massage and therapeutic exercise. Philadelphia: WB Saunders.

Meek S. (1993) Effects of slow stroke back massage on relaxation in hospice clients. IMAGE: J Nurs Scholarship 25(1):17–21.

Melzack R, Wall PD. (1965) Pain mechanisms: A new theory. Science 150:971–979.

Mennell JB. (1945) Physical treatment, 5th ed. Philadelphia: Blakiston.

Michlovitz SL. (1996) Thermal agents in rehabilitation, 3rd ed. Philadelphia: FA Davis.

Mitchell JK. (1904) Massage and exercise in system of physiologic therapeutics. Philadelphia: Blakiston.

Mobily P, Herr K, Nicholson A. (1994) Validation of cutaneous stimulation interventions for pain management. Int J Nurs Studies 31(6):533–544.

Mock HE. (1945) Massage in surgical cases. In A.M.A. handbook of physical medicine. Chicago: Council of Physical Medicine, p 95.

Morelli M, Seaborne D, Sullivan S. (1991) H-reflex modulation during manual muscle massage of human triceps surae. Arch Phys Med Rehab 72:915–919.

Nordschow M, Bierman W. (1962) Influence of manual massage on muscle relaxation: Effect on trunk flexion. Phys Ther 42:653–656.

Olson B. (1989) Effects of massage for prevention of pressure ulcers. Decubitus 2(4):32–37.

Owens M, Ehrenreich D. (1991) Application of nonpharmacologic methods of managing chronic pain. Holistic Nurs Pract 6(1):32–40.

Pemberton R. (1932) The physiologic influence of massage and the clinical application of heat and massage in internal medicine. In: Principles and Practices of Physical Medicine, Vol I. Hagerstown, MD: W.F. Prior.

Pemberton R. (1939) Physiology of massage. In: A.M.A. handbook of physical therapy, 3rd ed. Chicago: Council of Physical Therapy A.M.A., pp 78–87.

Pemberton R. (1945) Physiology of massage. In: A.M.A. handbook of physical medicine. Chicago, A.M.A. Council of Physical Medicine, p 141.

Pemberton R. (1950) Physiology of massage. In: A.M.A. handbook of physical medicine and rehabilitation. Philadelphia: Blakiston.

Robinson A, Snyder-Mackler L. (1995) Clinical electrophysiology: Electrotherapy and electrophysiological testing, 2nd ed. Baltimore: Williams & Wilkins.

Schneider EC, Havens LC. (1915) Changes in the blood flow after muscular activity and during training. Am J Physiol 36:259.

Severini V, Venerando A. (1967a) Effect on the peripheral circulation of substances producing hyperemia in combination with massage. Eur Medicophys 3:184–198.

Severini V, Venerando A. (1967b) The physiological effects of massage on the cardiovascular system. Europa Medicophys 3:165–183.

Smith L, Keating M, Holbert D, Spratt D, McCammon M,

Smith S, Israel R. (1994) The effects of athletic massage on delayed onset muscle soreness, creatine kinase, and neutrophil count: A preliminary report. JOSPT 19(2):93–99.

Sullivan S, Williams L, Seaborne D, Morelli M. (1991) Effects of massage on alpha motoneuron excitability. Phys Ther 71(8):555–560.

Suskind MI, Hajek NA, Hines HM. (1946) Effects of massage on denervated skeletal muscle. Arch Phys Med 27:133–135.

Travell JG, Simons DG. (1983) Myofascial pain and dysfunction: The trigger point manual. Volume I. Baltimore: Williams & Wilkins.

Travell JG, Simons DG. (1992) Myofascial pain and dysfunction: The trigger point manual. Volume II. Baltimore: Williams & Wilkins.

Wakim KG. (1949) The effects of massage on the circulation in normal and paralyzed extremities. Arch Phys Med 30:135.

Wakim KG. (1955) Influence of centripetal rhythmic compression on localized edema of an extremity. Arch Phys Med 36:98.

Wall PD. (1994) Textbook of pain. New York: Churchill Livingstone.

Watchie J. (1995) Cardiopulmonary physical therapy—A clinical manual. Philadelphia: WB Saunders.

Weinrich S, Weinrich M. (1990) The effect of massage on pain in cancer patients. Appl Nurs Res 3(4):140–145.

Wolfson H. (1931) Studies on effect of physical therapeutic procedures on function and structure. JAMA 96:2020–2021.

Wood EC, Kosman AJ, Osborne SL. (1948) Effects of massage upon denervated skeletal muscles of the dog. Phys Ther Rev 28:284–285.

Wright S. (1939) Physiological aspects of rheumatism. Proc R Soc Med 32:651–662.

Yamazaki Z, Idezuki Y, Nemoto T, Togawa T. (1988) Clinical experiences using pneumatic massage therapy of edematous limbs over the last 10 years. Angiology 2:154–163.

Part II

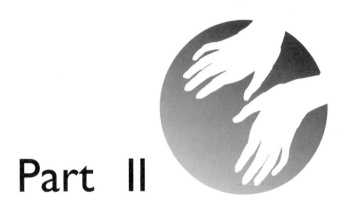

Practice

Chapter 5

A General Massage Sequence

The individual massage strokes described in Chapter 3 can be combined into a wide variety of massage sequences. Such a sequence is simply a collection of individual techniques put together with the intention of achieving a specific effect or series of effects. Of the many different massage sequences that are possible, the actual selection of techniques is, to a large extent, determined by the individual therapist. The massage sequences described in this text are by no means the only ones that should be practiced. Rather, these sequences have proven to be an effective combination of techniques for both general and local massage. Massage applied to the entire body is usually called "general massage," and massage applied to an individual body part is called "local massage."

Massage cannot be a substitute for exercise in restoring function; however, since massage improves the circulation of the blood and lymph, in this respect its effects are somewhat similar to those of exercise. In certain circumstances, therefore, when normal active physical exercise is not possible, and if the existing lesion is not a contraindication, general massage can be quite useful. For conditions that require long confinement to bed, daily massage of the entire body manually stimulates the general circulation and brings a sense of comfort and relaxation to the patient. For elderly people general massage may substitute for some of their former muscular activity, but again, it cannot replace active exercise programs, nor is it intended to. In most instances, massage to the entire body on a daily basis is not practical; still, massage only to the lower limbs is likely to be effective as the circulation of the lower limbs is very important in determining the efficiency of the general circulation.

A SEQUENCE AND TECHNIQUE FOR GENERAL MASSAGE

A good general massage may produce fatigue in the patient. A feeling of mild lassitude and the desire to rest immediately after general massage are signs of a successful treatment, and for this reason the patient should rest 1 to 1½ hours after treatment if that is possible. Significant fatigue should be avoided, and if the patient is not refreshed after a period of rest the duration of the treatment has been too long or the massage technique too vigorous. As a general guide, about 45 minutes to 1 hour is adequate for most general massage treatments. In the general massage sequence described here, a recommended number of repetitions is given for each stroke so that the treatment can be completed within this time frame.

Sequence for General Massage

Therapist on patient's right side:
  Right thigh and leg
  Right foot
Therapist on left side of patient
  Left thigh and leg
  Left foot
  Left arm, forearm, hand
Therapist on right side of patient
  Right arm, forearm, hand
  Chest and abdomen

To accomplish the relaxation and sedation usually desired in general massage, the change from one type of movement to another must be smooth and uninterrupted and a definite rhythm should be sustained through all movements. Certain adaptations of the Swedish remedial massage system seem to be well suited for this purpose. These movements are performed on an entire segment of each extremity without giving special attention to a particular muscle or muscle group. A type of massage sequence that follows specific muscle groups and muscles is more effective in the treatment of local injury or disease. That is described in Chapter 6.

The sequence of general massage should be such that the patient is not required to move or turn from side to side any more than is absolutely necessary. The therapist should change position as little as possible, and all movements should be efficient and quiet. The order of movements that facilitates such a program is described next and can be followed from the general massage sequence chart in the following section.

The sequence begins with the patient lying down facing the ceiling with the therapist on the patient's right-hand side. A small pillow or roll placed under the head or neck allows the therapist's hands to move smoothly around to the back of the neck and shoulder when treating the chest and neck. A similar pillow may be useful under the patient's knees, but it must be small or it will interfere with massage to the lower limb.

The patient turns to the prone position, and the treatment is concluded with massage to the back. (The therapist does not have to change position for this part of the treatment.)

This entire sequence may be reversed if the therapist prefers to begin on the left side of the patient. It is usually a matter of personal preference, though in some cases it may be that the layout of the room or treatment cubicle determines on which side of the patient it is best to begin massage.

GENERAL MASSAGE SEQUENCE

(The number in parentheses represents the number of repetitions for each stroke.)

1. Right Thigh
  1. Superficial stroking to the thigh (3)
  2. Palmar kneading to the quadriceps (3)
  3. Palmar kneading to the posterior surface of the thigh (3)
  4. Alternate palmar kneading to the thigh (3)
  5. Deep stroking to the thigh (3)

Right Leg and Knee
  1. Superficial stroking to the leg (3)
  2. Thumb pad kneading over the anterior tibial muscles (2)
  3. Kneading to the calf muscles (3)
  4. Alternate palmar kneading to the muscles of the leg (3)
  5. Stroking around the patella (4)
  6. Digital stroking over the popliteal space (4)
  7. Deep stroking with both hands to the entire leg (3)

Right Foot
  1. Superficial stroking over the dorsum of the foot (2)
  2. Thumb pad kneading over the dorsum of the foot (2)
  3. Deep thumb pad stroking to the plantar aspect of the foot (2)
  4. Deep palmar stroking to the plantar aspect of the foot (4)
  5. Deep digital stroking around the malleoli (4)
  6. Digital stroking of the Achilles tendon (4)
  7. Deep stroking to the leg and thigh (3)
  8. Superficial stroking to the right thigh, leg, and foot (4)
All these strokes are next applied to the left thigh, leg, and foot.

2. Left Arm, Forearm, and Hand
  1. Superficial stroking to the upper extremity (4)
  2. Alternate deep palmar stroking over the deltoid (10)
  3. Thumb pad kneading to the upper extremity (2)
  4. Palmar kneading to the arm and forearm (3)
  5. Alternate palmar kneading to the upper extremity (3)
  6. Thumb pad kneading to the dorsum of the hand (2)
  7. Thumb stroking to the palmar surface of the metacarpophalangeal joints (4)
  8. Thumb stroking over the thenar and hypothenar eminences (4)
  9. Thumb pad kneading to the thumb and fingers (2–3)
  10. Deep stroking to the upper extremity (3)
  11. Superficial stroking to the upper extremity (4)
All these strokes are next applied to the right arm, forearm, and hand.

3. Chest
  1. Superficial stroking to the upper chest (4)
  2. Deep stroking over the shoulders and around the neck (4)
  3. Digital kneading from the sternum to the shoulder (3)
  4. Alternate deep stroking from the shoulder to the sternum (4)
  5. Digital stroking around the neck (4)
  6. Deep stroking over the area of the jugular veins (4)
  7. Deep stroking around the neck (4)

Continued.

TECHNIQUE FOR A GENERAL MASSAGE SEQUENCE

Right Thigh

The therapist stands at the side of the table on the patient's right side.

Superficial Stroking to the Thigh

Both hands reach around the thigh, covering it as much as possible, and stroke from the anterior superior spine of the ilium to the knee. This stroke may be performed with the hands working alternately or simultaneously (Fig. 5–1). It is repeated four times.

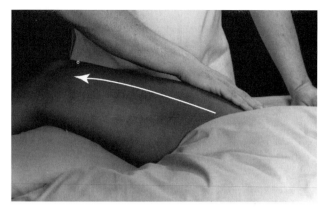

Figure 5–1. **Stroking to the thigh.**

GENERAL MASSAGE SEQUENCE *Continued*

4. Abdomen
1. Superficial stroking to the abdomen (4)
2. Deep stroking to the lower abdomen (4)
3. Deep stroking over the upper abdomen (4)
4. Palmar kneading over the colon (3)
5. Deep stroking over the colon (6)
6. Alternate palmar kneading over the entire abdomen (4)
7. Deep stroking to the lower abdomen (4)

5. Back and Hips
1. Superficial stroking to the back (4)
2. Deep palmar stroking to the back (3)
3. Finger pad kneading over the upper fibers of the trapezius (3)
4. Digital stroking over the upper fibers of the trapezius (4)
5. Kneading over the scapular region (3)
6. Alternate palmar kneading over the thoracic and lumbar regions (4)
7. Palmar stroking over the lumbar region (4)
8. Thumb pad kneading over the sacrum (4)
9. Alternate palmar kneading to the buttocks (2)
10. Deep kneading to the buttocks (2)
11. Alternate palmar kneading over the entire back (4)
12. Digital kneading to the erector spinae (1)
13. Deep palmar stroking to the erector spinae (4)
14. Deep palmar stroking to the back (1)

6. Face
1. Superficial stroking to the face (2)
2. Thumb pad kneading to the forehead (2)
3. Deep stroking to the forehead (3)
4. Alternate thumb pad kneading to the nose (3)
5. Deep stroking to the supraorbital ridge (4)
6. Deep stroking to the infraorbital ridge (4)
7. Digital kneading from the temple to the cervical spine (2)
8. Finger pad kneading from the temples to the shoulders (2)
9. Deep stroking over the area of the jugular veins (4)
10. Palmar kneading to the cheeks (2)
11. Thumb pad kneading to the chin and the jaw (3)
12. Deep stroking to the chin and the jaw (3)
13. Deep stroking over the jugular veins (4)
14. Superficial stroking to the face (2)

7. Scalp and Head
1. Finger pad kneading over the scalp (1)

8. Posterior Neck Region
1. Superficial and deep stroking over the upper fibers of the trapezius muscles (8)
2. Finger pad kneading over the upper fibers of the trapezius (3)
3. Deep stroking over the upper fibers of the trapezius (6)

Palmar Kneading to the Quadriceps

The stroke begins with the ulnar border of the right hand placed below the patella and the thumb on its lateral border. The fingers are placed on the medial border of the patella. The left hand picks up the distal portion of the muscle above the patella (Fig. 5–2A). The right hand strokes over the patella toward the left hand, as the ulnar border maintains firm contact during the upward pressure. The muscle is grasped between the thumb and the fingers using a lumbrical action to draw the tissues into the palms of the hands. The palmar surface of the fingers of the left hand pulls the muscles laterally as the surface of the abducted right thumb and palm simultaneously push the tissues medially (Fig. 5–2B). Then the surface of the palm and abducted thumb of the left hand push the muscles medially as the palmar surface of the fingers of the right hand pulls the tissues laterally (Fig. 5–2C). This push-pull movement is carried along the muscle, progressing from the distal part of the quadriceps to the proximal part. Movement is accomplished with gliding of the hands on the "pull" stroke of the kneading movement. This is not a pinching movement.

The thumb and fingers of each hand sustain their relationship to each other during the entire movement. The push and pull are accomplished chiefly by flexion and extension of the arms at shoulders and elbows as the movement progresses along the thigh. As the origin of the muscle is approached, the left hand is removed and the right hand gently "squeezes out" at the origin of the muscle (Fig. 5–2D) and returns to the lower border of the patella with a superficial stroke. These movements are repeated three times.

Palmar Kneading to the Posterior Thigh

The hip and knee are flexed slightly and the thigh rotated slightly externally. Both hands reach across the medial surface of the thigh, grasping the flexors at the knee (Fig. 5–3A), and perform the same movement that was done on the quadriceps muscle, except that the hands are held more transverse to the muscles as the hands progress along the muscle (Fig. 5–3B).

The movement is terminated a few inches below the hip joint. The left hand is removed; it crosses over the right hand to grasp the muscles above the knee (see Fig. 5–3C)

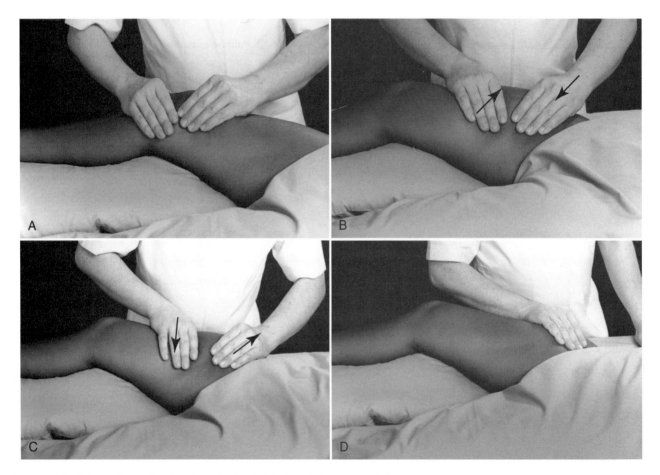

Figure 5–2. **Palmar kneading to the anterior thigh (quadriceps muscle).**

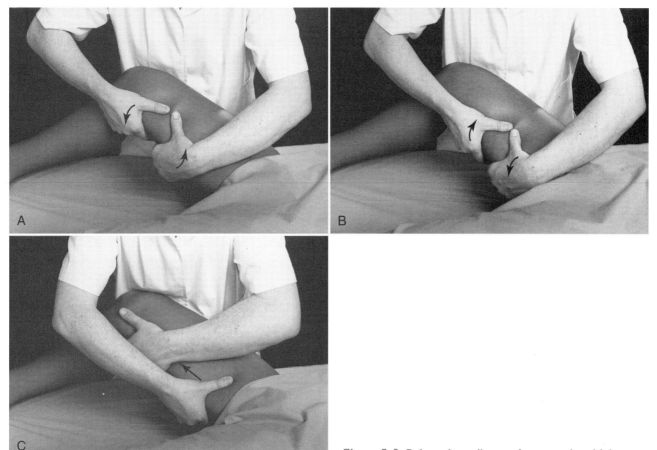

Figure 5–3. **Palmar kneading to the posterior thigh.**

and the right hand returns along the medial surface of the thigh with a superficial stroke. The movement is repeated three times.

Alternate Palmar Kneading to the Thigh

The hip may be slightly flexed and laterally rotated for this stroke, or it may be performed with the limb straight. Both hands grasp around the upper portion of the thigh (Fig. 5–4A); the hands perform the basic kneading technique, alternately rolling the muscles between the palms with firm pressure upward and relaxation while moving down the thigh toward the knee (Fig. 5–4B). Both hands return to the starting position with a deep stroke. This movement is repeated three times.

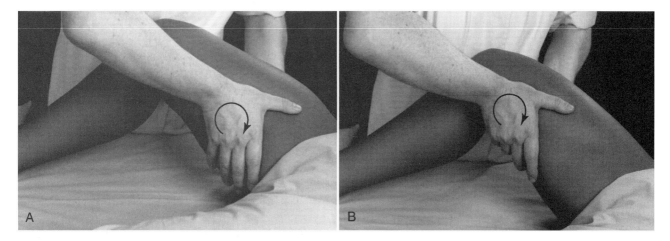

Figure 5–4. **Alternate palmar kneading to the thigh.**

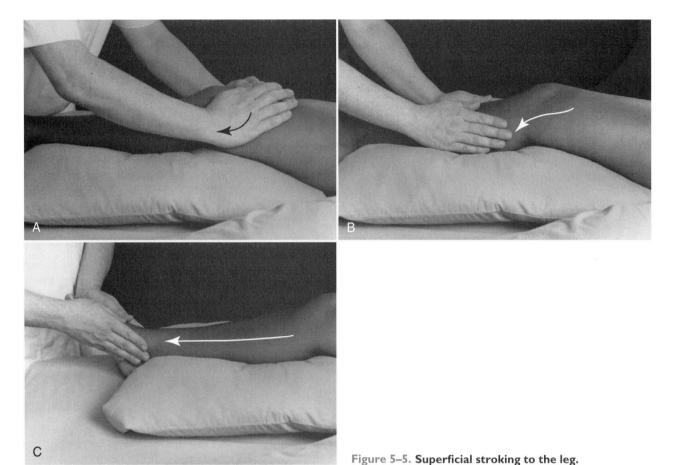

Figure 5–5. Superficial stroking to the leg.

Deep Stroking to the Thigh

Both hands grasp around the thigh just proximal to the knee joint, with the thumbs abducted and the fingers held together. Fingertips of opposing hands are in contact with each other on the posterior surface. With firm pressure of the entire palmar surface, the hands stroke upward to the upper portion of the thigh, then return to the knee with a superficial stroke. These movements are repeated three times.

Right Leg and Knee

The therapist continues to stand on the patient's right side but now is positioned at the far end of the table.

Superficial Stroking to the Leg

Both hands stroke from the knee to the ankle, covering the entire surface of the leg (Fig. 5–5). This movement is also repeated three times.

Thumb Pad Kneading over the Anterior Tibial Muscles

The thumb pad (distal phalanx) of each hand is placed in firm contact at the origin of the anterior tibial muscles; the remainder of the hand rests lightly on the surface of the leg (Fig. 5–6A). The thumbs move alternately in circles

applying pressure upward and outward. The hands glide to the more distal adjacent area as each circle is made. The movement progresses in this manner (Fig. 5–6B) to the ankle joint (Fig. 5–6C). The hands return to the starting position as the thumbs give deep stroking and the rest of the hand maintains light contact. The movements are repeated twice.

Kneading to the Calf Muscles

The right hand supports the slightly flexed knee joint at the medial border. The left hand grasps the lateral part of the muscle group just distal to the knee, and the muscles are pulled toward the lateral border of the leg with the palmar surface of the fingers exerting pressure (Fig. 5–7A). Then the palmar surface of the abducted thumb and thenar eminence push the muscles upward and toward the medial border of the leg (Fig. 5–7B). The fingers then glide distally, and these movements are repeated until the hand reaches the ankle (Fig. 5–7C). The hand returns to the knee with a deep stroke over the muscles. These movements are repeated three times.

The therapist then changes hands to massage the medial part of the muscle group. Supporting the knee with the left hand, the therapist repeats the procedure with the right hand three times.

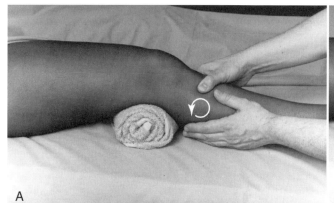

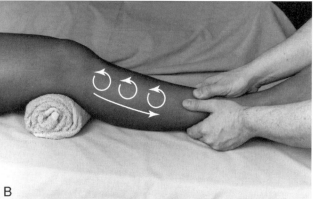

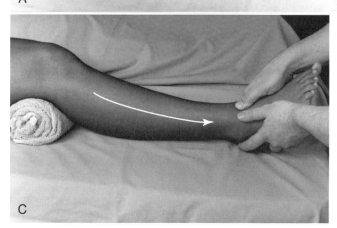

Figure 5–6. Thumb pad kneading over the anterior tibial muscles.

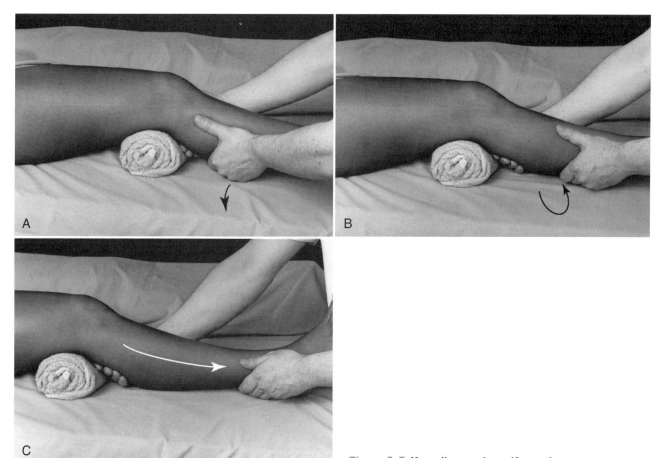

Figure 5–7. Kneading to the calf muscles.

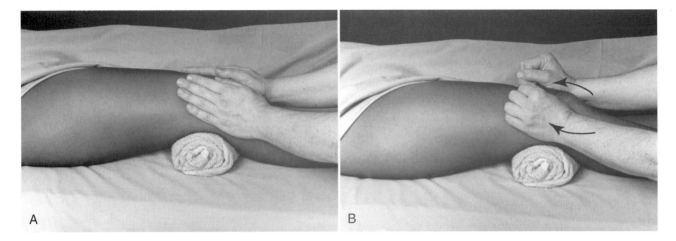

Figure 5–8. **Stroking around the patella.**

Alternate Palmar Kneading to the Muscles of the Leg

The basic kneading stroke is performed as both hands grasp around the muscles at the knee and alternately roll the muscles between the palms with firm pressure upward, working toward the ankle. The hands are returned to the knee with a deep stroke over the muscles. (This is the same technique used in alternate palmar kneading of the thigh—see Fig. 5–4.) These movements are repeated three times.

Stroking around the Patella

The heels of both hands are placed at the lower border of the patella; the palmar surfaces of the distal phalanges of the fingers are in contact with the skin above the superior border of the patella (Fig. 5–8A). The thenar eminences of both hands stroke firmly around the patella in a circular movement by allowing the fingers to flex while the tips maintain light contact (Fig. 5–8B). The heels of the hands

return to the beginning position with a superficial stroke distally, allowing the thumbs to glide lightly over the patella. These movements are repeated four times.

Digital Stroking over the Popliteal Space

The fingertips of both hands are placed together at the distal border of the popliteal space. Then they stroke firmly to the proximal border and return to the starting position with a superficial stroke. These movements are repeated four times.

Deep Stroking with Both Hands to the Entire Leg

Both hands begin the stroke at the ankle in a position similar to that shown in Figure 5–6C. Both hands then stroke firmly toward the knee, returning to their starting position with a light, superficial stroke. These movements are repeated three times.

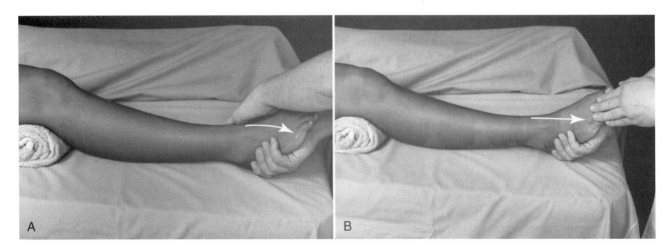

Figure 5–9. **Superficial stroking over the dorsum of the foot.**

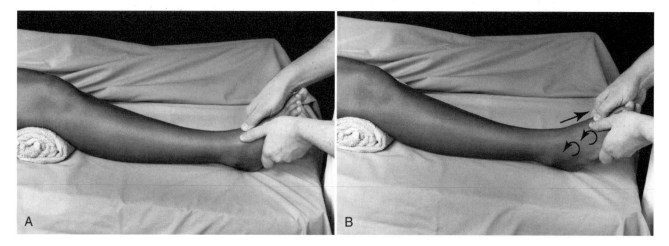

Figure 5–10. **Thumb pad kneading over the dorsum of the foot.**

Right Foot

With the therapist standing at the end of the table facing the patient, the massage continues to the leg and foot.

Superficial Stroking over the Dorsum of the Foot

The palmar surface of the right hand supports the sole of the foot, while the left hand strokes from the ankle (Fig. 5–9A) to the end of the toes (Fig. 5–9B), alternating over the lateral and the medial dorsal surfaces. These movements are repeated twice.

Thumb Pad Kneading over the Dorsum of the Foot

Each thumb pad (distal phalanx) is placed in firm contact with the dorsal surface of the foot, the fingers resting on the foot's plantar surface (Fig. 5–10A). Thumb pad kneading, as described for the anterior tibial muscle groups, is performed progressing from the ankle to the metatar-

sophalangeal joints (Fig. 5–10B). The thumbs return to the ankle position while applying deep stroking over the same area. The kneading is repeated in successive sections until the medial, dorsal, and lateral surfaces (i.e., the entire dorsum) of the foot are covered. These movements are repeated twice.

Deep Thumb Pad Stroking to the Plantar Aspect of the Foot

The thumbs are placed at the base of the toes, the right one at the medial border of the plantar surface, the left one at the lateral border. The fingers rest lightly on the dorsum of the foot (Fig. 5–11A). The thumbs stroke firmly in opposite directions from the borders of the foot, passing in the center (Fig. 5–11B). The stroking progresses from the base of the toes to the heel. The movement is performed chiefly by abducting and adducting the arms at the shoulder. The thumbs are removed, and the fingers maintain contact and return to the starting position with a superficial stroke. These movements are repeated twice.

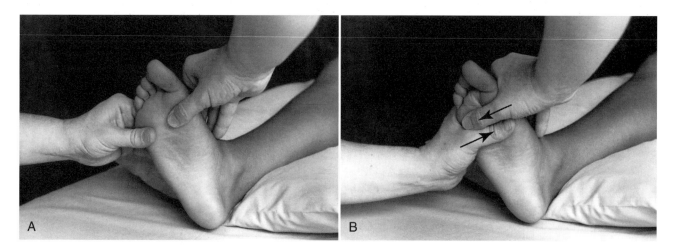

Figure 5–11. **Deep thumb pad stroking to the plantar aspect of the foot.**

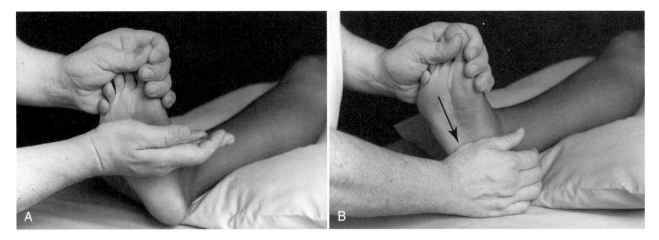

Figure 5–12. **Deep palmar stroking to the plantar aspect of the foot.**

Deep Palmar Stroking to the Plantar Aspect of the Foot

The therapist pivots to face across the end of the table. The left hand on the dorsum of the foot gives support. The ulnar border of the right hand is placed firmly on the plantar surface at the base of the toes (the hand is supinated as in Fig. 5–12A). As the hand strokes firmly down to the heel with deep pressure, it is pronated and made to fit well into the arch (Fig. 5–12B), finishing with the palm flat on the table. These movements are repeated four times.

Deep Digital Stroking around the Malleoli

The therapist pivots back to face the head of the table. Both hands are placed on the dorsum of the foot, with the tips of the fingers at the base of the toes, the index fingers together, and the thumbs crossed (Fig. 5–13A). The fingers perform deep stroking toward the ankle joint with firm pressure. At the ankle the hands separate with the fingers of the left hand stroking around the lateral malleolus as the fingers of the right hand stroke around the medial malleolus (Fig. 5–13B). The palmar surfaces of the fingers keep firm contact, fitting into the contour of the foot as they circle back to the dorsum of the foot and return to the base with a superficial stroke. These movements are repeated four times.

Digital Stroking of the Achilles Tendon

The wrists are flexed, and the radial sides of the index fingers stroke firmly upward on each side of the tendon (Fig. 5–14A). Without losing contact, the hands turn so that the ulnar side of the little fingers can stroke lightly downward to the heel (Fig. 5–14B). These movements are repeated four times.

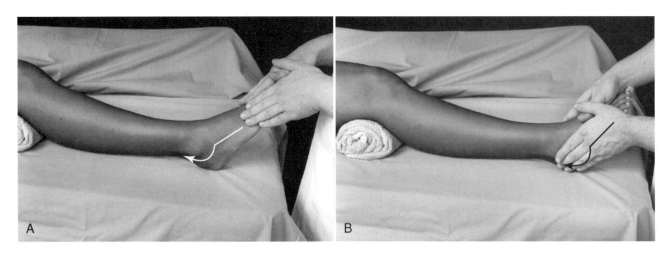

Figure 5–13. **Deep digital stroking around the malleoli.**

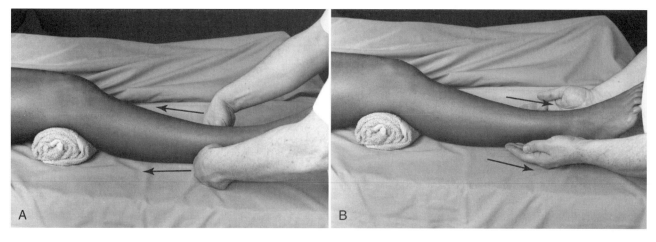

Figure 5–14. **Digital stroking of the Achilles tendon.**

Deep Stroking to the Leg and Thigh

The therapist returns from the foot to the side of the table, and the hands glide into position for deep stroking of the leg. Both hands perform deep stroking to the entire leg and thigh, returning to the foot with a superficial stroke. These movements are repeated three times.

Superficial Stroking to the Right Thigh, Leg, and Foot

The therapist stands at the right side of the patient. Superficial stroking movements are performed on all aspects of the right extremity, working from the hip down to the foot. These movements are repeated four times.

Left Thigh, Leg, and Foot

The therapist now moves around the end of the table to stand at the left side of the patient. All of the movements

described previously for the right lower limb are now repeated on the left side. All of the movements are the same, but the right- and left-hand positions are reversed.

Left Arm, Forearm, and Hand

The therapist continues to stand at the left side of the table but in a position that enables him or her to massage the upper extremity easily.

Superficial Stroking to the Upper Extremity

Both hands are placed on the deltoid muscle mass (Fig. 5–15A) and stroke together from the shoulder to the fingertips (Fig. 5–15B). This stroke may also be performed using an alternate hand technique if preferred. These movements are repeated four times.

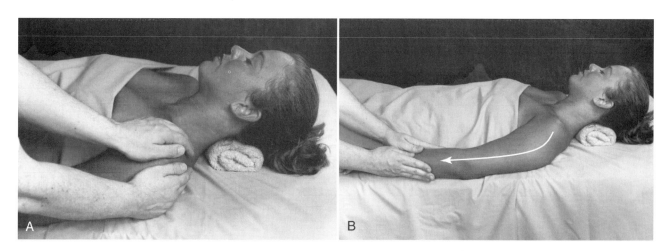

Figure 5–15. **Superficial stroking to the upper extremity.**

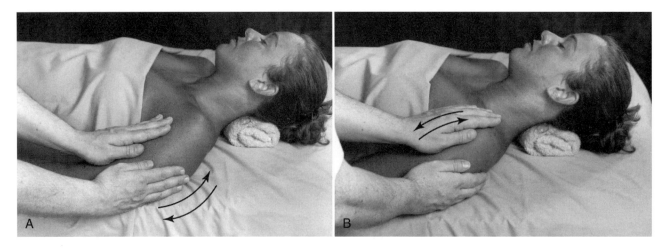

Figure 5–16. **Alternate, deep palmar stroking over the deltoid muscle.**

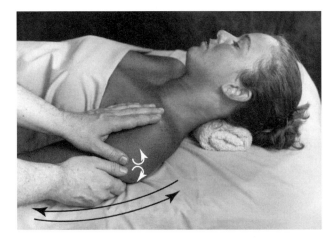

Figure 5–17. **Thumb pad kneading to the upper extremity.**

Alternate, Deep Palmar Stroking over the Deltoid Muscle

The hands are placed just distal to the borders of the deltoid muscle (Fig. 5–16A). The right hand, in firm contact, strokes upward over the posterior half of the deltoid. As the right hand returns with a superficial stroke, the left hand strokes upward over the anterior half of the deltoid (Fig. 5–16B). As it returns with a superficial stroke, the right hand starts its second stroke. These movements are repeated 10 times.

Thumb Pad Kneading to the Upper Extremity

Thumb pad kneading is performed to the entire surface of the limb in three sections—the anterior, lateral, and posterior surfaces (Fig. 5–17). Kneading is performed from the shoulder to the wrist, the hands returning with a deep

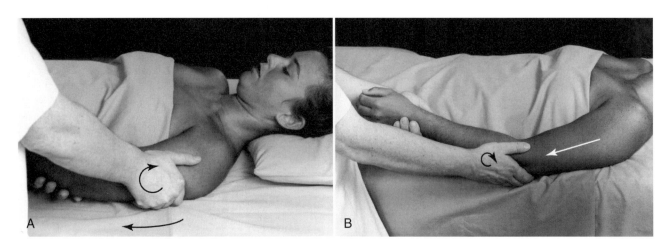

Figure 5–18. **Palmar kneading to the arm and forearm.**

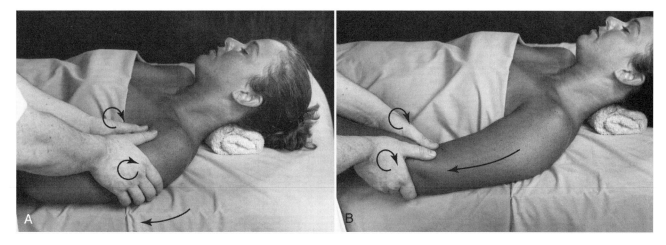

Figure 5–19. **Alternate palmar kneading to the upper extremity.**

stroke from the wrist to the shoulder. These movements are repeated twice.

Palmar Kneading to the Arm and Forearm

With the right hand the therapist performs palmar (compression) kneading as described for the leg while supporting the patient's arm with the left hand (Fig. 5–18A) and then allows the arm to rest on the table while the supporting hand passes to the wrist, giving support to the wrist while the forearm is kneaded (Fig. 5–18B). Tissues of the lateral part of the arm and forearm are kneaded by the right hand. The right hand returns to the shoulder, and the left hand returns to the elbow with a superficial stroke, and kneading of the arm and forearm is repeated. At the end of the second kneading, the left hand returns to the shoulder and the right hand returns to the elbow to support the arm in slight external rotation with the forearm in supination. Kneading to the medial tissues is then performed by the left hand as the right hand provides support. At the end of the second left-hand kneading, both hands return to the shoulder with a deep stroke (similar to that performed on the leg and thigh). These movements are repeated three times with each hand.

Alternate Palmar Kneading to the Upper Extremity

This movement is performed on the upper extremity in the same manner described for the leg, working from the shoulder to the wrist (Fig. 5–19A, B). On the last repeat, the hands do not return to the shoulder with a deep stroke but remain at the wrist to begin thumb pad kneading to the dorsum of the hand. These movements are repeated three times.

Thumb Pad Kneading to the Dorsum of the Hand

Thumb pad kneading is performed to the spaces between the metacarpals. The stroke begins at the wrist and progresses toward the metacarpophalangeal joints (Fig. 5–20). The movements finish with a deep stroking down the metacarpal spaces back to the wrist. The entire dorsum of the hand can be covered in this manner, working in the tissue spaces between the metacarpals. These movements are repeated twice.

Thumb Stroking to the Palmar Surface of the Metacarpophalangeal Joints

The patient's hand is held in supination and is supported on the fingers of both hands, with the left thumb at the

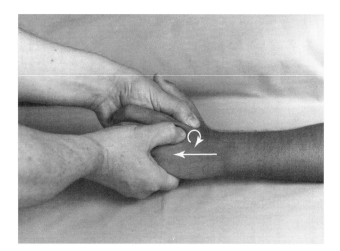

Figure 5–20. **Thumb pad kneading to the dorsum of the hand.**

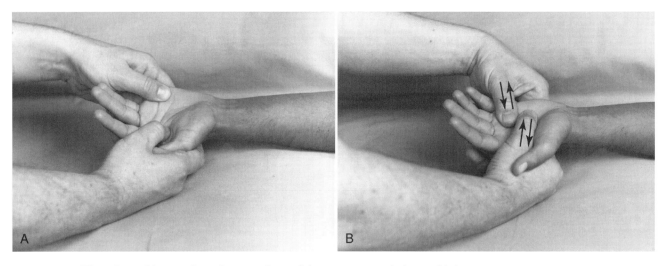

Figure 5–21. **Thumb stroking to the palmar surface of the metacarpophalangeal joints.**

medial border and the right thumb at the lateral border (Fig. 5–21A). The thumbs stroke toward and past each other (Fig. 5–21B) with firm pressure and return with light pressure, as described for the plantar surface of the foot. These movements are repeated four times.

Thumb Stroking over the Thenar and Hypothenar Eminences

The patient's hand is held in supination, supported on the fingers of both hands, with the left thumb on the hypothenar eminence and the right thumb on the thenar eminence (Fig. 5–22). The thumbs stroke alternately toward the wrist with firm pressure, returning with a light stroke. These movements are repeated four times.

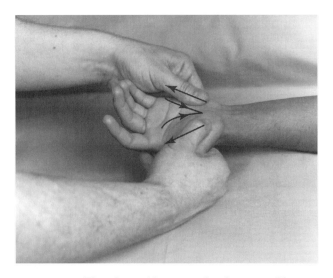

Figure 5–22. **Thumb stroking over the thenar and hypothenar eminences.**

Thumb Pad Kneading to the Thumb and Fingers

The hand is held in pronation and supported in the palm of the left hand. The right thumb, beginning at the metacarpophalangeal joint, kneads on a small area of the medial aspect of the little finger with firm pressure across the digit. The thumb passes lightly over the dorsum of the fingers and kneads on the lateral aspect. The thumb then strokes back lightly over the dorsum of the finger and repeats the movement in the area just distal. This procedure is continued to the tip of the finger (Fig. 5–23A). The thumb and the first finger then stroke firmly back to the base of the finger. The entire movement is performed twice on each finger. The thumb is massaged in the same manner, except that the right hand gives support while movements are performed with the left (Fig. 5–23B). These movements are repeated three times.

Deep Stroking to the Upper Extremity

Both hands stroke firmly upward from the wrist to the shoulder and return with a superficial movement. These movements are repeated three times. After the third deep stroke, the return stroke becomes the start of superficial stroking.

Superficial Stroking to the Upper Extremity

Both hands stroke alternately from the shoulder to the fingertips. These movements are repeated four times.

Right Arm, Forearm, and Hand

The therapist walks around the foot of the table and stands at the patient's right side near the right hand and repeats all of the previous strokes to the right limb. In each instance, the therapist's hand positions are now reversed.

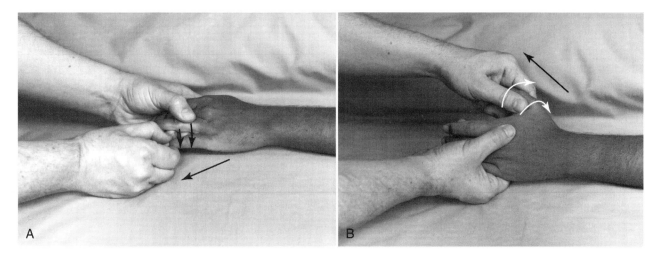

Figure 5–23. **Thumb pad kneading to the thumb and fingers.**

Chest

Superficial Stroking to the Upper Chest

The hands alternately stroke from the shoulders to the sternum. The relaxed hands stroke alternately from the left shoulder to the sternum, covering the area with a few overlapping strokes before moving to the right side without breaking contact (Fig. 5–24). Alternatively, the right hand may start from the patient's right shoulder, and, as it finishes the stroke at the sternum, the left hand starts the stroke from the left shoulder so that contact is not broken. These movements are repeated four times.

Deep Stroking over the Shoulders and around the Neck

Both hands, with the thumbs adducted, are placed with the fingertips at the mid to lower end of the sternum (Fig. 5–25A). The hands stroke simultaneously, the right hand passing lightly upward, then laterally and around the left

shoulder joint, and the left hand passing lightly upward, then laterally and around the right shoulder joint (Fig. 5–25B). Both hands continue the movement, stroking toward the midline of the body along the upper fibers of the trapezius (Fig. 5–25C).

After the fingers meet at the lower cervical spine, the hands stroke around the neck, firmly drawing the muscles forward (Fig. 5–25D). Pressure lightens as the hands stroke over the anterior surface of the neck and return to the starting position at the sternum. These movements are repeated four times.

Digital Kneading from the Sternum to the Shoulder

The fingertips of the left hand are placed at the sternum over the upper fibers of the left pectoralis major, and the right hand is placed over the left hand to reinforce it (Fig. 5–26A). The reverse hand position is equally acceptable. The kneading is then performed with the fingertips, moving in small clockwise circles with light pressure on the upward and outward part of the circle and firm pressure in the downward and inward part. Four circles are made, each succeeding one in an area nearer to the shoulder. As the fingertips reach the shoulder joint, the palm strokes around the joint (Fig. 5–26B), and the entire hand returns and strokes deeply as it returns to the sternum. These movements are repeated three times on the left side. With the hands in a reversed position (or same position) the movement is performed on the right side in counterclockwise circles (Fig. 5–26C). These movements are repeated three times on the right side.

Alternate Deep Stroking from the Shoulder to the Sternum

The hands are in the same position as in Figure 5–25A. With the entire palmar surface, the right hand strokes lightly to the left shoulder joint. The palm then strokes

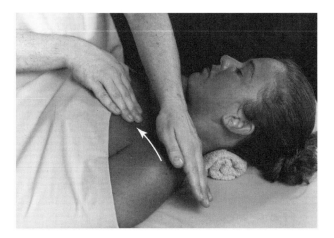

Figure 5–24. **Superficial stroking to the upper chest.**

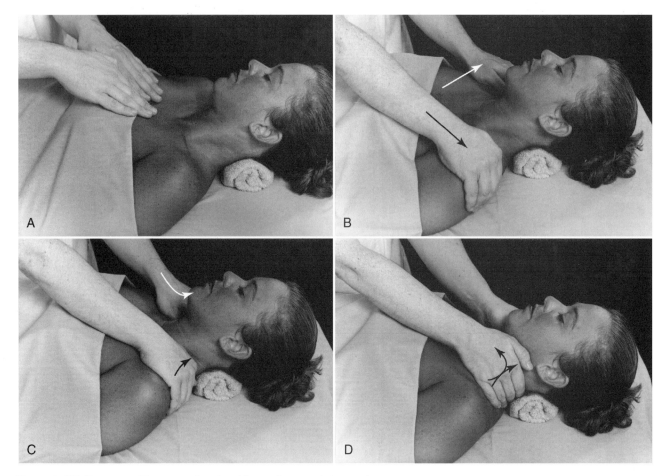

Figure 5–25. Deep stroking over the shoulder and around the neck.

around the joint and returns to the sternum with firm pressure (as in the previous movement). The movement is repeated on the right side. This alternate stroking is repeated four times.

Digital Stroking around the Neck

The hands start in the position shown in Figure 5–26A. The right hand strokes over the top of the left shoulder and in toward the midline of the body. When the fingertips reach the lower cervical spine they stroke upward until the palm is in contact with the neck. The hand then draws the muscles forward with firm pressure (Fig. 5–27A), exerts light pressure over the anterior surface of the neck and the clavicle, and then returns to the starting position. The stroking is then performed in the same manner on the right side (Fig. 5–27B). This alternate stroking is repeated four times.

Deep Stroking over the Areas of the Jugular Veins

With the thumbs widely abducted, the fingers (palmar surface) of the right hand are placed on the left side of the neck and those of the left hand are placed on the right side of the neck, with the borders of the index fingers at the lower tips of the ears (Fig. 5–28A). The hands stroke firmly downward to the base of the neck as the forearms are pronated and the arms abducted (Fig. 5–28B). The thumbs must not make any contact. With gradually lessening pressure, the hands continue the stroke to the tips of the shoulders (Fig. 5–28C). These movements are repeated four times.

Deep Stroking around the Neck

Repeat the movements for deep stroking over the shoulder and around the neck (above), but gradually reduce the pressure with each stroke, until the last stroke is performed as superficial stroking.

Abdomen

The therapist stands at the side of the table on the patient's right. The patient's knees are flexed and supported with a pillow.

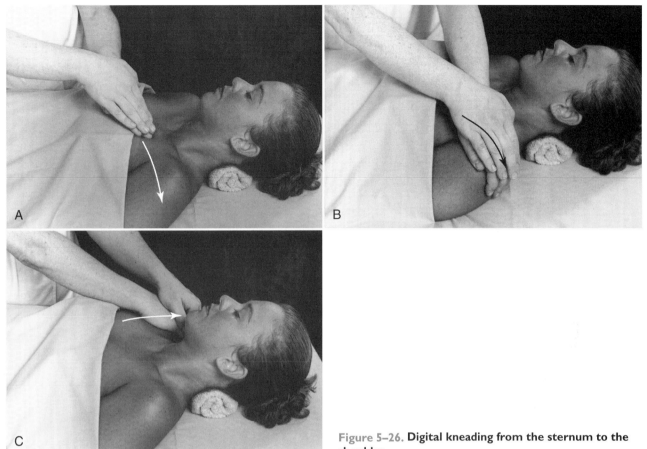

Figure 5–26. Digital kneading from the sternum to the shoulder.

Superficial Stroking to the Abdomen

With the thumb widely abducted, the right hand is placed over the lower border of the left ribs; the left hand is similarly placed over the lower border of the right ribs. Both hands stroke simultaneously or alternately to the symphysis pubis, covering the entire abdomen. The hands are lifted off at the end of the stroke and returned to the starting position without contacting the skin. These movements are repeated four times.

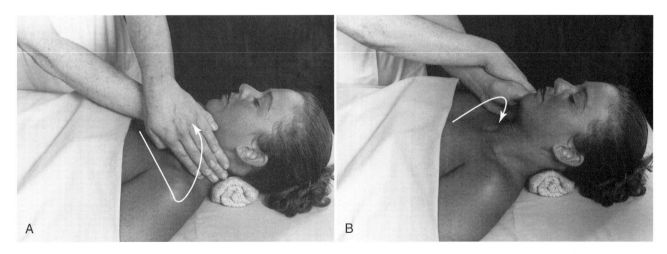

Figure 5–27. Digital stroking around the neck.

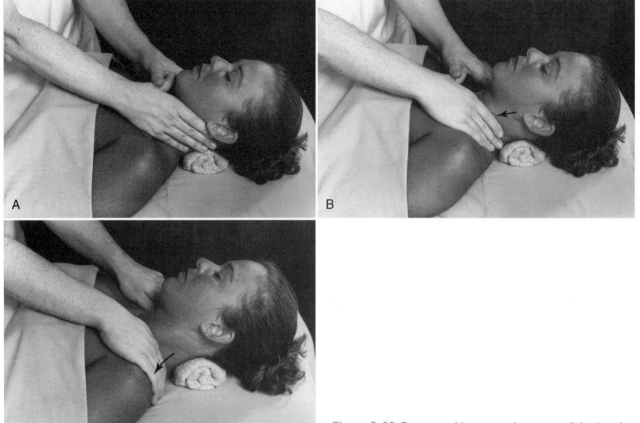

Figure 5–28. **Deep stroking over the areas of the jugular veins.**

Deep Stroking to the Lower Abdomen

The fingertips of both hands are placed side by side at the symphysis pubis. The right hand strokes lightly outward to the left anterior superior iliac spine while the left hand strokes to the right anterior superior iliac spine (Fig. 5–29A). Both hands continue stroking above and following the crest of the ilium around to the back toward the upper lumbar spine. The palms then stroke forward with firm pressure around the waistline (Fig. 5–29B) and over the abdomen to the symphysis pubis. (The purpose of this movement is to manipulate the abdominal musculature, not to exert pressure on the abdominal contents.) These movements are repeated four times.

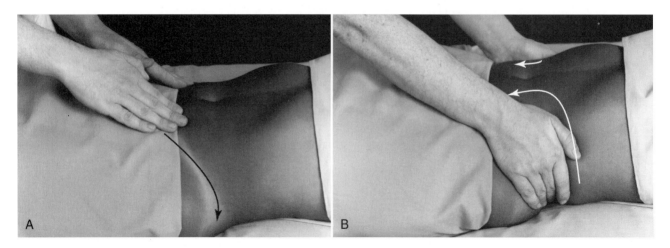

Figure 5–29. **Deep stroking to the lower abdomen.**

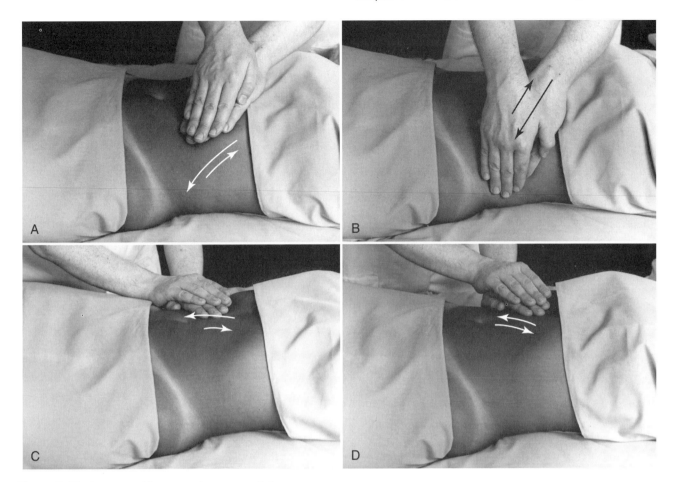

Figure 5–30. **Deep stroking over the upper abdomen.**

Deep Stroking over the Upper Abdomen

One hand is placed so that the fingers lie over the lower anterior border of the left ribs and the palm is at the base of the sternum; the other hand is placed over the top for reinforcement (Fig. 5–30A). The hands stroke lightly in the lateral direction over the ribs, then down over the upper abdominal muscles (Fig. 5–30B), and then return to the starting position with firm pressure over the upper abdomen. These movements are repeated four times on the left side.

One hand is then placed with the fingertips at the base of the sternum and the palm over the lower anterior border of the right ribs (Fig. 5–30C). Repeat the strokes described above on the right side (Fig. 5–30D). To have the palm in good contact on this side the wrist must be in full extension at the start of the stroke. These movements are repeated four times on the right side.

Palmar Kneading over the Colon

The right hand is placed over the lower right quadrant of the abdomen, so that the ulnar border of the hand lies along the pubic bone, just medial to the anterior superior iliac spine. The left hand reinforces the right hand. The ulnar

border of the right hand lifts up the tissues in a scooping movement, performed by pressure with the ulnar border of the hand, rolling the hand over to the thenar border as the palm is pushed toward the fingertips, which are kept in contact with the skin all during this scooping movement. The fingertips are then moved to a more proximal point on the ascending colon as the hand rolls back onto its ulnar border and the movement is repeated. Using this movement, the massage progresses over the abdomen, covering the areas of the ascending, the transverse, and the descending colon (Fig. 5–31A). The movement is changed slightly over the descending colon so that the firm pressure is applied with the thenar eminence of the palm and in a distal direction. The movement is completed with a firm stroke downward over the lower part of the area of the descending colon (Fig. 5–31B), with the hand passing lightly over the lower abdomen to the area of the lower border of the ascending colon (starting position). These movements are repeated three times.

Deep Stroking over the Colon

The fingertips of the right hand are placed at the lower border of the area of the ascending colon, the left hand

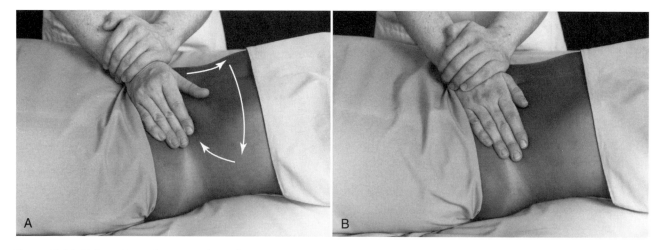

Figure 5–31. **Palmar kneading over the colon.**

reinforcing the right (Fig. 5–32A). The fingertips stroke firmly upward over the area of the ascending colon, across the area of the transverse colon (Fig. 5–32B), and downward over the area of the descending colon (Fig. 5–31C), then lightly over the lower abdomen to the starting point. These movements are repeated six times.

Alternate Palmar Kneading over the Entire Abdomen

At the right side of the abdomen, both hands, with the thumbs abducted, grasp the tissues and by alternate flexion and extension at the elbows and the shoulders progress across the abdomen with a kneading movement (Fig.

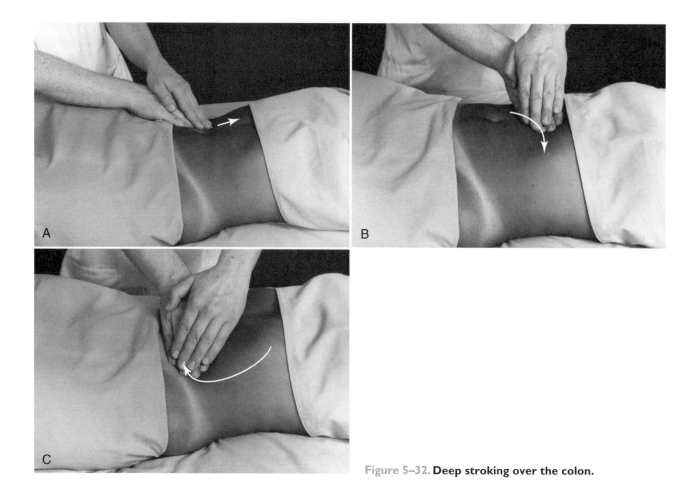

Figure 5–32. **Deep stroking over the colon.**

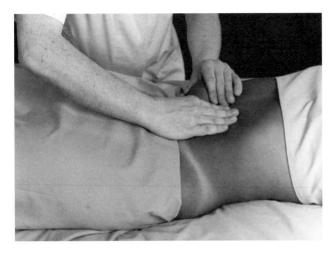

Figure 5–33. Alternate palmar kneading over the entire abdomen.

5–33). Both hands return together to the right side with a superficial stroke. These movements are repeated four times.

Deep Stroking to the Lower Abdomen

Repeat deep stroking to the lower abdomen (above), gradually reducing the pressure to eventually become superficial stroking. Repeat these movements four times.

Back and Hips

The therapist stands at the side of the table on the patient's left. The patient lies prone, with a pillow under the abdomen (lumbar spine region) and another under the ankles. The patient's head may be positioned in a number of ways, depending on what is comfortable.

Superficial Stroking to the Back

The right hand is placed over the right shoulder, and the left hand is placed over the left shoulder, with the thumbs just lateral to the spinous processes of the first cervical vertebra (Fig. 5–34A). Both hands, with thumbs abducted, stroke simultaneously to the sacrum, covering as much of the back as possible (Fig. 5–34B). The hands may return in the air to the starting position. These movements are repeated four times. At the end of the fourth stroke, the hands maintain contact so they are in position to start deep palmar stroking.

Deep Palmar Stroking to the Back

1. The fingers of both hands start the deep stroke at the lower border of the sacrum; the thumbs are crossed for reinforcement (Fig. 5–35A), and the hands stroke upward on each side of the spinous processes with firm pressure.

2. The hands separate at the neck and stroke over the top of the shoulder, as the thumbs stroke up to the first cervical vertebra on both sides of the spinous processes (Fig. 5–35B). The hands then stroke back, drawing the muscles back also, until the fingertips are at the top of the shoulder (Fig. 5–35C). At the same time, the thumbs stroke down on both sides of the cervical vertebrae. The hands, with thumbs adducted, then stroke laterally to the shoulder joint (Fig. 5–35D) and down the sides of the back to the waistline, and then toward the midline (Fig. 5–35E) and down until the fingertips are at the lower border of the sacrum. (Thumbs cross to reinforce as the hands start the downward stroke to the sacrum.)

3. The hands stroke upward and over the shoulders as in Step 2 (above) (Fig. 5–35A) and return the stroke

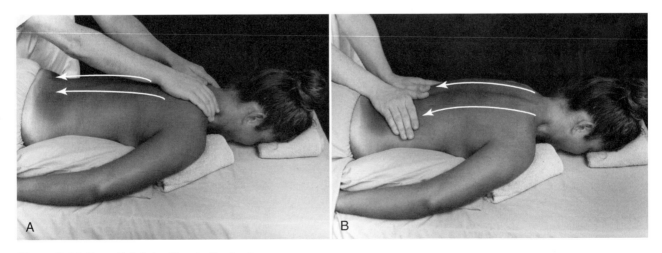

Figure 5–34. Superficial stroking to the back.

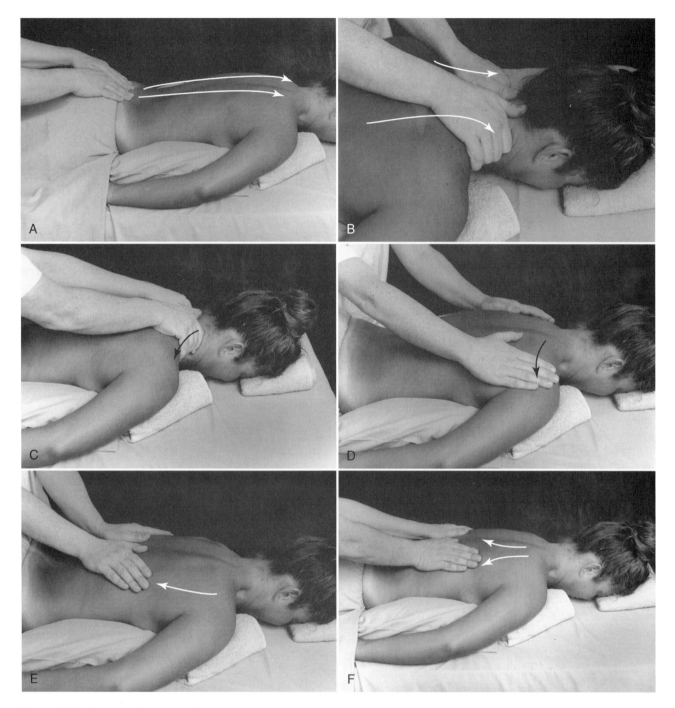

Figure 5–35. *See legend on opposite page*

downward until the fingertips are even with the axilla (Fig. 5–35F), then pass laterally and stroke to the sacrum, again as in Step 2.

4. The hands stroke upward and over the shoulder as in Step 2, return the stroke downward until the wrists are at the waistline (Fig. 5–35G), then pass laterally and stroke to the sacrum, again as in Step 2.

5. The hands stroke upward and over the shoulder as in Step 2, then return the stroke downward until the fingertips are at the waistline, then pass laterally and stroke to the sacrum (Fig. 5–35H), as in Step 2.

6. The hands stroke upward, as in Step 2, and return the stroke over the shoulder and then downward, with the hands spread to cover the entire back, and return to the sacrum (Fig. 5–35I).

These movements are repeated three times.

Finger Pad Kneading over the Upper Fibers of the Trapezius

The finger pads of the right hand, reinforced with the left hand, are placed at the upper cervical region of the upper fibers of the right trapezius muscle (Fig. 5–36A). They

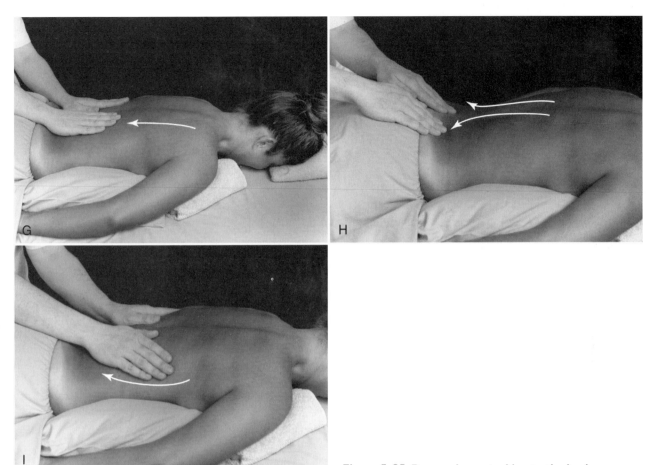

Figure 5–35. **Deep palmar stroking to the back.**

knead in small clockwise circles, progressing over to the acromion process (Fig. 5–36B). The fingers return to the starting position with a superficial stroke. These movements are repeated three times. The left side is kneaded in the same manner, except that circles are worked counterclockwise. Again, the movements are repeated three times.

Digital Stroking over the Upper Fibers of the Trapezius

The thumbs are placed on the borders of the upper fibers of the trapezius, lateral to the spinous processes of the upper cervical vertebrae. The palms of the hands are placed over the tops of the shoulders. Both hands stroke

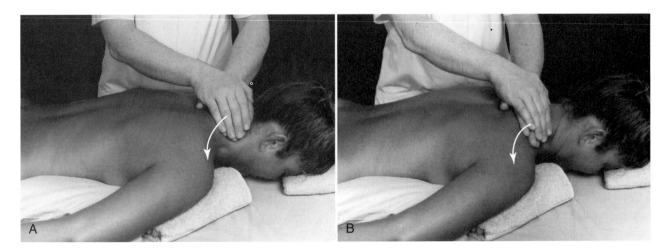

Figure 5–36. **Finger pad kneading over the upper fibers of the trapezius.**

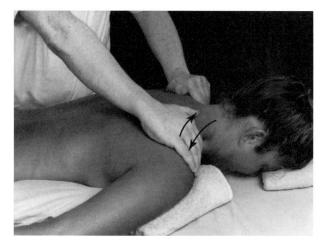

Figure 5–37. **Digital stroking over the upper fibers of the trapezius.**

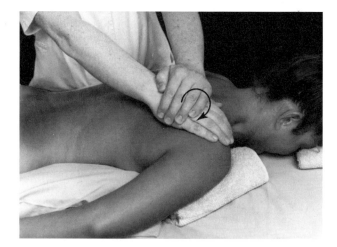

Figure 5–38. **Kneading over the scapular region.**

firmly to the acromions, picking up the muscle as the thumbs reach the lower cervical region (Fig. 5–37). The hands return with superficial strokes. These movements are repeated four times.

Kneading over the Scapular Region

Reinforced by the left hand, the right hand is placed with the palm above the spine of the right scapula and the thumb just lateral to the spinous process of the upper thoracic vertebra. The palm kneads in a clockwise circle over the upper scapular region (Fig. 5–38), then glides to make a second circle over the lateral border of the scapula, a third circle over the lower angle of the scapula, and a fourth circle over the medial border of the scapula. The movements are repeated three times.

Transition is made from one side to the other with no break in contact, the hand gliding across with a superficial stroke. To massage the left scapular region, the right hand

is placed with the palm above the spine of the left scapula and the ulnar border of the hand just lateral to the spinous processes of the upper thoracic vertebrae. The kneading is performed in the same manner as for the right side, except that the circles are made counterclockwise. These movements are repeated three times.

Alternate Palmar Kneading over the Thoracic and Lumbar Regions

Both hands are placed at the left side of the upper thoracic region. The left hand strokes across to the lateral border of the right dorsal region with firm pressure (Fig. 5–39A), and, as this hand returns to the left side the right hand strokes across to the right side. The muscles are kneaded by the alternate movement between the hands. As the right hand returns, the left hand again strokes to the right side. These strokes are repeated, the hands alternating in

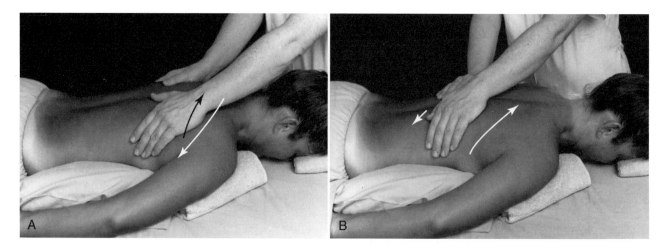

Figure 5–39. **Alternate palmar kneading over the thoracic and lumbar regions.**

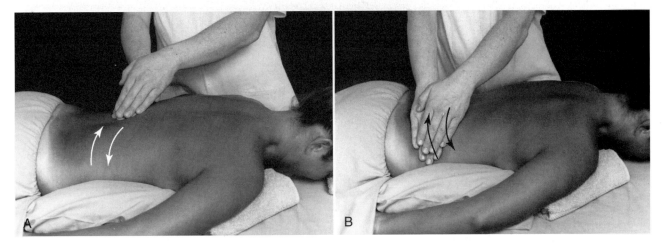

Figure 5–40. **Palmar stroking over the lumbar region.**

direction and progressing to the lower border of the lumbar region (Fig. 5–39B). Before the left hand completes the stroke at the lower lumbar area, the right hand is removed and is placed on the upper dorsal region to start the entire kneading sequence again. The movements are repeated four times.

Palmar Stroking over the Lumbar Region

The right hand, reinforced by the left, is placed over the lower ribs on the right side, the fingers extending along the ribs (Fig. 5–40A). The hand strokes lightly from the spine to the lateral lumbar region of the right side and returns below the ribs, stroking toward the spine with firm pressure (Fig. 5–40B). These movements are repeated four times. The left side is massaged in the same manner as the right, except that the right hand is placed with the fingertips at the spine for the initial stroke. These movements are repeated four times.

Thumb Pad Kneading over the Sacrum

The thumbs of both hands are placed at the upper border of the sacrum, with the palms in contact with the back just above the iliac crest (Fig. 5–41). The thumbs knead alternately in small circles with upward pressure, progressing to the lower border of the sacrum. The thumbs stroke upward with firm pressure for the return. The movements are repeated four times.

Alternate Palmar Kneading to the Buttocks

The ulnar border of the right hand is placed at the right gluteal fold, and the ulnar border of the left hand is placed in the area of the origin of the gluteal muscles. The muscle mass is then grasped and kneaded in an alternating movement similar to that described for the quadriceps. Pressure is applied in such a manner as to avoid separating the buttocks (Fig. 5–42). The left buttock is massaged in the same manner as the right. These movements are repeated twice on each side.

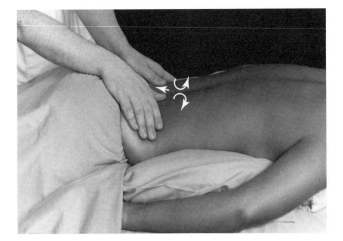

Figure 5–41. **Thumb pad kneading over the sacrum.**

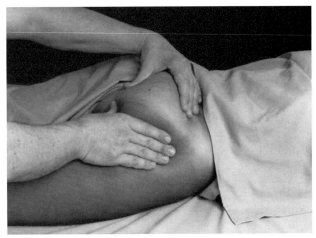

Figure 5–42. **Alternate palmar kneading to the buttocks.**

Deep Kneading to the Buttocks

The left hand supports the muscle, or the left hand may reinforce the right hand as the right hand performs deep kneading over the right buttock (Fig. 5–43) in the same manner as for kneading over the colon, except that the heel of the hand exerts firm pressure toward the midline throughout the movement, to avoid separation of the buttocks. This movement is repeated twice. The left buttock is kneaded in the same manner as the right, with the same number of repetitions.

Alternate Palmar Kneading over the Entire Back

This movement is the same as for Alternate Palmar Kneading over the Thoracic and Lumbar Regions (above), beginning at the upper scapular region and continuing over the entire back. These movements are repeated four times.

Digital Kneading to the Erector Spinae

This kneading of the tissues is performed between the thumb of one hand and the fingers of the other. The finger pads (distal phalanges) of the first and second fingers of both hands are placed just lateral to the spinous processes at the lower cervical region, and the distal phalanx of each thumb is placed an inch or two below the fingertips. (This relative position of fingers and thumb is maintained for each hand throughout the movement.) Using a circular motion and firm pressure, the fingers of the right hand draw a portion of the muscle downward; simultaneously the left thumb, also with firm pressure, presses a portion of the muscle upward; then the right thumb presses a portion upward as the fingers of the left hand draw a portion of the muscle downward, again using a circular motion. Progression from one area to the next is accomplished by gliding of the fingers during the period of firm pressure, while the thumb of the same hand superficially strokes the area to be covered next. (This kneading of the tissues between the thumb of one hand and the fingers of the other is produced by alternate flexion and extension at the elbows and the

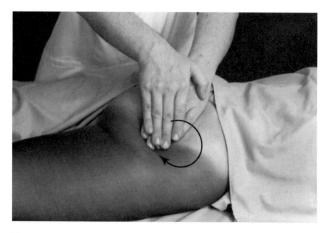

Figure 5–43. **Deep kneading to the buttocks.**

shoulders.) The kneading is continued to the sacrum. This movement usually is not repeated.

Deep Palmar Stroking to the Erector Spinae

The hands are used alternately in this stroke. The palm of the right hand is placed over the center of the spine at the cervical region and moves with a superficial stroke to the sacrum. As the right hand approaches the end of the stroke (Fig. 5–44A) the left hand starts another superficial stroke. The right hand returns in the air (Fig. 5–44B). These movements are repeated four times.

Deep Palmar Stroking

Repeat Deep Palmar Stroking to the Back (above), gradually reducing the pressure to finish with superficial stroking.

The number of repetitions indicated for each movement in the technique for general massage is the approximate number required to give a general massage within 1 hour, at the usual rate of speed for the movements (see Chapter 3). This must not be interpreted to mean that all general massage must be given for exactly 1 hour or that in all instances every movement must be performed in every area exactly the number of times suggested.

Face

Facial massage may be added to a general massage. Patients with insomnia frequently respond particularly well to facial massage, and it is a useful sedative in the treatment of headache. The movements are performed over a small area and should be gentle, so that a lubricant is not usually necessary. As always, the hands should be washed and thoroughly dried before treatment. A small amount of fine unscented talcum powder may be used if the skin is moist from perspiration.

The technique for facial massage that follows is a type recommended for sedation in the treatment of headache and insomnia. If general massage has not been given, the treatment should include the chest and upper back movements described previously for general massage, as well as face, head, and neck (described below).

The patient should be lying supine (recumbent) with the head supported on a small pillow or neck roll. The therapist stands facing the patient on either side of the table. All movements are performed with both hands in unison, with the exception of thumb pad kneading over the nose.

Superficial Stroking to the Face

1. The palms are placed side by side on the forehead, with the thenar eminences on either side of the midline. The fingers are flexed slightly to fit over the head, with the fingertips resting lightly on the top of the head (Fig. 5–45A). The palms stroke to the

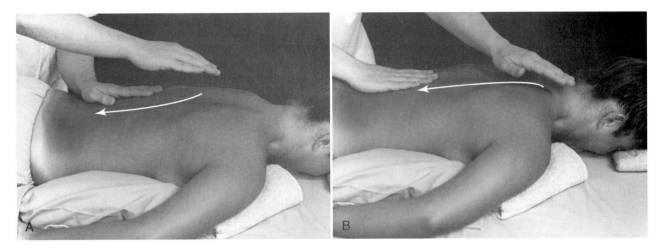

Figure 5–44. **Deep palmar stroking to the erector spinae.**

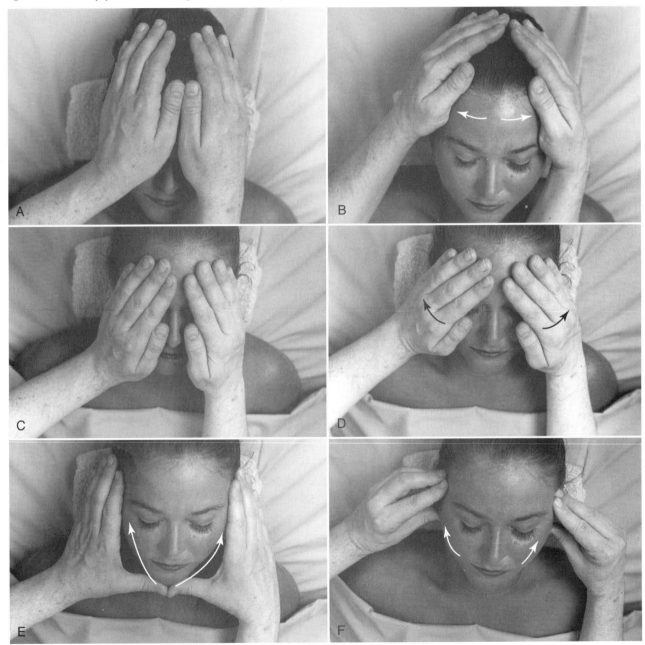

Figure 5–45. **Superficial stroking to the face.**

lateral borders of the forehead (Fig. 5–45B) and return to the starting position by moving through the air while the hands pivot on the fingertips. These movements are repeated twice.

2. The movements are the same as in Step 1 (above), except that the fingertips rest at the hairline so that the palms are placed over the cheeks (Fig. 5–45C, D). They are repeated twice.

3. The fingertips glide lightly from the hairline to the temples. The thumbs are placed together at the center of the chin (Fig. 5–45E). They stroke laterally along the border of the mandible to the tip of the ear (Fig. 5–45F) and return to the chin through the air. These movements are repeated twice.

4. The movements are the same as in Step 3 (above), except that the thumbs start under the chin and stroke under the jaw to the tip of the ear. The movements are repeated twice.

Thumb Pad Kneading to the Forehead

The fingertips of each hand keep contact at the temple, and the thumb pads are placed together at the center of the lower border of the forehead (Fig. 5–46A). The thumb pads knead simultaneously in small circles (Fig. 5–46B), continuing up to the hairline. They return in the air to the lower border of the forehead at more lateral areas and repeat the movements until the entire forehead is covered. The movements are repeated twice.

Deep Stroking to the Forehead

The fingertips of each hand are kept in contact at the temples, and the palms are placed with the radial borders

together on the forehead (Fig. 5–47A). The palms stroke laterally from the midline with firm pressure (Fig. 5–47B) and return through the air. The movements are repeated three times.

Alternate Thumb Pad Kneading to the Nose

The fingertips are kept in contact at the temples, and the distal phalanges of the thumbs are placed at the tip of the nose (Fig. 5–48A). Alternate thumb pad kneading is performed on the sides of the nose, up to the bridge. The thumbs pause with firm pressure in the hollows formed by the bridge of the nose and the medial part of the supraorbital ridge (Fig. 5–48B) before returning through the air. These movements are repeated three times.

At the end of the third kneading stroke, the thumbs keep contact at the hollows, ready to start the next movement.

Deep Stroking to the Supraorbital Ridge

This movement flows from the previous one without breaking contact. The thumbs stroke outward with firm pressure over the supraorbital ridge (Fig. 5–49) and return through the air. The movements are repeated four times.

Deep Stroking to the Infraorbital Ridge

The hands remain in the same position as for stroking the supraorbital ridge (above), allowing the thumbs to stroke over the infraorbital ridge (Fig. 5–50) and return through the air. The movements are repeated four times.

Digital Kneading from the Temple to the Cervical Spine

The thumbs remain in the air, and the fingertips (again without breaking the contact with the temples) simulta-

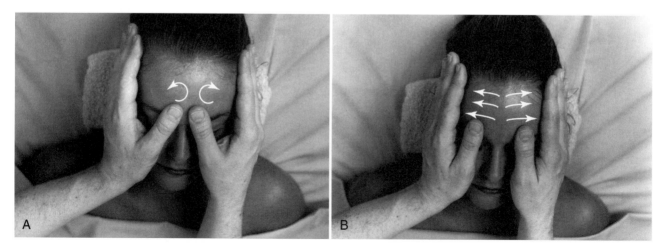

Figure 5–46. **Thumb pad kneading to the forehead.**

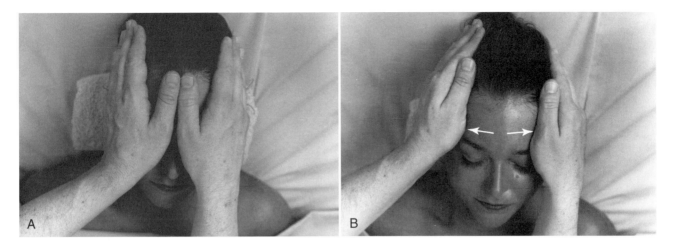

Figure 5–47. **Deep stroking to the forehead.**

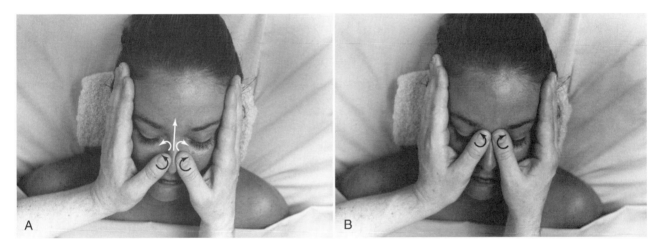

Figure 5–48. **Alternate thumb pad kneading to the nose.**

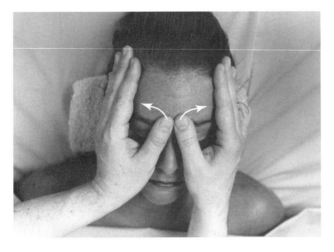

Figure 5–49. **Deep stroking to the supraorbital ridge.**

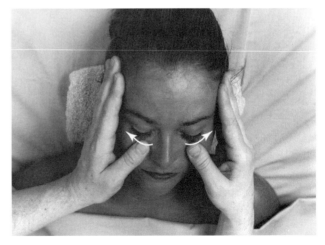

Figure 5–50. **Deep stroking to the infraorbital ridge.**

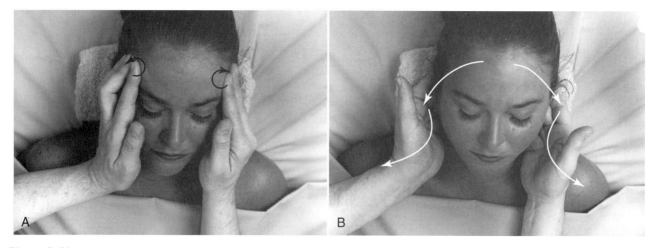

Figure 5–51. **Digital kneading from the temple to the cervical spine.**

neously knead in small circles, starting at the temples (Fig. 5–51A) and, following the hairline, continue along the back of the ears until the fingers meet at the cervical spine (Fig. 5–51B).

Without breaking contact, the fingers stroke with firm pressure down the cervical spine to the seventh cervical vertebra. The thumbs then make contact with the anterior borders of the trapezius, and the stroking is continued with the thumbs and fingers over the upper fibers of the trapezius, gradually reducing pressure to the tips of the shoulders. The hands again return to the temples through the air. These movements are repeated twice.

Finger Pad Kneading from the Temples to the Shoulders

The fingertips knead in small circles from the temples (Fig. 5–52A), passing in front of the ears to the mastoid processes. The strokes continue over both sternocleido-

mastoids and the upper fibers of the trapezius muscles (Fig. 5–52B) to the tips of the shoulders. The hands then return through the air. The movements are repeated twice.

Deep Stroking over the Area of the Jugular Veins

This stroke is the same as that described for Deep Stroking over the Areas of the Jugular Veins under Chest (Fig. 5–28). These movements are repeated four times.

Palmar Kneading to the Cheeks

The fingertips rest lightly on the forehead while the palms rest lightly on the cheeks and knead in circles, three times in a forward direction (Fig. 5–53A) and three times backward (Fig. 5–53B). The palms do not move over the skin but with gentle pressure move the tissues over the bony surface underneath. The movements are repeated twice.

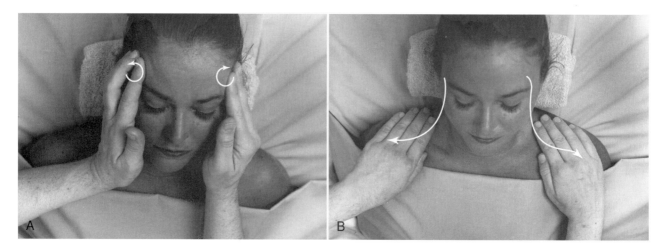

Figure 5–52. **Finger pad kneading from the temples to the shoulders.**

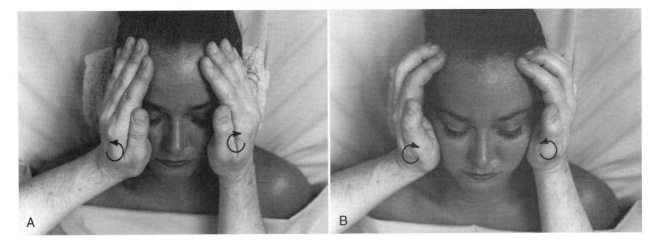

Figure 5–53. **Palmar kneading to the cheeks.**

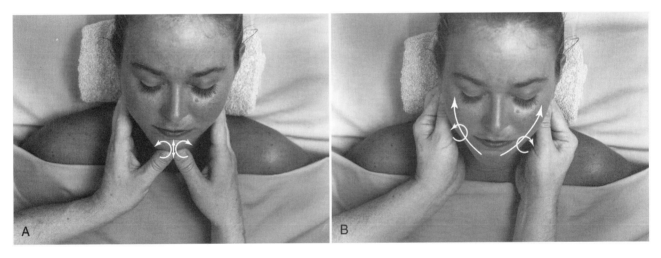

Figure 5–54. **Thumb pad kneading to the chin and the jaw.**

Thumb Pad Kneading to the Chin and the Jaw

The fingertips glide lightly to make contact below the ears. The thumbs are placed together at the center of the lower border of the chin (Fig. 5–54A) and knead simultaneously in small circles upward to the lower lip, returning with superficial stroking to knead over more lateral areas of the chin. They continue this kneading over the mandibles to the tips of the ears (Fig. 5–54B). These movements are repeated three times.

Deep Stroking to the Chin and the Jaw

Keeping the fingers in contact, the thumbs return to the chin as at the start of the previous movement. They then stroke with firm pressure from the chin (Fig. 5–55) to the

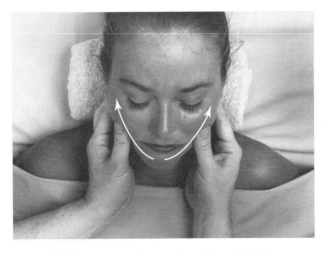

Figure 5–55. **Deep stroking to the chin and the jaw.**

tips of the ears, to return through the air. These movements are repeated three times.

Deep Stroking over the Jugular Veins

Without breaking contact after the preceding movement, the therapist repeats the procedures described for Deep Stroking over the Shoulders and around the Neck, under Chest (Fig. 5–28). Repeat these movements four times.

Superficial Stroking

The movements are those described for Superficial Stroking to the Face (Fig. 5–45).

Scalp

Finger Pad Kneading over the Scalp

The thumbs are placed at the temples with the fingers spread apart and the fingertips placed on either side of the medial line of the scalp. The fingers knead with firm pressure in small circles, in sections, until the entire head is covered. The fingertips keep contact with the skin and move the scalp over the bony surface. The pressure must be released before the fingertips are moved to each surrounding area, to avoid pulling the hair.

Posterior Neck Region

Superficial and Deep Stroking over the Upper Fibers of the Trapezius Muscles

The thumbs are placed on the borders of the upper fibers of the trapezius muscles on both sides, just lateral to the spinous processes of the upper cervical vertebrae. The palms of the hands are in contact over the tops of the shoulders. Both hands stroke lightly to the acromions, picking up the muscle as the thumbs reach the lower cervical region. The hands return to the starting position with a superficial stroke. This movement is performed eight times, with increasing pressure, so that by the fifth stroke

the therapist is applying deep stroking; the hands return to the starting position with superficial stroking.

Finger Pad Kneading over the Upper Fibers of the Trapezius

The fingertips of the right hand, reinforced by the left hand, are placed at the upper cervical region of the left trapezius muscle. As usual, the fingers knead in small clockwise circles, exerting heavier pressure over one half of each circle. Kneading progresses to the acromion process. The fingertips return to the starting position with a superficial stroke. These movements are repeated three times. The right side is kneaded in the same manner, except that the circles are made counterclockwise. These movements are repeated three times.

Deep Stroking over the Upper Fibers of the Trapezius Muscles

This movement is performed in the same manner described for Superficial and Deep Stroking over the Upper Fibers of the Trapezius Muscles (above), except that the pressure starts deeply and is gradually lessened to superficial stroking. These movements are repeated six times.

SUMMARY

The massage sequence described in this chapter is designed to cover the entire body in a single treatment session. The massage would take about 45 minutes to an hour to complete in the average patient. The actual sequence is, of course, made up of a series of individual massage strokes. As mentioned previously, there are many ways in which these basic massage strokes can be combined into a general massage sequence. This is simply one example of many possibilities. In fact, the suggested massage sequences for each region of the body described in this chapter can be used as a method of performing local massage. This concept is addressed in more detail in the next chapter.

Chapter 6

Local Massage Sequences

A variety of massage strokes can be a very useful part of a total treatment plan for the management of local trauma or disease. Local injury or disease can affect many different tissues, including skin, muscles, tendons, joints, nerves, and blood vessels. A therapist must have a thorough knowledge of the anatomy and physiology of the structures involved and an understanding of the pathologic conditions in the tissues to be treated, if the treatment is to be as effective as possible. Muscles may be atrophied, decreased in tone, fibrotic, flaccid, or in spasm. Tissues may be edematous; joint effusion and inflammation may limit movement and produce pain. Normal limb motion may also be limited by adhesions or contractures; the tendons may be adherent to the surrounding structures; and the circulation may also be impaired. Each of these potential problems must be evaluated and treated by techniques selected according to the changes present and the desired effects. Massage techniques are simply one of many different options for the management of local trauma or disease. The best results are most likely to be achieved when the appropriate manual techniques, including massage, are combined with a suitable rest or exercise program and appropriate electrophysical agents (modalities).

The individual techniques described in Chapter 3 can be used separately or in combination with each other and with many other treatment approaches. The important point is to gain a thorough understanding of the patient's problem and how it affects the tissues. Once this is properly understood choosing a suitable massage technique is relatively easy. It is simply a question of matching the needs of the tissues with the known effects of the massage technique. For example, if tendon and muscle contractures are limiting joint motion, the mobilizing effects of kneading, wringing, picking up, and deep frictions might be very helpful, especially when combined with other treatments such as exercise and appropriate electrophysical agents. It is therefore quite proper for an experienced therapist to develop his or her own particular combination of massage techniques (a sequence) to be used as part of a treatment plan for local trauma or disease.

Modern rehabilitation practice now encompasses many different treatment concepts, including soft tissue massage. Many of today's treatment concepts have been developed over the past 50 years, and this has significantly increased the treatment options available to therapists.

It is important to recognize that there are many different ideas about massage strokes and their sequencing. Many of these systems of massage were extremely popular in the early part of this century and were effective then, as, indeed, they are today; however, the development of modern rehabilitation methods has produced more effective procedures than massage alone. For this reason, massage is rarely used as a sole treatment today; in fact, one could argue that massage is best combined with other treatments to give a more rounded approach to the management of the patient's problem. It is quite appropriate to select suitable techniques from those detailed in Chapter 3 and to combine them with any of a number of complementary techniques. This may well result in a "minisequence" of strokes designed to achieve a specific effect. The rest of this chapter is devoted to a local massage sequence based on Hoffa's concept of local massage. Although this system can be used alone, it can also be combined with other suitable treatments. A modified version is presented here to provide suggestions about how this approach might be used. For purposes of completeness, all important areas of the body are discussed. Each area can be considered separately, and, when appropriate, they may be combined.

THE HOFFA SYSTEM

Hoffa's original work, *Technic der Massage,* was published in four editions, the last one in 1903. The system developed by this eminent surgeon follows an anatomic pattern and is based on a knowledge of physiology. The movements are applied to certain muscles or muscle groups; this contrasts with some other systems that apply strokes either to an entire extremity or to a certain area of the body. Hoffa classified the essential massage strokes as effleurage (stroking), petrissage (kneading), and friction, vibration, and tapotement (percussion) and stated that these are only the framework on which an experienced therapist with good judgment may build up an effective treatment for a given patient's problem. He emphasized the value of massage for increasing venous and lymphatic circulation. One must keep in mind, however, the context in which he developed his system and, in particular, the range of treatment options available at the time and the state of medical knowledge. (The rehabilitation professions as we currently know them did not exist.)

The Movements

According to Hoffa *effleurage* (stroking) is employed to stimulate circulation in the small veins in the muscles, and particularly in the large veins or venous plexuses that lie in the grooves between the individual muscles. This is accomplished by making the hand conform closely to the contours of the part as the thumb and finger tips simultaneously proceed along these interstices. *Petrissage* (kneading) is used chiefly to increase the circulation in the muscles and to remove "products" in a manner analogous to that of friction. *Friction* movements are applied chiefly to break down pathologic exudates, deposits, and thickenings in tissue around joints and tendons, and to help remove the waste products through the lymphatic system. *Vibration* and *tapotement* (percussion) are recommended to increase blood supply, reduce nerve irritability, and increase contraction of muscle fibers. These techniques are probably of little value in the treatment of local trauma, but they do have some specific uses for certain lesions; for example, vibration techniques can be very useful in treating some respiratory problems.

CLASSIFICATION AND DESCRIPTION OF LOCAL MASSAGE MOVEMENTS

The following classification and description of massage strokes is a modification of the Hoffa system of massage. In general, all of these descriptions match those defined in Chapter 3.

Stroking (Superficial or Deep)

1. The direction of the deep stroke is always the direction of venous blood and lymph flow.

2. The stroke is applied to the entire length of the muscle or muscle group, beginning at the insertion and continuing to the origin.

3. The hand returns over the same area with light pressure (superficial stroking).

4. The hand is made to conform to the shape of the muscle or muscle group, attempting to reach around and lift up the bulk of the muscle or group. The palmar surfaces of the entire hand or the distal phalanges of the fingers (finger pads) or of the thumb (thumb pad) are used, according to the size of the muscle.

5. The pressure is regulated according to the bulk of the muscles: light at the beginning of the deep stroke, increasing over the bulkiest part of the muscles, and diminishing at the end of the stroke, finishing with a "squeeze-out" movement. In performing the squeeze-out movement, the grasping surfaces of the hand are gradually approximated more closely as the muscle bulk decreases and the hand approaches the origin of the muscle. As the hand reaches the point of origin, it is pronated. The bulk of the tissue being massaged is thus squeezed out of the hand, and the hand is in position to start the return stroke.

6. The movements should be performed rhythmically.

7. The rate of movement should be that described previously under general massage (see Chapter 5).

Kneading

The kneading movements in the Hoffa system are performed with one or both hands (single-handed or two-hand kneading) or with the distal phalanges of the thumb and index and middle fingers of one or both hands (digital kneading/finger pad or thumb pad kneading). Single-handed kneading is used on muscles that are not too large to be grasped in one hand. For very large muscles two-handed kneading can be used. Digital kneading is used on narrow or flat muscles that cannot be grasped easily by the entire hand. As in stroking, the hand must conform to the size and shape of the muscles and make firm contact. The movement begins at the insertion of the muscle and is carried through to the origin.

Single-Handed Kneading

1. The hand is placed at the insertion of the muscle with the palmar surface of its ulnar border in firm contact (Fig. 6–1A).

2. The hand grasps around the bulk of the muscle and lifts it as much as possible from the underlying tissues (Fig. 6–1B).

3. The fingers and ulnar border of the hand follow along one border of the muscle or muscle group, and the thumb follows along the opposite border (see Fig. 6–1B).

4. The movement is one of grasping and releasing the tissues, and it is carried through to the origin of the muscle, finishing with a squeeze-out movement (Fig. 6–1C).

5. The thumb and fingers work simultaneously, but the pressure must be diminished as they approach each other, to prevent pinching.

6. Care must be used to keep the bulk of the muscle well back in the palm of the hand between the thenar eminence and the metacarpal pad of the palm (see Fig. 6–1A).

7. At the origin of the muscle, the hand is brought over into pronation and returned to the starting position with a superficial stroke over the area (Fig. 6–1D, E).

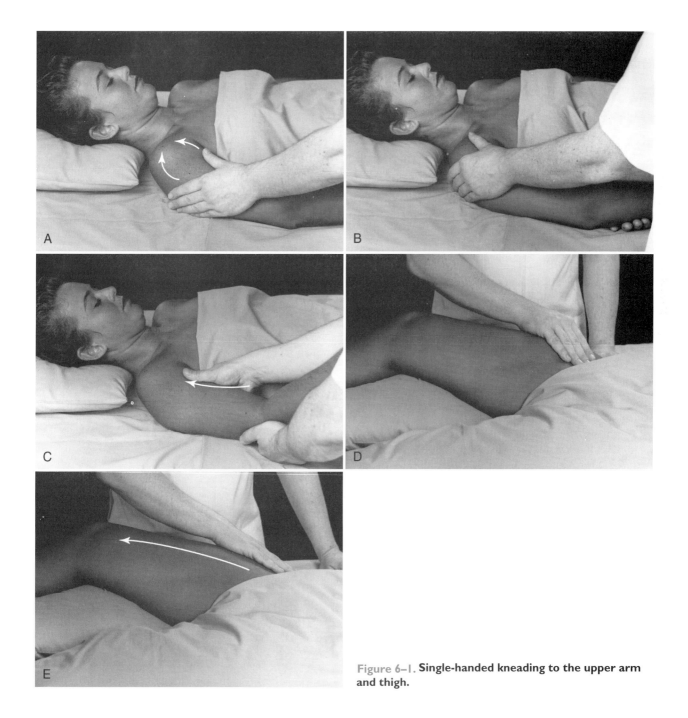

Figure 6–1. **Single-handed kneading to the upper arm and thigh.**

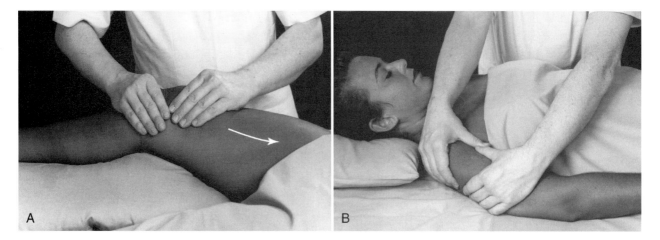

Figure 6–2. Two-handed kneading to the thigh and upper arm.

Two-Handed Kneading

1. One hand is placed at the insertion of the muscle, as in single-handed kneading; the other hand is placed just proximal to it (Fig. 6–2A).

2. Both hands grasp around as much of the muscle as possible. The palmar surface of the fingers of the left hand pulls the muscles laterally as the surface of the abducted right thumb and palm simultaneously pushes the tissues medially. Then the surface of the palm and abducted thumb of the left hand pushes the muscles medially as the palmar surface of the fingers of the right hand pulls the tissue laterally (Fig. 6–2B). Progression from the distal to the proximal part of the muscle is accomplished with a gliding of the hands on the pull stroke of the kneading movement. This procedure is very similar to the technique of wringing described in Chapter 3.

This is not a pinching type of movement. The thumb and fingers of each hand are meant to be kept in the same relationship to each other during the entire movement. The push and pull are accomplished chiefly by flexion and extension of the arms at the shoulders and elbows. At the origin, the proximal hand is removed and the distal hand finishes with the squeeze-out movement (see Fig. 6–1D, E) and returns to the starting position with a superficial stroke, as in single-handed kneading.

Two-Handed Digital Kneading

The muscle is grasped at its insertion by both hands (between the thumb and the index and middle fingers of each hand). The palmar surface of the left fingers pulls the tissues toward the therapist while the right thumb pushes the adjacent tissues away. Then the right fingers pull the tissues while the left thumb pushes the adjacent tissues (Fig. 6–3). Progression from origin to insertion is accom-

plished with a gliding of the fingers on the pull movement. Again, this is also not a pinching movement. The thumb and fingers of each hand are kept in the same relation to each other during the entire movement. The push and pull are accomplished chiefly by flexing and extending of the arms at the shoulders and elbows. The return stroke is performed with the fingers of the distal hand. This movement is used on muscles of small bulk. Care must be taken to ensure that the hands are held as nearly parallel to the length of the muscles as possible and so as to have as much contact as possible.

Friction

Deep friction and the indications for its use are described in Chapter 3. Deep friction is a technique that is applicable in local massage for the treatment of scars and adhesions of muscles, tendons, and joints.

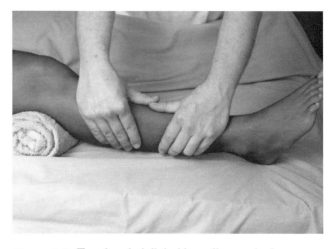

Figure 6–3. Two-handed digital kneading to the leg.

TECHNIQUE FOR LOCAL MASSAGE

The technique of local massage described next and its application to the anatomic sections of the body are modified from the Hoffa system. In the application of the massage strokes to the anatomic sections of an extremity the proximal portion should be treated first and then the more distal segment or segments. Then, special attention may be given to areas that require additional treatment. The stroking and kneading movements may be adapted to conform to the muscles of any body area. In the beginning of treatment, stroking precedes the kneading movement, and periods of stroking and kneading (or stroking and friction) should alternate according to the pathologic condition being treated, the desired effect, and the result

being obtained from the massage. The final stroke should always be superficial stroking.

The order in which massage is given to the various muscle groups of each anatomical section depends on the condition being treated and the ability of the patient to be moved into the required positions. It may be necessary to alter the techniques of the movements slightly, to avoid unnecessary changes of the patient's position. In general, the position of the patient should be changed as little as possible. The techniques, as described, are those that should be followed when it is possible to place the patient in the ideal position to perform each stroke. Under most circumstances, the patient should lie recumbent while receiving massage treatment. The entire local sequence suggested here is summarized at this point, so that the reader can gain a clear understanding of its structure.

Local Massage Sequence

Upper Extremity

Right Arm

Right Upper Arm
1. Deltoid muscle group
2. Extensor muscle group (triceps and anconeus)
3. Flexor muscle group (biceps, brachialis, and coracobrachialis)

Right Forearm
1. Muscle group
2. Lateral muscle group

Right Hand
1. Muscles of the radial border
2. Muscles of the ulnar border
3. Volar surface
4. Dorsal surface

Right Thumb and Fingers
1. Dorsal surface

Left Upper Extremity **(repeat all movements to the left upper extremity)**

Lower Extremity

Right Thigh
1. Inner hamstring group (semimembranosus and semitendinosus)
2. Outer hamstring group (biceps femoris)
3. Tensor fasciae latae
4. Quadriceps muscle group
5. Adductor muscle group

Right Leg
1. Anterior tibial muscle group
2. Peroneal muscle group
3. Calf muscle group (gastrocnemius and soleus)

Right Foot
1. Medial border
2. Lateral border
3. Dorsal surface
4. Plantar surface

Right Toes

Left Lower Extremity **(repeat all movements to the left lower extremity)**

Head and Trunk

Back
1. Erector spinae muscle group
2. Trapezius and scapular muscle group
3. Latissimus dorsi

Abdomen
1. Stroking over the entire abdomen
2. Stroking over the area of the colon
3. Kneading over the area of the colon

Face

TECHNIQUE FOR A LOCAL MASSAGE SEQUENCE

Right Arm

The therapist stands at the side of the table, on the patient's right. The patient lies supine, with the right arm slightly abducted. The arm is divided into three muscle groups: deltoid, extensors, and flexors.

Deltoid Muscle Group

Stroking. The hands stroke alternately. Beginning at the insertion of the muscle (Fig. 6–4A), the thumb of each hand passes up the midline of the muscle; the fingers of the left hand follow the posterior border of the muscle and curve around the origin to the center (Fig. 6–4B); the fingers of the right hand follow the anterior border in the same manner (Fig. 6–4C). Each hand returns to its starting position with a superficial stroke (Fig. 6–4D).

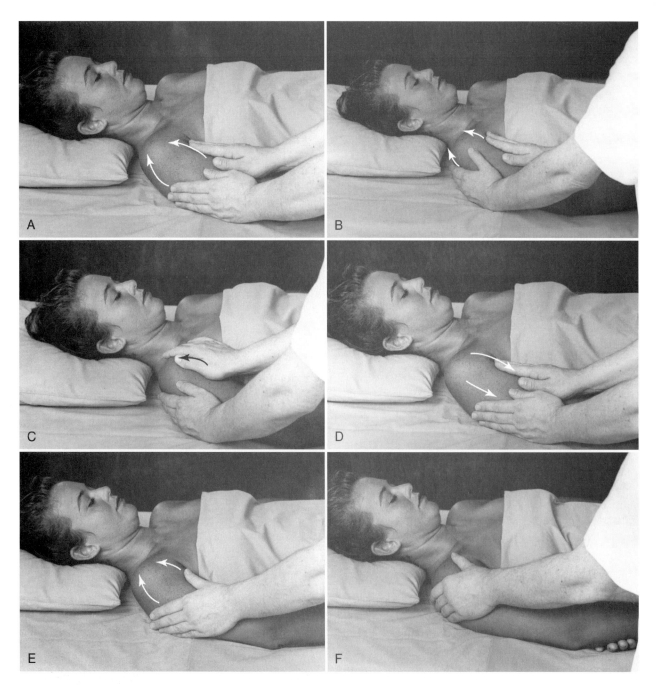

Figure 6–4. **Local massage to the deltoid muscle group. Figure continued.**

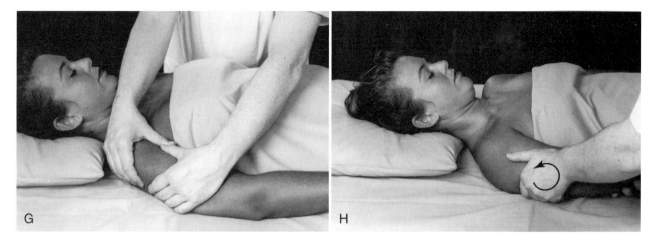

Figure 6–4. *Continued*

If the muscle is small, the entire muscle may be stroked with the left hand, as the right hand supports the inner side of the upper arm. The fingers of the left hand follow the posterior border of the muscle, and the thumb follows the anterior border (Fig. 6–4E); they meet at the acromion in a squeeze-out movement (Fig. 6–4F). The left hand returns to its starting position with a superficial stroke.

Kneading. Two-handed kneading is performed to the entire muscle, with the patient's arm partially abducted. Kneading progresses from the insertion to the origin of the muscle (Fig. 6–4G). The left hand does a squeeze-out movement at the origin and returns to the starting position with a superficial stroke, as the right hand returns through

the air. Single-handed kneading may be performed with the left hand if the muscle is small; the right hand gives support to the arm (Fig. 6–4H).

Extensor Muscle Group (Triceps and Anconeus)

Stroking. The right hand supports the elbow; the left hand grasps around the muscle group at the insertion. The thumb follows the lateral border and the fingers the medial border of the triceps, as the hand strokes over the muscle (Fig. 6–5A). At the end of the stroke, the thumb passes around the posterior border of the deltoid while the fingers move into the axilla, as the hand performs a squeeze-out movement (Fig. 6–5B). The hand then returns to the starting position with a superficial stroke.

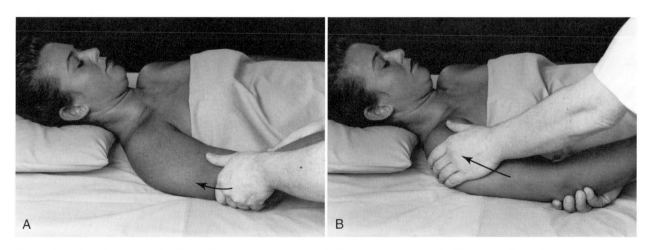

Figure 6–5. **Local massage to the extensor muscle group (triceps and anconeus). Figure continued.**

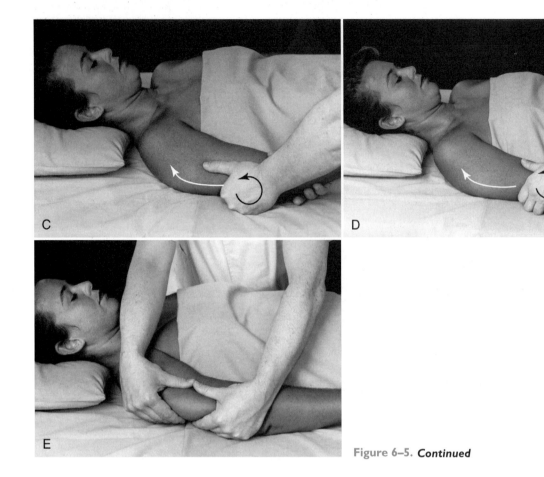

Figure 6–5. *Continued*

Kneading. Single-handed kneading is performed over the same area as the stroking (Fig. 6–5C, D), and the hand returns with a superficial stroke. Two-handed kneading may be used if the muscle group is large. The patient's arm is partially abducted, and both hands grasp the triceps, the left hand at the insertion and the right hand just proximal to it (Fig. 6–5E).

Flexor Muscle Group (Biceps, Brachialis, and Coracobrachialis)

Stroking. The left hand supports the elbow, and the right hand grasps the muscle group at its insertion below the elbow joint (Fig. 6–6A). The thumb follows the lateral border and the fingers the medial border of the flexor muscle group, as the hand strokes over the muscles. At the end of the stroke, the thumb passes around the anterior border of the deltoid, while the fingers move into the axilla as the hand performs a squeeze-out movement (Fig. 6–6B). The hand then returns to the starting position with a superficial stroke.

Kneading. Single-handed kneading is performed over the same area as the stroking (Fig. 6–6C). Two-handed kneading may be used if the muscle group is large. Hand

positions are the reverse of those described for two-handed kneading of the triceps group (see Fig. 6–5E).

Right Forearm

The forearm is divided into two muscle groups: medial and lateral.

Medial Muscle Group

The patient's elbow is slightly flexed with the forearm in supination while the arm rests on the table. A pillow may be used to support the arm if necessary.

Stroking. The left hand supports the forearm at the wrist. The right hand starts the stroking by grasping around the medial half of the forearm at the wrist (Fig. 6–7A). The thumb then passes up the midline of the forearm to the elbow and over the medial condyle as the fingers pass up along the ulna and over the medial aspect to meet the thumb in a squeeze-out movement (Fig. 6–7B). The hand returns to the wrist with a superficial stroke.

Kneading. Single-handed kneading is performed over the same area as the stroking (Fig. 6–7C, D), the hand returning with a superficial stroke.

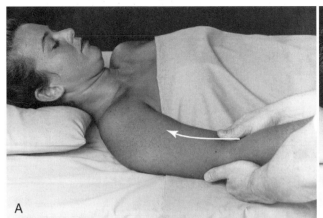

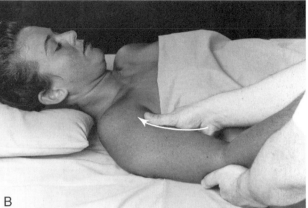

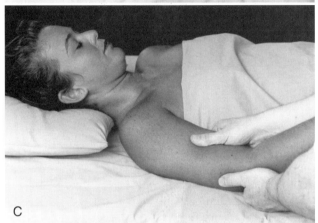

Figure 6–6. **Local massage to the flexor muscle group (biceps, brachialis, and coracobrachialis).**

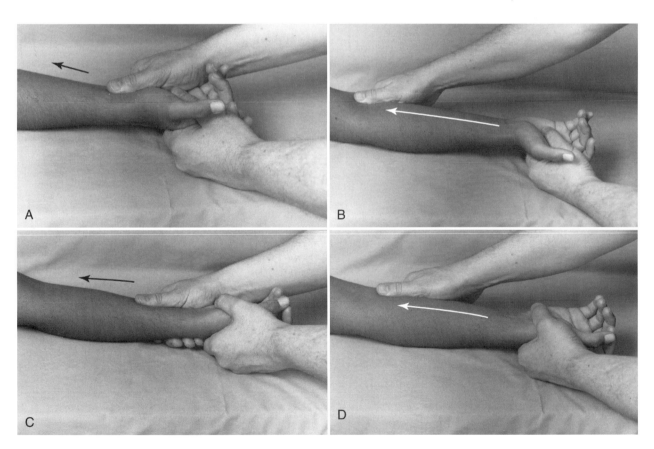

Figure 6–7. **Local massage to the medial forearm muscle groups.**

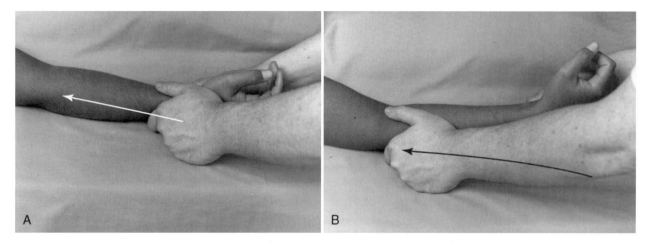

Figure 6–8. **Local massage to the lateral forearm muscle groups.**

Lateral Muscle Group

Stroking. The right hand supports the wrist. The left hand starts the stroke by grasping around the lateral half of the forearm (Fig. 6–8A). The thumb then passes up the midline of the forearm to the elbow and over the lateral condyle as the fingers pass along the radius and over the lateral condyle to meet the thumb in a squeeze-out movement (Fig. 6–8B). The hand returns to the wrist with a superficial stroke.

Kneading. Single-handed kneading is performed over the same area as the stroking. The hand returns with a superficial stroke.

Right Hand

Muscles of the Radial Border

The patient's forearm and hand are in supination, with the thumb abducted and the forearm comfortably supported on the table.

Stroking. The therapist's right hand supports the patient's hand. The left hand grasps the radial half of the hand at the metacarpophalangeal joint. The thumb then passes up the midline of the palm (Fig. 6–9), around the thenar eminence to the wrist. The fingers pass up the midline of the dorsal surface of the hand to join the thumb at the wrist with a squeeze-out movement. The hand returns with a superficial stroke.

Kneading. Single-handed kneading is performed over the same area as the stroking (see Fig. 6–9). The hand returns with a superficial stroke in the usual manner.

Muscles of the Ulnar Border

Stroking. The therapist's left hand supports the patient's hand. The right hand grasps the ulnar half of the patient's

hand at the metacarpophalangeal joint line. The thumb then passes up the midline of the palm (Fig. 6–10A) around the hypothenar eminence to the wrist. The fingers pass up the midline of the dorsal surface of the hand to meet the thumb at the wrist with a squeeze-out movement. The hand returns with a superficial stroke.

Kneading. Single-handed kneading is performed over the same area as the stroking (Fig. 6–10B), and the hand returns with a superficial stroke.

Volar Surface

The patient's hand is supinated.

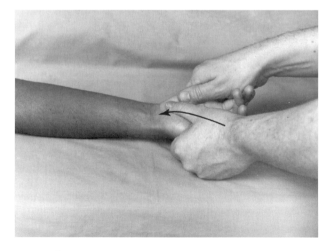

Figure 6–9. **Local massage to the muscles of the radial border of the hand.**

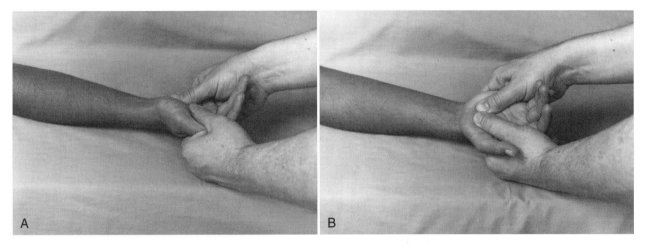

Figure 6–10. **Local massage to the muscles on the ulnar border of the hand.**

Stroking. The patient's hand is supported by the therapist's right hand while the thumb of the left hand strokes over each of the following areas: the thenar eminence from the first metacarpophalangeal joint to the wrist (Fig. 6–11A); the interosseous and the lumbrical muscles from the metacarpophalangeal joints to the wrist (Fig. 6–11B); and the hypothenar eminence, from the fifth metacarpopha-

langeal joint to the wrist (Fig. 6–11C). The thumb returns with a superficial stroke after each movement.

Kneading. The thumb pad kneads in small circles over the same areas and in the same order as indicated in the stroking (see Fig. 6–11), returning each time with superficial strokes.

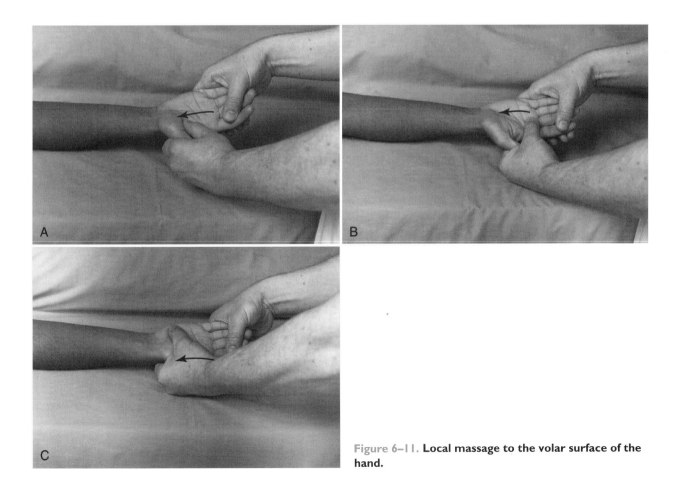

Figure 6–11. **Local massage to the volar surface of the hand.**

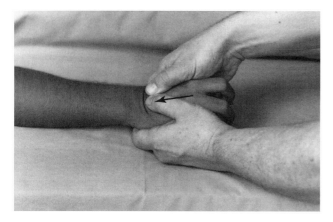

Figure 6–12. **Local massage to the dorsal aspect of the hand.**

Dorsal Surface

The patient's hand is in pronation. In effect, the therapist will be stroking in the interosseous spaces between the metacarpals, with pressure directed to the interosseous muscles.

Stroking. The patient's hand is supported by the therapist's left hand. The thumb of the right hand strokes over the ulnar side of the first metacarpal, just proximal to the first interphalangeal joint, continuing to the wrist (Fig. 6–12). The thumb pad then returns with a superficial stroke along the radial side of the second metacarpal to its first

interphalangeal joint; it strokes over this same area to the wrist. The thumb then slides over so that it can return along the ulnar border of the second metacarpal to the first interphalangeal joint and then strokes over the same area to the wrist. The same procedures are performed on the third and fourth metacarpal areas and the radial side of the fifth metacarpal.

Kneading. The thumb pad kneads in small circles along each interosseous muscle from the insertion to the wrist, following the routine described for stroking.

Right Thumb and Fingers

Dorsal Surface

The patient's hand is pronated. The patient's hand is supported on the volar surface by the finger tips of the left hand (Fig. 6–13A). These fingers also support the phalanges as needed to prevent flexion during these movements. The right thumb and index finger first stroke, then knead the thumb and each succeeding finger in the following manner:

Thumb Stroking. The thumb and the index finger grasp around the tip of the patient's digit (Fig. 6–13A). The index finger passes up the radial side of the digit to the metacarpophalangeal joint as the thumb passes up the ulnar side (Fig. 6–13B, C) and continues the stroke into the metacarpal-interosseous space (Fig. 6–13D). The thumb

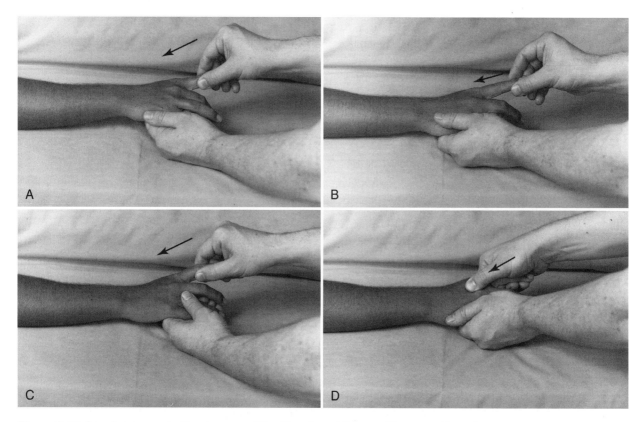

Figure 6–13. **Local massage to the dorsum of the thumb and fingers. Figure continued.**

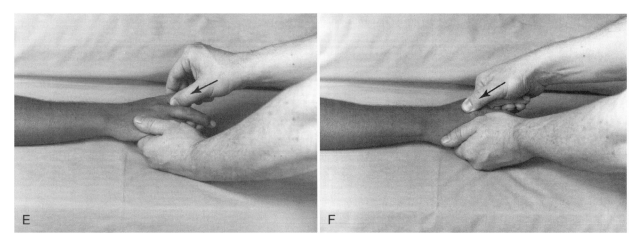

Figure 6-13. *Continued*

and the finger return to the tip of the digit with a superficial stroke.

Thumb Pad Kneading. The finger supports, while the thumb pad kneads over the same area it stroked (Fig. 6–13E, F). The thumb and the finger return to the tip of the digit with a superficial stroke. The therapist's hand is then supinated so that the thumb can knead on the radial side of the patient's digit while the index finger supports the ulnar side. The thumb and the finger return to the tip of the digit with a superficial stroke.

Volar Surface

The patient's hand is positioned in supination.

Stroking and Kneading. The patient's hand is supported on the dorsal surface by the finger tips of the left hand (Fig. 6–14A). The right thumb and index finger first stroke (Fig. 6–14A, B), then knead (Fig. 6–14C, D) the thumb and all the fingers in a manner similar to that performed on the dorsal surface, except that the massage begins with the little finger and progresses toward the thumb.

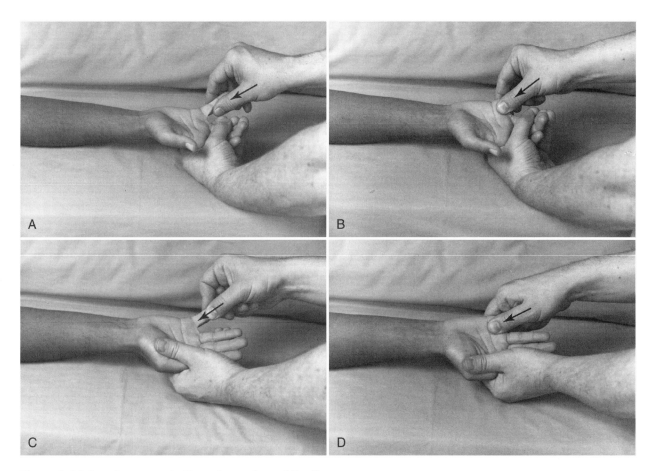

Figure 6–14. **Local massage to the volar surface of the fingers.**

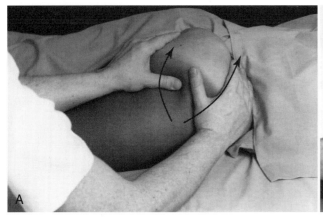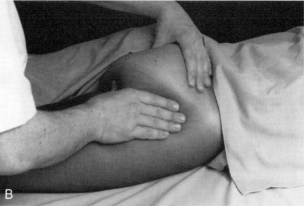

Figure 6–15. **Local massage to the right buttock.**

Left Upper Extremity

The therapist stands by the side of the table on the left side of the patient. The movements described for the right upper extremity can be used on the left side by simply reversing the hand positions described in the text.

Right Buttock

The therapist stands at the side of the table on the patient's right. The patient is prone, with pillows under the abdomen and the ankles; the head may be turned to either side for comfort, if required, or supported in the midline.

Gluteal Muscle Group

Stroking. The left hand starts the stroke at the insertion of the gluteus maximus into the fascia lata (Fig. 6–15A) and follows the fibers of this muscle to its origin at the sacrum, coccyx, and ilium (along the gluteal fold). The right hand follows the fibers of the gluteus medius from its insertion at the greater trochanter to its origin on the crest of the ilium (see Fig. 6–15A). The hands stroke alternately and return with a superficial stroke. If the muscles are large, each one may be stroked separately. In this instance, the thumbs of the hands pass up the midline of the muscle being stroked.

Kneading. Two-handed kneading is performed over the same area as the stroking (Fig. 6–15B). At the end of the stroke, the right hand performs a squeeze-out movement and returns with a superficial stroke, as the left hand returns through the air.

Right Thigh

The therapist stands at the side of the table on the patient's right. The patient lies prone, comfortably supported. If preferred, a pillow may be placed under the shins and ankle regions, so long as it does not interfere with the treatment.

Inner Hamstring Group (Semimembranosus and Semitendinosus)

Stroking. While the right hand supports the extremity the left hand begins at the insertion of the muscles just below the medial condyle of the tibia and grasps around the muscle group (Fig. 6–16A). The thumb strokes up the midline of the thigh as the fingers follow the medial border of the muscle group to meet the thumb at the gluteal fold in a squeeze-out movement (Fig. 6–16B). The hand returns with a superficial stroke.

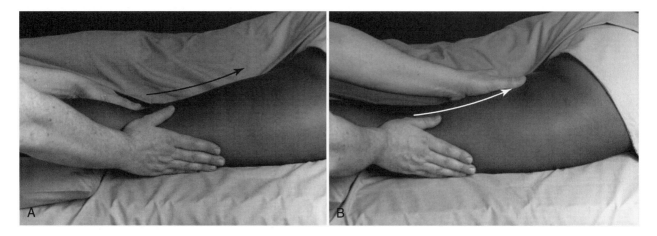

Figure 6–16. **Local massage to the inner hamstring muscle group (semimembranosus and semitendinosus).**

120

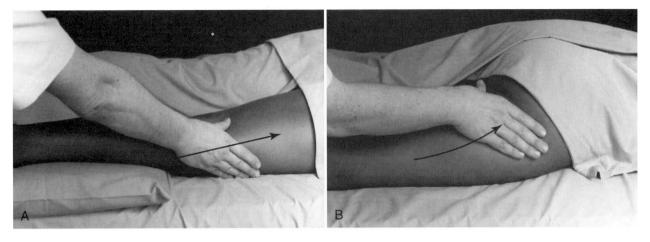

Figure 6–17. **Local massage to the outer hamstring group (biceps femoris).**

Kneading. Two-handed kneading is performed over the same area as the stroking.

Outer Hamstring Group (Biceps Femoris)

Stroking. The left hand supports the extremity. The right hand begins at the insertion of the muscle on the head of the fibula, grasping around the muscle. The thumb passes up the midline of the thigh (Fig. 6–17A), the fingers following the lateral border of the muscle to meet the thumb in a squeeze-out movement (Fig. 6–17B). The hand returns with a superficial stroke.

Kneading. Two-handed kneading is performed over the same area as the stroking. Single-handed kneading may be used for both inner and outer hamstring groups if the muscles are small.

(*Note:* The stroking and kneading movements to both inner and outer hamstring muscles may also be performed with the patient lying supine or on one side, if the patient is unable to assume the prone position. In the supine position, one hand supports the knee in slight flexion while the other hand performs the movement.)

Tensor Fasciae Latae

The therapist stands at the side of the table on the patient's right. The patient is now repositioned to supine lying. A small pillow or roll may be placed under the knee if preferred.

Stroking. The right hand gives support to the thigh at the medial side of the knee, and the left hand starts the stroke at the insertion of the tensor fasciae latae (Fig. 6–18A), on the head of the fibula. The thumb follows the anterior border of the fascia and muscle, and the fingers follow the posterior border of the fascia and muscle as the hand strokes toward the origin. As the hand approaches the muscular portion it spreads out to stroke over the muscle to its origin (Fig. 6–18B) and finishes with a squeeze-out movement. The hand returns with a superficial stroke.

Kneading. Two-handed kneading is performed over the same area as the stroking. Single-handed kneading may be used if the muscle is small.

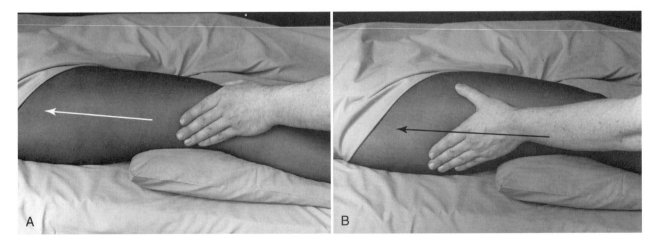

Figure 6–18. **Local massage to the tensor fasciae latae.**

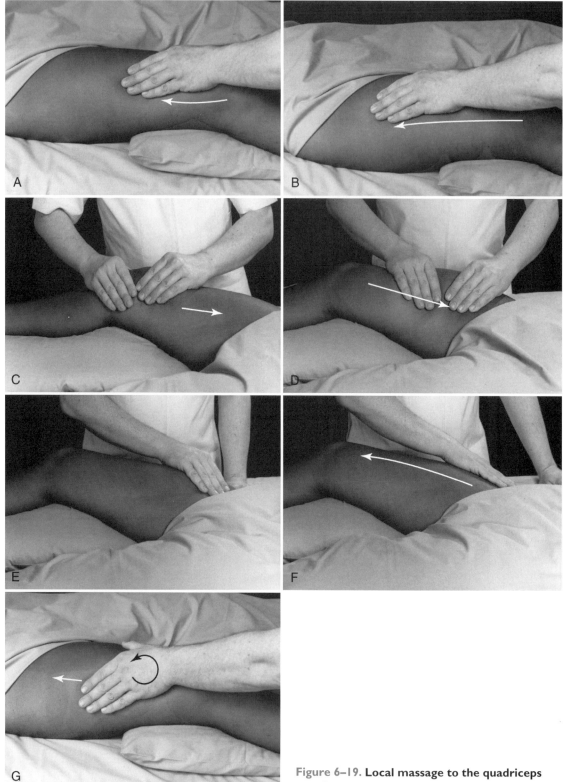

Figure 6–19. **Local massage to the quadriceps muscle group.**

Quadriceps Muscle Group

The therapist stands at the side of the table on the patient's right. The patient lies supine. A pillow or roll may be placed under the knee and the limb allowed to roll out a little into external rotation if preferred.

Stroking. The right hand supports the extremity at the knee. The left hand is placed below the patella at the insertion of the muscle, with the thumb at the medial side and the fingers at the lateral border of the patella. The hand passes lightly over the patella, grasps around the muscle (Fig. 6–19A), and strokes to the muscle origin, where the

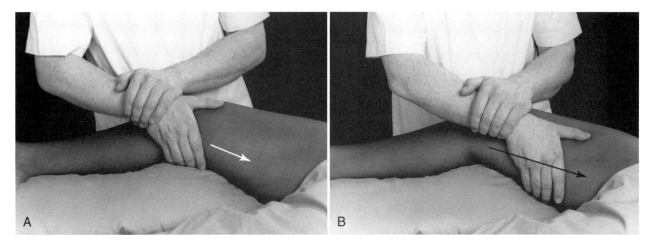

Figure 6–20. **Local massage to the adductor muscle group.**

thumb and fingers meet in a squeeze-out movement (Fig. 6–19B). The hand returns with a superficial stroke.

Kneading. The right hand is placed at the lower border of the patella and passes lightly over it; the left hand picks up the muscle above the patella (Fig. 6–19C), and both hands knead the entire muscle, to its origin (Fig. 6–19D). The right hand performs a squeeze-out movement (Fig. 6–19E) and returns with a superficial stroke (Fig. 6–19F). The left hand returns through the air. Single-handed kneading may be performed with the left hand while the right hand supports the extremity (Fig. 6–19G).

Adductor Muscle Group

Stroking. The right hand, reinforced by the left hand, starts the stroke at the insertion of the muscle group on the medial condyle of the tibia by grasping around the entire group (Fig. 6–20A). The thumb passes along the anterior border of the muscle group, and the fingers follow the posterior border toward the origin, finishing with a squeeze-out movement (Fig. 6–20B). The hand returns with a superficial stroke. *Note:* Theoretically, this stroke should end at the origin of the muscle, close to the symphysis pubis, but, for obvious ethical and practical reasons, it should be completed a few inches below the inguinal ligament. In fact, it is best to remain below the midpoint of the femoral triangle in both male and female patients.

Kneading. Two-handed kneading is performed over the same area as the stroking, observing the same restrictions over the femoral triangle. The right hand performs a squeeze-out movement at the end of the kneading and returns with a superficial stroke. The left hand returns through the air. Single-handed kneading may be used on a small adductor mass; the left hand can reinforce the right hand.

Right Leg

The therapist stands at the foot of the table, facing the patient. A rolled towel is particularly useful to support the knee and still allow the therapist's hands to work around the knee. A small pillow can also be used for this purpose.

Anterior Tibial Muscle Group

Stroking. The right hand is placed slightly distal to the ankle joint, and the right hand supports the ankle by grasping the foot at the arch. The left thumb passes along the anterior border of the tibia, and the index finger follows the lateral border of the muscle group (Fig. 6–21A) to the anterior surface of the head of the fibula, meeting the thumb in a squeeze-out movement. The other fingers maintain light contact with the skin throughout the movement. The hand returns to the starting position with a superficial stroke.

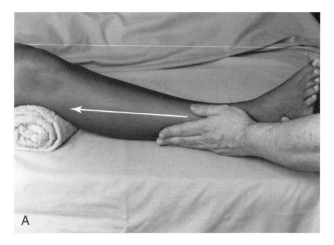

Figure 6–21. **Local massage to the anterior tibial muscle group. Figure continued.**

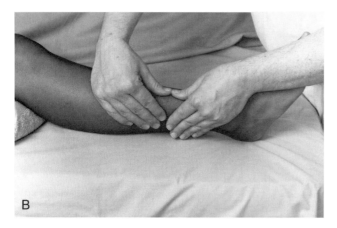

Figure 6–21. Continued

Kneading. Two-handed digital kneading is performed over the same area as the stroking. The therapist may stand at the foot of the table and turn his or her body so as to reach across the tibia to knead the muscles. The right hand is placed proximally and the left hand distally (Fig. 6–21B). The left hand performs the squeeze-out movement at the

end of the procedure, returning with a superficial stroke, while the right hand returns in the air.

Alternatively, the therapist may move to the right side of the table (facing the patient) and perform two-handed kneading with the left hand placed proximally and the right hand distally. The right hand gives the squeeze out at the end of the movement and returns with a superficial stroke while the left hand returns in the air.

Peroneal Muscle Group

Stroking. The left hand is placed distal to the lateral malleolus while the right hand supports the ankle by grasping the foot at the arch (Fig. 6–22A). The left thumb follows the anterior border of the muscle group, while the index finger follows along the posterior border of the muscle group (Fig. 6–22B) to the posterior surface of the head of the fibula, meeting the thumb in a squeeze-out movement. The hand returns to the starting position with a superficial stroke. The other fingers maintain light contact with the skin throughout the movement.

Kneading. Two-handed digital kneading is given over the same area as the stroking. Procedures are similar to those

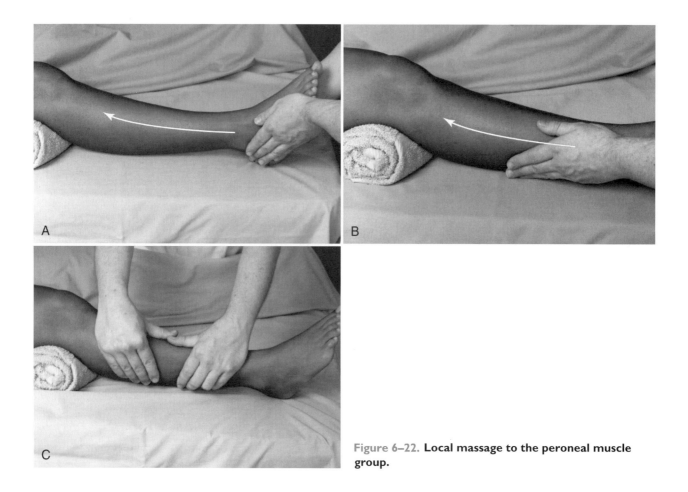

Figure 6–22. Local massage to the peroneal muscle group.

described for two-handed digital kneading of the anterior tibial muscle group (Fig. 6–22C).

Calf Muscle Group (Gastrocnemius and Soleus)

The therapist stands at the side of the table on the patient's right. The patient is comfortably supported, lying prone.

Stroking. The left hand is placed on the heel and the right hand stabilizes the leg at the knee (Fig. 6–23A). The left thumb follows along the lateral border of the Achilles tendon and passes up the lateral border of the muscle group as the fingers follow along the medial border of the tendon and muscle group. The hand grasps around the muscle group and strokes toward the origins of the

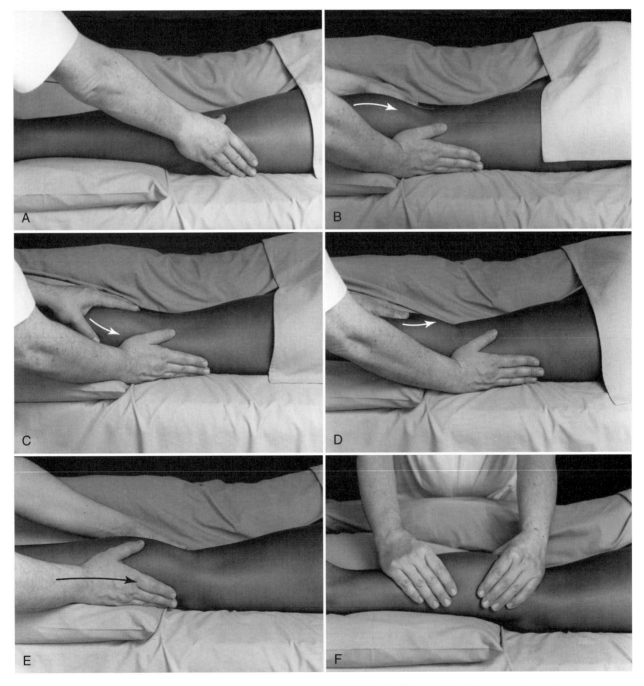

Figure 6–23. **Local massage to the posterior muscle group of the leg (calf muscles). Figure continued.**

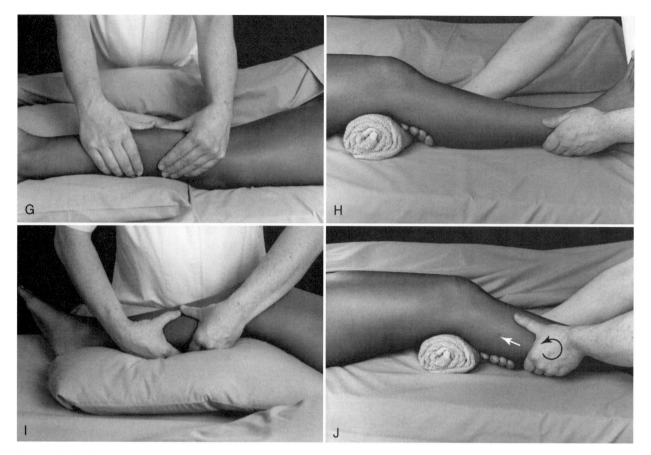

Figure 6–23. Continued

gastrocnemius. The first stroke ends in a squeeze-out movement over the medial head (Fig. 6–23B); the second stroke ends in a squeeze-out movement over the lateral head (Fig. 6–23C). Additional strokes continue to alternate. The hand returns to the starting position with a superficial stroke.

If the muscle group is too large to be grasped in one hand, it may be massaged in two sections. The medial side of the muscle group is stroked with the left hand, as the right hand supports the knee (Fig. 6–23D). The left thumb passes up the midline of the muscle group, and the "squeeze out" is performed at the medial head of the gastrocnemius. The lateral side of the muscle group is stroked with the right hand, as the left hand supports the knee (Fig. 6–23E). The squeeze out is given at the lateral head of the gastrocnemius.

Kneading. Two-handed kneading is performed to the same area as the stroking (Fig. 6–23F). The left hand returns to the starting position with a superficial stroke, and the right hand returns in the air. If the muscle group is very large,

two-handed kneading is given over each half of the muscle group (Fig. 6–23G). Alternatively, if the muscle group is small, single-handed kneading may be used over the whole muscle group. In this case, the left hand kneads as the right hand supports the extremity.

If it is not possible for the patient to lie prone, this muscle group may be massaged with the patient supine. With the patient in this position, one hand supports the knee in slight flexion while the other performs the stroking movement (Fig. 6–23H).

Two-handed kneading is given with the therapist standing at the side of the table on the patient's right. The patient's thigh is rotated laterally so that both hands can grasp the muscle group easily (Fig. 6–23I). If the muscle group is small, single-handed kneading may be given with the left hand, as the right hand supports the knee in slight flexion (Fig. 6–23J).

Right Foot

The therapist stands at the foot of the table facing the patient. The patient lies supine with a pillow supporting the knee.

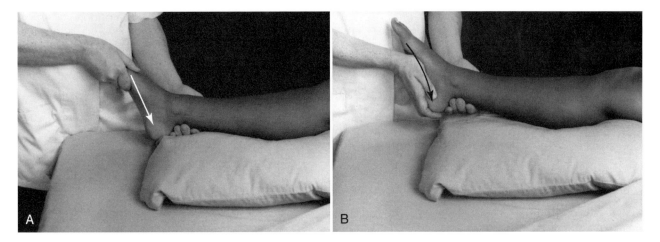

Figure 6–24. **Local massage to the medial border of the foot.**

Medial Border

Stroking. The left hand supports the ankle on the lateral side, just proximal to the heel (Fig. 6–24A), while the right hand grasps the medial half of the foot at the toes. The thumb passes up the midline of the dorsum of the foot and below the medial malleolus, as the fingers pass up the midline of the plantar surface and around the heel to meet the thumb in a squeeze-out movement (Fig. 6–24B). The hand returns to the starting position with a superficial stroke.

Kneading. Single-handed kneading is given over the same area as the stroking. The hand returns to the starting position with a superficial stroke.

Lateral Border

Stroking. The right hand supports the ankle on the medial side just proximal to the heel, while the left hand grasps the lateral half of the foot at the toes (Fig. 6–25A). The thumb passes up the midline of the dorsum of the foot and below the lateral malleolus. At the same time, the fingers pass up the midline of the plantar surface and around the heel to meet the thumb in a squeeze-out movement (Fig. 6–25B). The hand returns to the starting position with a superficial stroke.

Kneading. Single-handed kneading is performed over the same area as the stroking. The hand returns to the starting position with a superficial stroke.

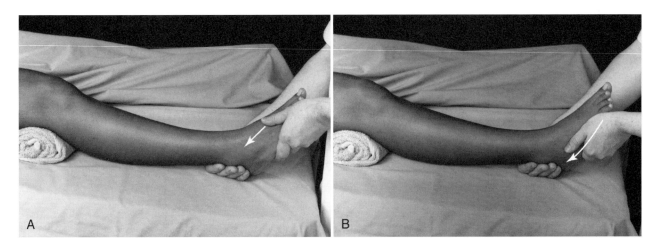

Figure 6–25. **Local massage to the lateral border of the foot.**

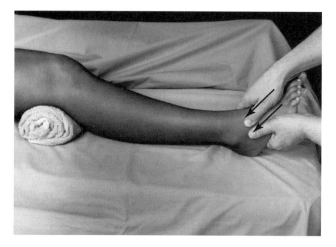

Figure 6–26. **Local massage to the dorsum of the foot.**

Dorsal Surface

Stroking. The fingers of both hands are placed on the plantar surface of the foot to support it. The thumbs perform short, alternate strokes between the first and second metatarsal bones, progressing from the base of the toes to the ankle. Both thumbs together return to the starting position with a superficial stroke. They repeat the movements in each metatarsal space (Fig. 6–26).

Kneading. Kneading is given with one thumb moving in small circles over the same area as the stroking. The right thumb kneads over the first and second metatarsal spaces, and the left thumb kneads over the third and fourth metatarsal spaces. The thumb returns to the starting position with a superficial stroke.

Plantar Surface

Stroking. The left hand supports the foot by grasping the forefoot and toes so that the dorsal surface of the foot fits into the palm of the left hand (Fig. 6–27A). The fingers of the right hand are flexed at the metacarpophalangeal and the proximal interphalangeal joints. The proximal phalanges are placed in firm contact at the base of the toes (see Fig. 6–32A). The hand strokes *firmly* toward the heel (Fig. 6–32B). As the movement progresses, the right hand is rolled into pronation (Fig. 6–32C), and the fingers are extended to allow the heel of the hand to fit into the longitudinal arch of the foot. The right hand is removed and returns through the air to the starting position.

Right Toes

If there is reason to massage the toes, stroking and kneading procedures similar to those described for the thumb and fingers are appropriate (see Fig. 6–13). *Note:* If

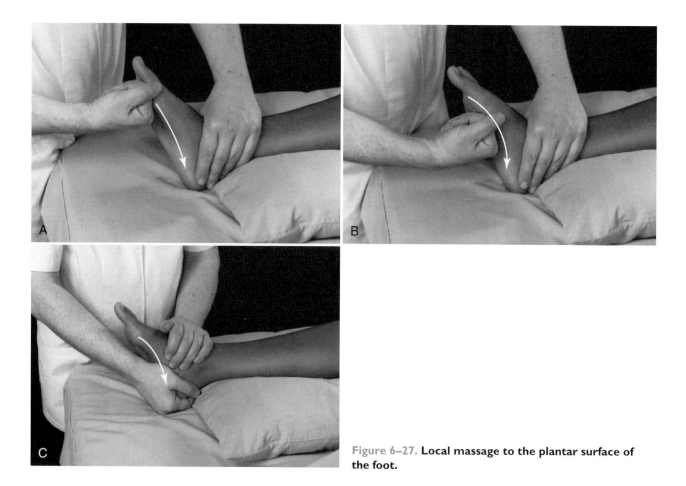

Figure 6–27. **Local massage to the plantar surface of the foot.**

massage to the lower extremity is contemplated after a cast has been bivalved for treatment of the extremity, all of the movements that can be done with the patient lying prone should follow one another. Then, after the patient has been turned to the supine position, all of the movements that can be done in that position should again follow.

Left Leg

The therapist stands at the patient's left side. The movements are performed as described for the right leg, except that the right hand is substituted for the left and the left hand for the right.

Back

The therapist stands at the side of the table on the patient's left side. The patient is positioned comfortably, lying prone with pillows under the abdomen and ankles and towel rolls under the shoulders. Local massage to the back may be performed to three basic muscle groups—the erector spinae group, the trapezius and scapular group, and the latissimus dorsi—although of course some parts of these

muscles are often massaged at the same time. With the exception of stroking to the erector spinae group, all movements are given at one time to one side of the back.

Erector Spinae Muscle Group

Stroking. The thumbs are placed at the sides of the spinous processes of the upper cervical vertebrae, and the fingers are placed in the supraclavicular fossae (Fig. 6–28A). Both thumbs stroke down firmly over the cervical region and at the seventh cervical vertebra are lifted and crossed. The fingers are then drawn backward lightly toward the seventh cervical vertebra (Fig. 6–28B), and the palms stroke firmly over the erector spinae muscles from the seventh cervical vertebra to the sacrum.

The hands then separate and with thumbs adducted stroke with light pressure over the iliac crests (Fig. 6–28C) to the inguinal region and return to the sacrum (Fig. 6–28D). The hands then stroke back over the erector spinae muscles to the seventh cervical vertebra, the thumbs again being lifted and crossed. Light pressure is used for the return stroke.

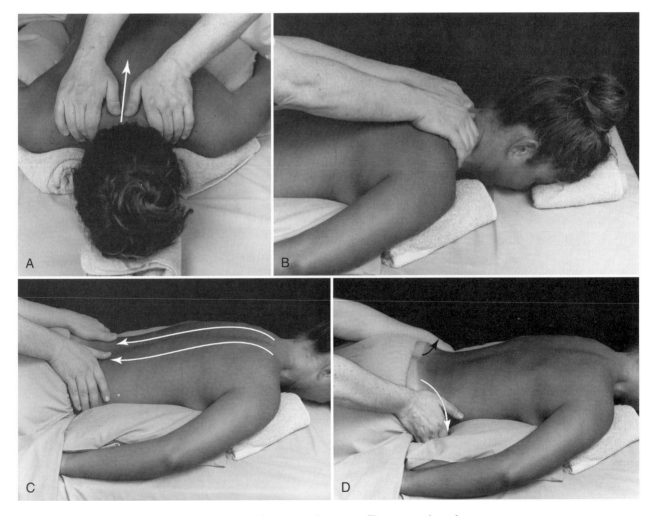

Figure 6–28. **Local massage to the erector spinae muscle group. Figure continued.**

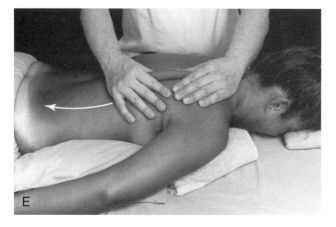

Figure 6–28. *Continued*

Kneading. Two-handed digital kneading is performed, first to the right side and then to the left side, beginning at the cervical region and continuing to the sacrum (Fig. 6–28E). The right hand returns with a superficial stroke as the left hand returns through the air.

Trapezius and Scapular Muscle Group

Stroking. Starting on the right side, the right hand is placed over the upper fibers of the trapezius muscle with the thumb at the lateral border of the upper cervical spinous processes. The hand grasps around the upper fibers of the right trapezius muscle and strokes to the acromion. As the right hand completes the movement the left hand begins at the origin of the middle fibers of the trapezius muscle (Fig. 6–29A) and strokes across with the thumb abducted over toward the acromion. Then the right hand, with the thumb abducted, is placed with the thumb beside the spinous processes, and the ulnar border at the border of the lower trapezius fibers (at the level of the twelfth thoracic vertebra). From this position, the hand strokes outward to the acromion. As it reaches the acromion, the left hand starts the first stroking movement, over the upper fibers of the trapezius. The right hand then strokes over the middle fibers (Fig. 6–29B), then the left hand strokes over the lower fibers. The movements are performed in the same manner on the left side, except that the left hand substitutes for the right and the right hand for the left.

Kneading. The movement starts on the right side.

Upper fibers. Two-handed digital kneading is given over the same area as the stroking. The right hand returns with a superficial stroke as the left hand returns through the air.

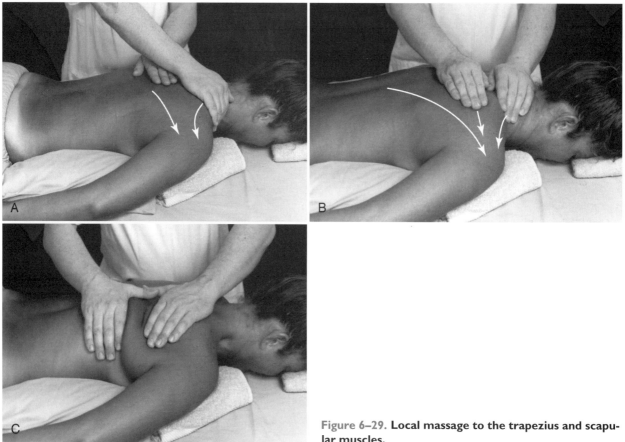

Figure 6–29. Local massage to the trapezius and scapular muscles.

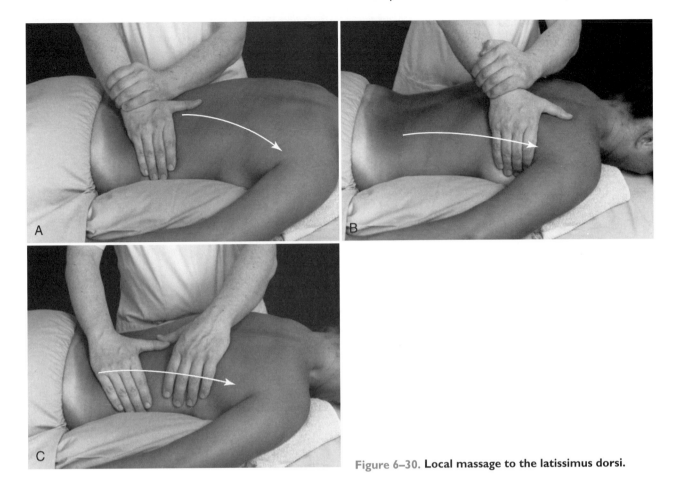

Figure 6–30. **Local massage to the latissimus dorsi.**

Middle and lower fibers. Two-handed kneading is performed over both areas (Fig. 6–29C). The right hand returns with a superficial stroke while the left hand returns through the air.

The movements are performed in the same manner on the left side, except that the left hand substitutes for the right, and the right hand for the left.

Latissimus Dorsi

Stroking. Starting on the right side, place the right hand (reinforced by the left hand) with the thumb at the lateral border of the spinous processes of the lumbar area and the ulnar border on the crest of the ilium (Fig. 6–30A). The thumb follows along the medial border of the muscle, while the fingers follow along the lateral border. The hand turns into pronation as the fingers meet the thumb in the axilla in a squeeze-out movement (Fig. 6–30B). The hand returns with a superficial stroke.

Kneading. Two-handed kneading is performed over the same area as the stroking (Fig. 6–30C). The right hand returns with a superficial stroke as the left hand returns through the air. If the muscle is too large to be covered with one hand, the stroking and kneading may be performed in two sections. The movements are given in the same manner

on the left side, except that the left hand substitutes for the right, and the right hand for the left.

Abdomen

The therapist stands at the side of the table on the patient's right. The patient is supine, with the head and knees supported by pillows.

Stroking over the Entire Abdomen

Starting with the fingertips of both hands at the symphysis pubis (Fig 6–31A), the hands stroke over the rectus abdominis muscle to its origin (Fig. 6–31B). The hands then stroke laterally with light pressure (Fig. 6–31C), the fingers passing over the lower ribs. As the hands continue the lateral stroking over the dorsal part of the fibers they turn (Fig. 6–31D) so that the fingertips stroke toward the spine.

The hands then return over the same area with a firm stroke to the transverse abdominal muscles (Fig. 6–31E) and a light stroke down the rectus abdominis to the symphysis pubis. The stroking to the rectus abdominis and the lateral stroking are repeated, but the return stroke is given over the oblique abdominal muscles (Fig. 6–31F) toward the symphysis pubis.

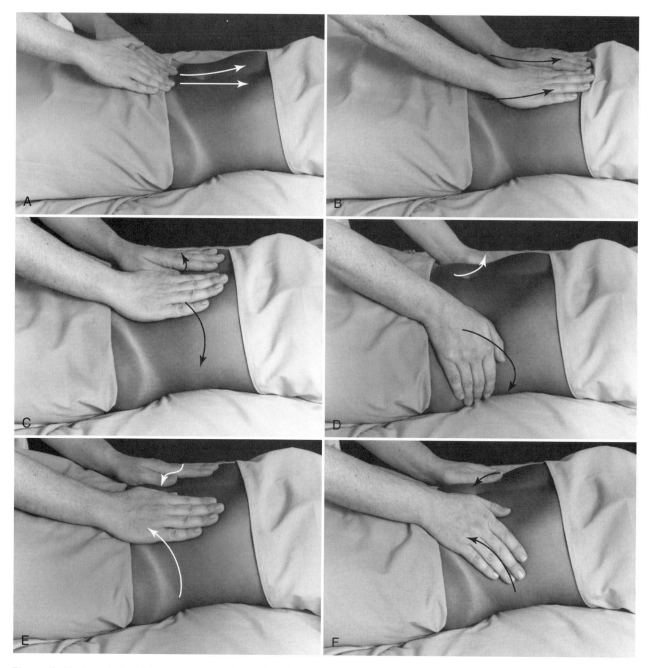

Figure 6–31. **Local stroking massage to the entire abdomen.**

Stroking over the Area of the Colon

The fingertips of the right hand, reinforced by the left hand, are placed over the area of the cecum (Fig. 6–32A). They stroke upward with firm pressure over the area of the ascending colon (Fig. 6–32B), across the abdomen over the area of the transverse colon, and downward over the area of the descending colon. The hands return with a superficial stroke across the lower abdomen to the starting point (Fig. 6–32C).

Kneading over the Area of the Colon

The fingertips of the reinforced right hand are placed about 2 inches above the area of the distal part of the descending colon (Fig. 6–33A). The fingertips are kept in contact with the skin as in friction movements. A circular movement with firm pressure is repeated several times in this one area and then followed by a firm stroke (Fig. 6–33B) over the area of the distal portion of the colon toward the rectum. With a light stroke, the hand returns to a point about 2 inches proximal to the starting point and repeats the movements. Progression is made in this manner over the rest of the areas of the descending colon, the transverse colon, and the ascending colon (Fig. 6–33C). It is important to perform this stroke in the direction specified, although this appears to be opposite the normal direction of peristalsis. Performed in this manner, the kneading tends to clear the colon rather than cause congestion.

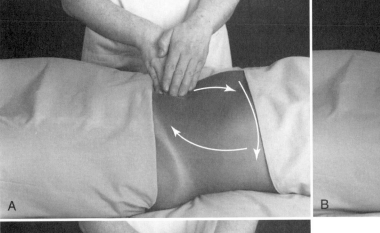

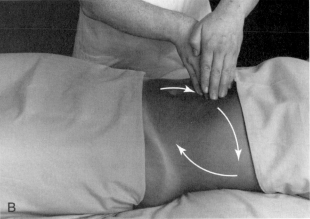

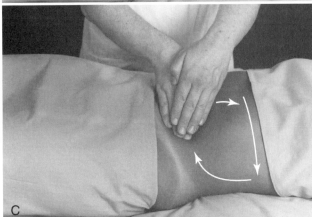

Figure 6–32. **Local stroking massage over the colon.**

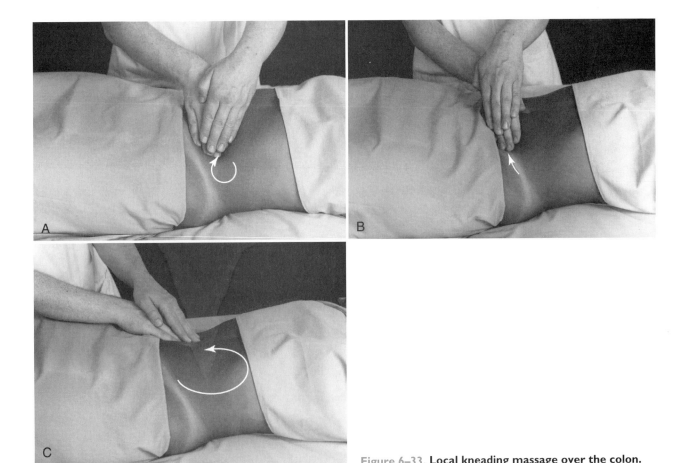

Figure 6–33. **Local kneading massage over the colon.**

133

Face

The therapist stands or sits at the head of the table. The patient lies supine with a small pillow or neck roll to support the head. The following technique for massage of the face is based on the principles of the Hoffa method to the extent that the strokes are applied to individual muscles or muscle groups and the stroking movements follow the general longitudinal direction of the muscle fibers. It must be kept in mind that the muscles of facial expression are small and delicate. They have little mass and are thin and located immediately over bony surfaces. A significant part of their structure is attached to the subcutaneous layers of the facial skin. For these reasons, the pressure of the massage strokes must be very light, particularly when the massage is being given to flaccid muscles. This type of massage is particularly applicable for facial paralysis and may aid in preventing contractures and resolving fibrosis. It also provides significant sensory stimulation to the tissues, and this may assist in the recovery process if this is possible. This type of massage can also be readily taught to the patient. In this manner, treatment can be administered more frequently, and at home.

In general, each stroke passes from insertion to origin, following the normal muscle action. Whenever possible, paralyzed muscles are supported in the position of normal function as the massage is being performed. Support may be given by one hand or by the fingers (Fig. 6–34).

Both stroking and kneading are performed with the distal phalanges of the digits being used. One or more fingers, either or both thumbs, or the thumb and one or more fingers may be used so as to conform to the shape, size, and location of the muscles (see Fig. 6–34). The muscles and muscle groups that are massaged are the frontalis (see Fig. 6–34A), orbicularis oculi (see Fig. 6–34B, C), nasalis (see Fig. 6–33D), muscles that elevate the corners of the mouth and wrinkle the nose (see Fig. 6–34E), orbicularis oris (see Fig. 6–34F), muscles that depress the corners of the mouth (see Fig. 6–34G), and the platysma (see Fig. 6–34H). At the finish of the local massage movements to the face, both hands perform superficial stroking from the chin to the temples (see Fig. 6–34I).

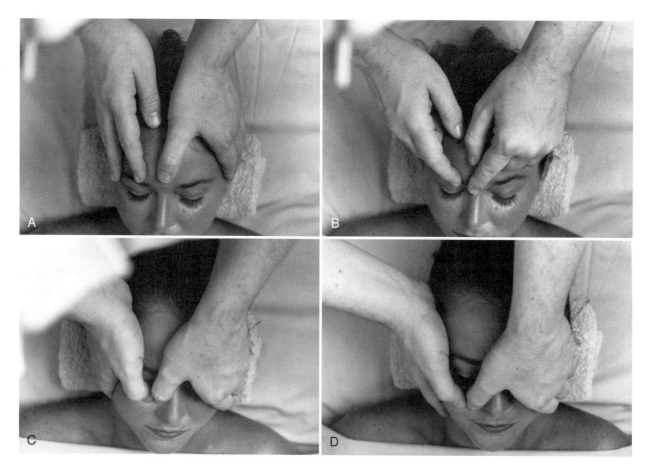

Figure 6–34. **Local massage to the muscles of the face. Figure continued.**

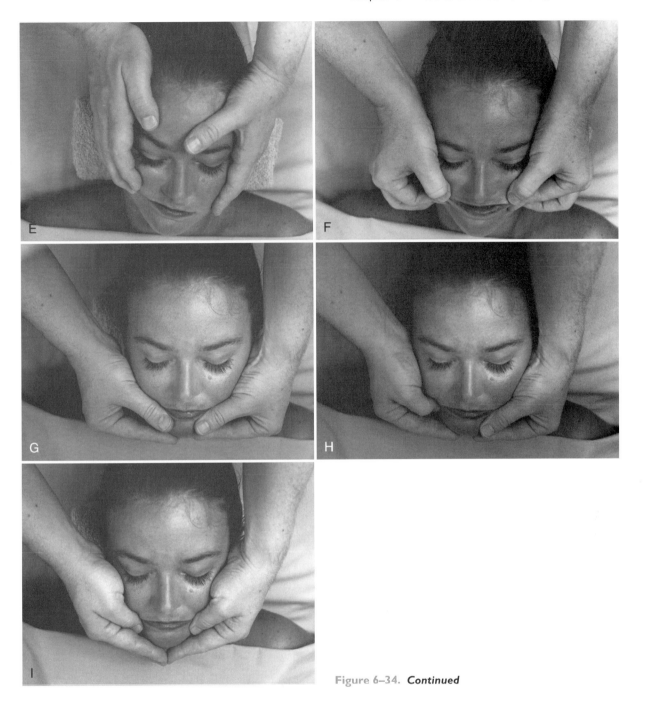

Figure 6–34. *Continued*

Chapter 7

Soft Tissue Massage Techniques as an Evaluation Tool

The human hand is one of the wonders of nature. It is capable of immense dexterity and sensitivity, yet it also possesses tremendous strength and functional ability. Not surprisingly, then, control of all aspects of hand function is vested in large areas of the sensory and motor cortex of the brain. Unlike any other species, humans have the enormous advantage of an advanced brain that is able to control an amazingly versatile hand. This has surely given humans a significant advantage in evolutionary development.

Two major functions—sensory and motor—can be assigned to the hand. Sensory functions include the gathering of all of the information received by the multitude of sensory receptors in the various parts of the hand. These sensory signals are relayed to the brain and interpreted as the experience of touching. A wide variety of information can be perceived in this manner, including object recognition, temperature, and texture, among others. A more encompassing sensory experience is also associated with the hands. This may be loosely termed "psychic" sensitivity. Of course, all sensation is perceived at the cortical level; however, the special sensitivity of the hands may allow some persons greatly increased awareness and integration of the sensory experience provided by touching. There can be little doubt that the act of touching can produce very significant responses in both parties. This may be one reason why soft tissue massage has proven such a potent therapeutic tool over the millennia and why so many people still have great faith in the laying on of hands.

Although palpation is a very important part of the examination of a patient, the value of massage strokes as an evaluation tool has not been sufficiently appreciated. Palpation does play a major role in the examination of most body functions and certainly enjoys a prominent position in the evaluation and treatment of musculoskeletal disorders. The fact that such information gathered by palpation appears to be less objective than that gathered by instruments reflects more on the limitations of the instrumentation than on the powers of human observation. There is clearly great potential for soft tissue massage manipulations in the evaluation of all aspects of musculoskeletal function. The potential value of the sensory information received during the performance of the major groups of massage strokes will now be briefly discussed.

SUPERFICIAL STROKING

Superficial stroking gives initial information about the skin and superficial muscle groups. Contour, texture, tissue, tone, and temperature may reveal acute or chronic changes in these tissues. Tissues of one area can be compared with those of adjacent areas to see if the changes are local or generalized. In particular, the sites of trigger points and pressure points can often be identified by using such strokes. Areas of altered skin resistance, temperature, and compliance—factors secondary to local and regional autonomic changes—are the keys to locating these points. Information gathered by superficial stroking can also be used as a reference point after specific therapeutic procedures are applied. Changes noted later on superficial stroking provide subjective and objective data on the effect of the procedures used.

Superficial stroking is helpful in measuring centrally induced, generalized muscle tension. It also provides time for the patient to adapt to the therapist's "touch" and to become accustomed to the increased sensory input. Such strokes have traditionally been used to relax the patient, though some patients who are "tactilely defensive" may require a modified approach. It is important that the patient's entire body and the specific areas to be treated be relaxed; relaxation can be enhanced and evaluated by superficial stroking.

The varied responses to sustained or interrupted contact probably indicate selective stimulation of tonic or phasic receptors and integrated central potency of one or the other. We know no good rules at this time for predicting which type of stimulation will have the greatest potency; however, experience indicates that sustained contact and rhythmic movement are soothing and relaxing for most people.

DEEP STROKING

Deep stroking (including effleurage), performed slowly over large areas, moves fluid in lymphatic and venous channels. It permits the therapist a sense of the relative contribution of interstitial fluid to local and regional swelling. As the superficial layers are assessed and more specific information is desired, kneading and lifting strokes can identify specific muscles or segments of muscles, both superficial and deep. These strokes can also be used to outline specific vascular pathways, tendons, ligaments, and related structures.

Special variations of these strokes, such as skin rolling and skin dragging, are useful for identifying specific localized changes. These techniques are similar to the basic strokes of connective tissue massage. Local connective tissue changes not explained by known pathologic conditions must be viewed with caution. Skin dragging used for low back assessment could produce undesired autonomic changes if carried into adjacent reflex zones and repeated several times.

KNEADING STROKES

The nature of kneading and lifting strokes gives them a unique role, particularly in muscle assessment. Local or generalized muscle tightness or atrophy of these structures can be identified as specific structures are isolated and mobilized. During treatment the therapist can come back to an area that earlier resisted being mobilized or lifted, to judge the effectiveness of treatment. In this way massage becomes a more dynamic part of treatment. A muscle might be unable to function effectively because of contracture of its tendon sheath. When this problem is reduced by applying deep friction, the muscle becomes more mobile and capable of more active movement. Thus, both assessment and treatment are accomplished.

PERCUSSION AND VIBRATION

Percussion and vibration are techniques used primarily in the treatment of pulmonary disorders (see Chapter 9).

Generally performed over the chest wall—and specifically over the ribs and intercostal muscles—these techniques also provide indirect evidence of inflation and compliance of lungs and infiltration or adherence of lungs and surrounding structures. Selective or precisely placed percussive techniques are utilized to test reflex responses of muscles and can be used to stimulate specific ligaments and tendinous structures. Rebound pain on percussion may often have specific meaning for certain orthopedic conditions.

DEEP FRICTION STROKES

Friction strokes provide the best localized, most specific information about certain connective tissue structures. The compliance and adherence of connective tissue can be assessed. The fascial compartments and sheaths of muscle, joint capsules, tendon sheaths, and related structures can be assessed, and local or generalized changes in these structures can be identified and rated. Transverse friction can be used to assess joint capsule mobility, especially around superficial joints. Transverse friction is generally more effective than longitudinal friction in producing plastic deformity of the target tissues. It may be necessary at times to combine the technique with passive movement or selected positioning to align specific structures to provide appropriate presentation and tension of the tissue. The perception of pain is altered and plastic lengthening of connective tissue can be achieved by repeated oscillatory movement of an adherent structure and the surrounding receptor structures.

SUMMARY

All the strokes mentioned here have value both as a part of the art of massage and as an assessment tool in other therapeutic areas. If care is taken to relate findings to specific anatomic structures, much of what normally passes as subjective information may prove to be more objective—and therefore more useful.

The therapist can come back during treatment to an area that earlier resisted being mobilized or lifted to judge the effectiveness of treatment. In this way massage becomes a more dynamic part of treatment. A muscle might be unable to function effectively because of contracture of its tendon sheath. When this problem is reduced by applying deep friction or some other stroke, the muscle may become more mobile and, thus, capable of increased active motion. The increased range of movement may be pain free. Thus, both assessment and treatment are accomplished.

Chapter 8

Massage for Specific Purposes

COLLEEN LISTON, Ph.D.

In this chapter, the use of massage in preventing and treating sports injuries across all age groups, for the elderly and dying, and for infants, will be presented. Background information and the techniques used for each are outlined. Descriptions of techniques already covered in preceding chapters will be referred to, and their application in sports, for the elderly, the dying, and infants will be described.

SPORTS MASSAGE

Historically, definitions in textbooks on massage have referred to repairing movement (Rawlins, 1930), healing (Basmajian, 1985; Krieger, 1973; Major, 1954), and mechanical stimulation of the tissue through the application of pressure and stretching (Beard & Wood, 1964; Wood & Becker, 1981).

In Homer's *Odyssey* (ca. 8th century B.C.) the use of massage in conjunction with athletic pursuits was first reported (Graham, 1902). Herodotus, in the 5th century B.C., and Hippocrates (ca. 460–375 B.C.) wrote of massage being given to prepare competitors for strenuous tests of strength. It was purported to make the tissues more supple and prevent ruptures and strains. Gladiators were massaged after strength tests and games to relieve pain and bruising, to stroke away swelling, and to refresh them. "Anointers"—medical practitioners or, more commonly, slaves—massaged wrestlers before and after they competed.

Sports massage—sometimes called "apotherapy"— was revived from its Greek origins with gymnasts, wrestlers, and gladiators in the 20th century and was referred to in two French books, by Coste (1906) and Ruffier (1907), as *"massage sportif."* The value of sports massage in hastening recovery from muscle fatigue has been confirmed

Effects of sports massage

- Decrease training damage
- Improve training consistency
- Help prevent muscle and tendon injuries
- Promote acute injury healing
- Promote complete healing to prevent acute problems from becoming chronic
- Promote healing of long-standing injury (break down adhesions to restore mobility)
- Reduce muscle spasm to promote restoration of normal muscle function
- Encourage a relaxed mental attitude
- Enhance confidence
- Enable athlete to stay in the game longer

by numerous investigators (Kamenetz, 1985). Sports massage is gaining recognition as an important preventive and treatment modality as more people of all ages are involving themselves in sports and fitness training. Investigations into its efficacy and uses continue, and a leading masseur at the Australian Institute of Sport has written a book about self-massage techniques for athletes (Clews, 1990).

Rhythmic application of pressure and stretching to the soft tissues of the body results, first, in stimulation of exteroceptors, both deep and superficial; second, proprioceptors in tendons and muscles; and third, interoceptors in the deeper tissues and the organs. The cycle of "tight→tear→tighter→more tearing" can be avoided.

The effects of massage techniques that can be employed in sport are physical, physiological, and psychological and are achieved through reflex and mechanical mechanisms described earlier in this text.

In the management of athletes in various endeavors, facilitation of capillary circulation and lymph flow not only enhances nutritive supply and removal of waste products but ensures that swelling and induration are reduced, adhesions broken down, contracted tendons and ligaments stretched, and the skin warmed and mobilized on the underlying tissues (Drinker, 1939; Drinker & Yoffey, 1941; Graham, 1913; Kleen, 1921; Krogh, 1929; Ladd et al., 1952; Maggiora, 1891; Pemberton, 1945; Starling, 1894; Wakim et al., 1949).

Some forms of massage provoke reflex effects such as vasodilatation or constriction of the capillaries, relaxation or stimulation of voluntary muscles, and pain relief or exacerbation with varying sensory input variations (Bugaj, 1975; Ebner, 1956; Jacobs, 1960; MacKenzie, 1923; Mattson Porth, 1986; Mennell, 1945). Peripheral vasodilatation and increased peripheral blood flow have been noted by Skull (1954). Acetylcholine is released, and histamine and histamine-like substances produce vasodilatation.

The literature does not support the use of lubricants, creams, or gels. For deeper techniques oily substances may reduce friction too much, rendering the tissues too slippery to grasp, and the treatment ineffective. Local counterirritation results as any agents that penetrate are absorbed by the blood in the cutaneous capillaries. A pleasant warmth and glow may be produced as a result, but the only effect on deeper tissues is reduction of blood flow in them as circulation to the skin increases. The penetrating substances are, however, quickly removed from the local area, so they do not have any lasting or systemic effects (Tappan, 1988).

It is important that anyone who performs sports massage remember that it does not take the place of stretching and warm-up exercises. Massage should be an adjunct to these activities, which are very important preparation for any athletic effort.

Table 8–1 provides a list of massage techniques useful for sports massage and a brief statement of their major effects and indications. It can serve as a guide for selecting the most appropriate technique for a given condition. The techniques themselves have been described elsewhere in this text.

The general contraindications to massage are set forth in Chapters 3 and 4; they will not be repeated here. When there is an acute injury, the regimen of rest, ice, compression, and elevation (RICE) must be instituted immediately. Massage should not be used for complete tears, in the first 48 hours after a muscle injury, or when pain is severe. A part that exhibits any signs of inflammation (for example, an accumulation of fluid in muscle tissue with a "dent" in it indicating intramuscular bleeding [such as a "corked" thigh]) should be treated with the greatest caution, and rest is essential.

Table 8.1	SPORTS MASSAGE: TECHNIQUES, EFFECTS, AND INDICATIONS	
TECHNIQUE	LIKELY EFFECTS	INDICATIONS
Swedish remedial massage		
Effleurage	Lymphatic drainage, relaxation	Edema, physical tension, psychological
Stroking	Relaxation or stimulation	stress, immobility and lethargy
Petrissage (kneading, wringing, picking up, ironing, skin rolling)	Stimulation of blood flow removes waste and provides nutrients, deep movement of soft tissues	Retention of waste products, poor circulation, immobility, adhesions, contractures
Frictions (circular)	Break down of adhesions	Adhesions, contractures
Tapotement (hacking, pounding, beating)	Stimulation of peripheral nerve endings and circulation	Poor circulation, inactive stretch reflex
Cyriax frictions		
Transverse	Prevention and breakdown of adhesions, movement, traumatic hyperemia, pain relief	Subacute muscle and ligamentous lesions, chronic adhesions, tenosynovitis, tendinitis, vaginitis
Connective tissue massage		
Basic section	Stimulation of somatic and autonomic nervous systems, reflex effects produce vascular changes	Peripheral vascular disease, adhesions, circulatory insufficiency
Long and short strokes		
Balancing strokes		
Acupressure/Shiatsu (finger pressure to points)	Homeostasis, balance of Ch'i (Ki) (energy)	Pain, functional disorders
Trigger point		
Icing	Reduce muscle reflex responses, muscle relaxation, pain reduction	Local pain, muscle tension, referred pain
Stretching		
Pressure		
Myofascial release		
Stretching	Reduce constriction and pain	Fascial and muscle restriction, pain

Sports massage techniques are no different from those used for other applications. Judicious selection and application of the massage techniques presented in Table 8–1 will provide optimal benefit for participants in many sports. An understanding of structure and function is important, as are the ability to perform a full assessment of the musculoskeletal system, diagnose dysfunction, and identify changes in postural alignment and soft tissue tension, and to plan safe, effective intervention. The choice of the most efficacious technique depends on experience and practice.

Goals of sports massage are (1) prevention of injury (achieved by maintaining the optimal resting length of muscles); (2) lasting beneficial effect for acute and chronic injuries (Hannaford et al., 1988); and (3) pain prevention. To ensure these aims are met, it is recommended that the following regimen be adopted: (1) Massage becomes part of the training routine. It is performed before and as part of warm-up and for prevention or treatment, as necessary. (2) Deep techniques are included for muscles, ligaments, and tendons that are vulnerable. These may include trigger point techniques (including myofascial stretching), connective tissue massage, and Cyriax-type of deep transverse frictions. And (3) Conditioning massage using petrissage (kneading) techniques and tapotement (percussion).

The massage techniques need to be learned and practiced on unaffected persons before the therapist applies them therapeutically. Before anyone attempts to perform any massage technique he or she must understand the expected effects and the indications for its use. The age and psychological and physical status of the client must be considered. Safety precautions and contraindications should also be part of the rationale for selection of techniques. The soft tissue should be assessed by observation and palpation to detect any color, temperature, or texture change and frank edema or induration. Objective assessment of function, muscle length and strength, and joint mobility and range plus pain charting provide relevant information.

The summary in Table 8–1 gives information relevant to massage application. Specific massage techniques may be chosen for swelling, adhesions, contractures, pain, or some other sign or symptom. Massage is best used as part of a complete treatment program. It may follow or precede application of a hot or cold pack, therapeutic ultrasound, or electrical stimulation and may facilitate joint mobilization or manipulation. Exercise regimens should be complementary to sustain the effects achieved by massage.

Pre- and post-treatment measurement of swelling (for example, circumference or fluid displacement techniques), joint range and muscle tension (by goniometry and similar measurement methods), and muscle strength (by dynamometry or charting) is recommended, as is recording areas of skin temperature change and color. These objective signs, as well as detailed information about dysfunction and discrepancies (e.g., leg length) provide evidence of the effects of the massage. Re-evaluation tells

the therapist whether to continue the same treatment or whether alternative modalities may better achieve the desired outcomes. Those working with athletes are ideally placed to use massage for prevention before the workout, for acute and chronic injuries, for restoration of normal soft tissue states, and to improve the client's level of performance.

Pre-event Massage

To promote speed, power, and endurance and to prevent injury it is reasonable to use massage to (1) break down adhesions, (2) increase cell nutrition, (3) increase circulation, and (4) reduce muscle spasm. An ideal time to give massage is 20 to 30 minutes before warm-up—specifically stretching the body parts that will be subjected to the greatest stress in the event (Calder, 1990). Before the massage, a brisk "needle" shower to stimulate peripheral nerve endings should begin with warm water at about 45°C and end with cold water (25°C). Ending with a cool shower leaves the sensory receptors stimulated and the core temperature at a normal level (Tappan, 1988). The massage should not itself increase the core temperature of the body yet should warm the body parts that benefit most from the warm-up and specific stretching that follow. This is particularly important for marathon events, as they are associated with greater risk of increased core body temperature, especially in warm climates and on days when humidity is high. In these instances, warm-up time is reduced and the only objective means of assessing the effect on the core temperature is a rectal thermometer.

With the client lying prone in a comfortable resting position, effleurage is given to the back, starting lightly and progressing deeper to facilitate relaxation. Deep petrissage techniques such as kneading can be used for large muscle groups such as the trapezius, erector spinae, latissimus dorsi, and rhomboids. Picking up and wringing of the upper fibers of the trapezius, double flat-handed ironing upward and inward across the trunk muscles to the spine, and skin rolling and frictions on either side of the spinous processes complete the massage to the back. If there are signs of increased tension and symptoms of pain or discomfort, those can be targeted. Other techniques include frictions to tendons, ligaments, and musculotendinous junctions. Massage to muscles more actively involved in specific sports—for example in the upper limbs of swimmers, throwers, and tennis players or the lower limbs of runners, footballers, and hurdlers—should be applied selectively (Nekrasov & Chuganov, 1991).

Interested athletes may be taught to give themselves massage in the muscle groups they use most. While self-massage for the lower limb is relatively easy, it is more difficult for the upper limb as only one hand is available. A good deal of imagination is required to self-massage the back and buttocks, such as rubber balls on the floor or a mechanical or electrically powered cushion or oriental style set of wooden balls strung together (Clews, 1990; Prentice, 1986; Tappan, 1988).

Brisk tapotement, for example hacking, is best used at the conclusion of the massage session because it provides general stimulation of the nervous system. Furthermore, it creates a sense of well-being and ensures that the athlete is ready to participate. That is, the massage should enhance the preparation of the body *and* the mind for warm-up and stretching before strenuous exercise.

Massage for Sports Injuries

Though prevention is preferred, injury may occur despite the best preparation. A discussion of the use of massage in the management of acute and chronic injuries will be presented before moving on to strategies for massage after competition or exercise.

Acute Injuries

For ligament and tendon injuries it is preferable to encourage the development of an orderly fibrillary network early. In this way, strong, pliable connective tissue can be established, and the injured tissue restored to its correct length. Too often, structures heal shorter than they should and are thus rendered vulnerable to more extensive and repeated injuries. Deep transverse frictions, like those taught by James Cyriax, can be used to "spin" the fibers (Cyriax, 1980). As outlined in the section on Cyriax frictions (Chapter 3), the spinning is analogous to separating the individual strands in a piece of string rolled under the finger. The fibrillary network is present 48 hours after injury, and if not encouraged to recover in a flat position, curls tightly, leading to shortening of the overall structure (Stearns, 1940). Fibroplasia can be prevented by inhibiting an inflammatory reaction (Ketchum, 1977).

Unfortunately, deep frictions are rarely completely effective, so other mechanisms are required, such as stretching and electrophysical agents, to reduce formation of tight scar tissue resulting from fibroplasia (Akeson et al., 1977; Noyes et al., 1974). Immobility has been shown to lead to scar tissue in soft tissue structures and pain when movement recommences (Cooper, 1986; Mason & Allen, 1941; Noyes, 1977; Tipton et al., 1970; Woo et al., 1975). Others (Akeson et al., 1977; Stearns, 1940; Vailas et al., 1981) have found that it is likely that movement prevents scar formation in three ways. First, proteoglycan synthesis is stimulated; second, the mechanical stress of movement promotes orderly laying down of new collagen fibers; and third, any intermolecular cross-linking that results in tight, short collagen fibers is prevented. In addition, the connective tissue is lubricated through the movement, and fibers are kept separated to ensure efficient remodeling of the structure.

Fresh ligament sprains (i.e., minor ruptures or tears of the ligamentous fibers) respond well to less vigorous frictions applied immediately to passively maintain mobil-

ity in the ligament. Light transverse frictions can be applied when the fibroblasts are newly formed and before they become firmly attached. Vigorous deep frictions are more appropriate to chronic sprains. They induce the numbing effect of hyperemia (Chamberlain, 1982) by enhancing the blood supply to the area so that Lewis' substance P is destroyed more rapidly. As a result, pain is reduced during the treatment, which usually takes 15 to 20 minutes, and for up to half an hour after that (Tappan, 1988). Any adhesions that bind the ligaments to the underlying bone can similarly be broken down to facilitate more normal healing, as in acute injuries. The importance of movement during healing has been stressed. Prevention of the formation of scar tissue and maintenance of the length of involved structures cannot be overemphasized.

The techniques applied for tenosynovitis and tendinitis require the tendon to be stretched to provide a base on which to move the sheath (as described in Chapter 3). It is not within the scope of this text to discuss other modalities, but it is interesting to note that severe pain associated with scar tissue in tendons may be treated with steroid infiltration. Nevertheless, injecting steroids has no effect on the breaking down of scarring and promotion of optimal healing (Cyriax, 1977).

Chronic Injuries

Because the circulation brings in nutrients and removes waste products, it is proposed that general deep massage is most effective for treating chronic muscle injuries. Compression of the tissues with relaxed palms spreads the fibers, intensifies the hyperemia, and increases blood flow to and from the area. Broad thumb strokes may be used to feel along muscle fibers to assess for adhesions, and they can be applied just as effectively across the muscle fibers. The thumb is used because it is more sensitive than other areas, such as the heel of the hand. Normal muscle spreads, but where there are adhesions the whole muscle moves away and snaps back after the stroke, especially during work across the fibers.

For therapeutic effects, similar deep thumb stroking, with the thumbs working side by side or following one another, may be used to stimulate flow of lymph and induce hyperemia in deeper tissues. An elbow, one or more fingers, or the heel of the hand may be useful when moving along the muscle fibers. The bulk of the patient's tissues and his or her acceptance of the technique being applied determine the depth of the massage. Other massage and associated techniques that may be useful in the treatment of chronic sports injuries include deep transverse (Cyriax) frictions, as already discussed, connective tissue massage, acupressure/shiatsu, trigger point stimulation, and myofascial techniques, which are all presented elsewhere in the text.

For muscle spasm, gentle stretching after the application of cold or heat may reduce pain. Stretching *torn* muscle only increases pain, induces greater spasm in intact muscle fibers, and may lead to further tearing. In muscle spasm the physiological response is capillary restriction, which reduces blood flow. Restriction of normal circulation means that the flow of nutrients and oxygen to the area is limited and waste products in the soft tissue are retained. An adverse cycle is thereby set up: more spasm leads to more pain and less tissue flexibility. This cycle can be interrupted by massage. If the joint range is affected, for example when two-joint muscles (muscles on either side of the joints involved) are involved, structures above and below the joint should be treated, including both agonistic and antagonistic muscle groups and their associated tendons (Wiktorsson-Möller et al., 1983).

Delayed muscle soreness is a phenomenon that is not necessarily associated with fatigue. It occurs most frequently after unaccustomed exercise, as after prolonged training or after competing in a full day of events (or even after a day gardening at the end of winter). It is commonly described as a dull aching pain accompanied by tender, stiff muscles, and it can affect everyday functional activities such as squatting, walking, climbing, and running (Ebbeling & Clarkson, 1989). It has been reported that studies of the pathophysiological parameters of delayed muscle soreness have found muscle trauma, especially after activities that involve eccentric muscle work. Tonic muscle spasm has been a common finding, and in many cases of delayed soreness the connective tissue has been damaged (Abraham, 1977; Armstrong, 1984; Armstrong, 1990; Ebbeling & Clarkson, 1989; Ferstat & Davidson, 1990; Hasson et al., 1989; Maxwell et al., 1988). Some clinical trials have found that massage may provide a faster and more graded recovery from delayed muscle soreness as compared with no treatment (Dolenger & Morien, 1993; Ferstat & Davidson, 1990; Hill & Richardson, 1989; Maxwell et al., 1988; Smith et al., 1994; Wiktorsson-Möller et al., 1983).

Connective tissue massage for chronic sports injuries may help because it can relieve pain and increase the microcirculation in vascular beds. Kaada and Torsteinbo (1989) measured the concentration of plasma beta-endorphins before and 5, 30, and 90 minutes after 30 minutes of connective tissue massage and found a 16% increase in the beta-endorphin levels from 20.0 to 23.2 pg/0.1 ml ($P = .025$). It occurred maximally 5 minutes after the end of the massage and persisted about 1 hour. The finding that pain can be relieved by stroking over reflex areas ("head zones"), especially on the trunk, has been presented in the section on Connective Tissue Massage (Baker & Taylor, 1954; Ebner, 1956, 1962; Kisner & Taslitz, 1968; Langen, 1959; Mahoney, 1957). For management of sports injuries, where areas in the muscle are bound down, flat, long pulls on the connective tissue are likely to be effective. For more local problems, shorter hooking strokes may be used (Counsilman & McAllister, 1986; Hannaford et al., 1988; Scher, 1988).

Studies of autonomic activity—heart rate, blood pressure, galvanic skin resistance, peripheral skin temperature—reflect increased sympathetic activity when connective tissue massage is applied (Burch & De Pasquale, 1965; Kisner & Taslitz, 1968; Lazarus et al., 1963; Wang, 1958). Furthermore, when psychological parameters were included, one study by McKechnie and colleagues (1983) established that symptoms that may be associated with tension are alleviated when connective tissue massage is applied. They reported slowing of the heart rate, increased skin resistance, and decreased levels of muscle tension ($P = <.001$). The subjects were more relaxed and were prepared to discuss their physical problems more openly.

It is interesting to note the overlap in the reflex zones stroked in connective tissue massage and acupuncture points that when stimulated have been reported to relieve symptoms for the same pathologic states and conditions. In Chapters 11 and 12, where special and Eastern systems of massage such as Japanese shiatsu and Chinese acupuncture/pressure are presented, the relationship between the effects attributed to connective tissue massage and those attributed to the techniques used in these other systems will be highlighted.

Training and Postevent Massage

Slow stroking of the soft tissues and kneading of muscles are widely used, particularly by the Russians. These techniques are applied for 10 to 30 minutes to enhance relaxation, both in training sessions and on the day of an event. The rationale is that these massage techniques improve performance capability and assist in recovery. Calder (1990) reports that enhanced performance was the outcome for athletes engaged in a wide range of sports who were given massage. These results were published by a number of researchers in the Soviet Sports Review (Dubrovski et al., 1992). The greatest gains were reported in strength. It has also been found that massage techniques are two to three times more likely than rest to promote recovery; this corroborates earlier claims about the importance of mechanical stimulation.

To achieve this outcome 30 to 60 minutes of massage is recommended. After strenuous activities (such as weight lifting and cross-country skiing), light techniques may be given up to 8 hours later; after less strenuous activities such as high jumping or 100-meter sprints, deeper techniques may be given 1 or 2 days later (Arbuthnot, 1992; Banner, 1993; Crampton & Fox, 1987; Hanten & Chandler, 1994; Lowden et al., 1991). Physiological and psychological states should return to pre-performance levels during the recovery phase (Blake et al., 1989; Danneskiold-Samsøe et al., 1982). Thus, plasma myoglobin, hormone and enzyme levels, and metabolic rate can be restored. In other words, there has been a return to homeostasis (Arkko et al., 1983; Barr & Taslitz, 1970). Future research on the psychophysiological effects of massage will benefit from the exponential increase in the sensitivity levels for indices used to determine these states.

Massage can be used to enhance a feeling—both emotional and psychological—of well-being and relaxation. There are few age- or gender-specific considerations for any type or application of massage in sport. Massage is best combined with other techniques and modalities, such as stretching, passive and active movements, proprioceptive neuromuscular facilitation, free and resisted exercise, ice, heat, electrical stimulation, and hydrotherapy.

MASSAGE FOR THE ELDERLY AND THE TERMINALLY ILL

Increasing medical mechanization and pharmacologic advances contribute to dehumanizing patient management. The isolation and lack of physical contact perceived by many patients may promote a search for ways to provide closer human contact, for example, touch and massage. Physical therapists have a license to touch, and massage has a legislated place in the practice of physical therapy in most countries. Other health care practitioners also use massage in providing care for their patients. For patients of all ages judicious use of massage can ameliorate the discomfort of invasive techniques and provide a sense of reassurance and caring.

Massage is particularly useful for relaxation and pain relief for elderly or dying persons. Of course, not all terminally ill patients are elderly. However, the constantly changing needs of the patient must be considered (Levine, 1982). The person's tolerance, age, and skin condition (dryness, tightness, fragility) must be taken into account when massage is performed. For well elderly persons, these are the only reservations to be considered; otherwise, any and all techniques are suitable. The importance of touch as a means of communication, to impart a sense of well-being and confidence, should not be ignored or underestimated. The average person has approximately 18,000 cm² of skin, a very sensitive area for touch. Massage creates delightful sensations (in most cases) that can have a soothing or stimulating effect, promotes increased flexibility and elasticity in the skin and underlying tissues, and improves interactions between patient and therapist (Montague, 1978; Pratt & Mason, 1981). Hippocrates (ca. 460–375 B.C.) wrote of mobilizing the body's natural recuperative powers (White, 1988).

In massage the hands stimulate sensory receptors in the skin and the resultant stimuli pass along afferent fibers to the spinal cord and thence through the autonomic and the central nervous system. The aforementioned effects occur in the segmentally related body zones. Barrow suggested an explanation for the visceral effects that may accompany the reflex effects of massage (Graham, 1913).

Touching another person communicates an intention—in the case of therapeutic touch and massage, to heal, recruit, balance, or share inherent energy or promote relaxation (Krieger, 1979, 1981; Regan & Shapiro, 1988).

An increase in hemoglobin has been reported (Krieger, 1973; Krieger, 1976; Pemberton, 1945), as has release of acetylcholine and histamine (as well as histamine-like substances) (Skull, 1945). Furthermore, Siegel (1986) believes that it is possible to activate the body's immune system through loving, healing touch and self-healing.

The massage techniques that can be used for frail elderly and dying persons include effleurage, stroking, and light kneading. Often the most valuable technique is pressure, as in stationary kneading or squeeze kneading. Attention to the feet, hands, and face may be all that is acceptable. Indeed, those who cannot tolerate even the lightest brush of a sheet often may be physically and emotionally comforted by gentle pressure to the face and scalp. Reflexology techniques have been used to good effect for patients who have terminal cancer. Terminally ill patients have specific needs: (1) control of pain, which may be preventing sleep, restricting eating, or interfering with communication; (2) material comfort, which is provided by a bed and/or chair, privacy, and physical attention from care givers; (3) psychological comfort (including respect for personal dignity) which comes from attentive care givers who provide appropriate information, the presence of loved ones, physical contact, and the opportunity to express feelings.

Principles of reflexology have the potential to address these needs. A practitioner—a family member, friend, or care giver—can provide physical contact in a private place with the patient in a preferred position in bed or in a chair. It will be understood from the section on reflexology that the relaxing and pain-relieving effects are achieved through stimulation of the proprioceptors, the sympathetic nervous system, and improved circulation, both physiologically and functionally, as in the flow of energy (Dobbs, 1985).

The willingness, tolerance, and needs of frail elderly and dying persons should guide the application of massage. The use of massage in palliative care is growing rapidly, and is performed by many different health care professionals (Burke et al., 1994; Doehning, 1989; Feltham, 1991). The basic techniques can easily be adapted and taught to family members and care givers. Less important than the technical skill of the hands is the caring intention of the person performing the massage.

BABY AND INFANT MASSAGE

Massage for babies is well-recognized as an ideal way to promote tactile communication. It has a beneficial effect on development, alertness, and emotional status (Leboyer, 1976; Prudence, 1984; Rice, 1975; Schneider, 1982) and can continue to any age. It strengthens the bonding process and helps establish a warm, positive, parent–child relationship. Baby massage has been used in varying forms for centuries and is being accepted in societies that have not traditionally valued the power of touch.

It is beneficial to use massage on all babies and infants, whether or not they have problems. Benefits to both parents and baby include pleasure, confidence, communication, relaxation, reassurance through skin contact, development of body awareness, and calmness (McClure, 1989; Tiquia, 1986).

Massage is particularly useful in the following situations:

- For a colicky baby who cries when being fed. Often the baby continues to be tense and irritable long after the cause of the colic has been identified and treated.

- For an anxious baby who dislikes rapid changes of position, does not need much sleep, and is hypersensitive to external stimuli.

- For an irritable baby who often exhibits abnormal neurologic signs, hyperactivity, and persistent primitive reflexes.

- For infants with disorders such as earache, urinary tract infection, or gastric reflux.

Infants who undergo surgery can be included in this category, as can the preterm infant. These babies need to learn that touch is pleasurable. Some of their early experiences—monitoring devices and various life support and other invasive procedures—have been uncomfortable. Indeed, a number of studies provide evidence of the benefits of massage for the preterm infant, such as improved weight gain, fewer facial grimaces, less fist clenching, and enhanced development of the sympathetic nervous system (Field et al., 1986; Kuhn et al., 1991; Ottenbacher et al., 1987; Scafidi et al., 1993; Solkoff et al., 1975). Babies who are not particularly active can be stimulated, rather than relaxed, with massage that alternates light tickling with gentle, firm pressure.

Preparations should include ensuring a peaceful atmosphere (no phones or loud sounds but calm, soothing music may be beneficial); subdued lighting; appropriate room temperature (no drafts); and the availability of a natural massage oil, e.g., almond or apricot. A preferred time to massage is when both parent and baby are relaxed and the baby is not hungry. Parts of the body not being massaged may be covered with a blanket if necessary to maintain body temperature. Massage should begin with the baby positioned supine on the parent's or therapist's lap to provide eye contact, and in this position massage to the front of the body can be completed.

Since the baby will undoubtedly move around during the massage, it is important that the techniques be adapted to accommodate this and therefore cannot be rigidly prescribed or applied.

Massage flows from head to toe, covering all of the body, back and front. The technique applied should be gentle stroking, and the position adapted to wherever the baby is most comfortable at any given time.

Head and Face

Stroke the crown of the head with the thumbs using circular movements. Then, with the fingertips stroke from the head down along the sides of the face. Include the eyebrows, nose, cheeks, jawbone, and around the ears.

Shoulders, Arms, and Hands

Stroke across the shoulders, rounding them forward, and down the arms to the hands. Encircle the baby's arm with the hands and gently squeeze each arm from shoulder to wrist, then massage the baby's hands and fingers using your thumb and forefinger. Stroking the back of the hand with the thumb encourages it to open. Finish each stroke by taking the hands off of the body.

Chest and Abdomen

Using both hands stroke the chest from the center following the line of the ribs to the side of the body. Abdominal discomfort may be relieved by using circular, clockwise strokes around the umbilicus. Then follow the course of the large bowel.

Legs, Feet, and Ankles

Give long strokes along the legs from thigh to toes on all surfaces, then massage by gently squeezing, as with the arms. Massage the ankles; then support the ankle and use the thumb to massage the sole of the foot firmly. Stroke each toe. Stroke the soles firmly with the thumbs. Rubbing the soles of the feet together is pleasant and calming for the baby.

Back

Starting from the neck, stroke down the back with a flat hand, then gently massage with the fingertips in a circular motion down either side of the spine to the buttocks. The baby may be prone or lying on one side. Stroke all over the back in a circular motion, as in finger kneading.

Buttocks

Jiggle the buttocks and use finger and thumb squeezing.

Suckling

Stimulating the rooting reflex causes the baby to open the mouth and nuzzle, searching for the nipple. This may be achieved by gently stroking from the cheek to the mouth. Such gentle touch may help a baby who is having difficulty suckling.

Close body contact can be provided through activities other than massage, such as breast feeding, bottle feeding with the baby cuddled against the bare chest, a cuddle in bed with parent(s), carrying in a front pack, and having a bath with parent(s). All of these activities will help to foster close bonding between the baby and parent(s) and provide a strong basis for the emotional and physical development of the child.

References

Sports Massage

Abraham N. (1977) Factors in delayed muscle soreness. Med Sci Sports 9(1):11–20.

Akeson WH, Amiel D, Mechanic GL, Woo SL, Harwood ML. (1977) Collagen cross-linking alterations in joint contractures: Changes in the reducible cross-links in periarticular connective tissue collagen after nine weeks of immobilisation. Connect Tissue Res 5:15–19.

Arbuthnot H. (1992) The role of sports massage in the preparation of elite athletes. Sportsmed News, July, pp 7.

Arkko PJ, Pakarinen AJ, Kari-koskinen, O. (1983) Effects of whole body massage on serum protein, electrolyte and hormone concentrations, enzyme activities and haematological parameters. Int J Sports Med 4:265–267.

Armstrong RB. (1984) Mechanisms of exercise-induced delayed onset muscular soreness: A brief review. Med Sci Sports Exercise 16(6):529–535.

Armstrong RB. (1990) Initial events in exercise-induced muscular injuries. Med Sci Sports Exercise 22(4):429–435.

Baker LM, Taylor WM. (1954) The relationship under stress between changes in skin temperature, electrical resistance and pulse rate. J Exp Psychol 48:361–366.

Banner KA. (1994) World Triathlon Championships—Manchester 1993—sports massage. NZ J Sports Med, Autumn: 15.

Barr JS, Taslitz N.(1970) The influence of back massage on autonomic functions. Phys Ther 50:1670–1691.

Basmajian JV. (ed) (1985) Manipulation, traction and massage, 3rd ed. Baltimore: Williams & Wilkins.

Beard G, Wood EC. (1964) Massage principles and techniques. Philadelphia: WB Saunders.

Blake B, Anthony J, Wyatt F. (1989) The effects of massage treatment on exercise fatigue. Clin Sports Med 1:189–196.

Bugaj R. (1975) The cooling, analgesic, rewarming effects of ice massage on localised skin. Phys Ther 55:11.

Burch GE, De Pasquale A. (1965) Methods for studying the influence of higher central nervous centers on the peripheral circulation of intact man. Am Heart J 70:411–422.

Calder A. (1990) Sports Massage. In Draper J. (ed.): Third Report on National Sports Research Program July 1988–June 1990. Canberra: Australian Sports Commission CPN, pp 44–51.

Chamberlain GJ. (1982) Cyriax's friction massage: A review. J Orthop Sports Phys Ther 4(1):16–22.

Clews W. (1990) Sports massage and stretching. Sydney: Bantam.

Cooper B. (1986) Massage of the forearms for male gymnasts. Sports Sci Med Q 2(3):4–6.

Counsilman J, McAllister B. (1986) Breaking up shoulder problems. Swim Tech Feb/Apr:14–18.

Crampton J, Fox J. (1987) Regeneration vs burnout: Prevention is better than cure. Sports Coach 10(4):7–10.

Cyriax J. (1977) Deep massage. Physiotherapy JCSP 63(2):60–61.

Cyriax J. (1980) Textbook of orthopaedic medicine, 10th ed, Vol 2. London: Baillière Tindall.

Danneskiold-Samsøe, B., Christiansen E, Lund B, Anderson RB. (1982) Regional muscle tension and pain ("fibrositis"). Scand J Rehab Med 15:17–20.

Dolgener FA, Morien A. (1993) The effect of massage on lactate disappearance. J Strength Condition Res 7(3):159–162.

Drinker CK. (1939) The formation and movements of lymph. Am Heart J 18:389.

Drinker CK, Yoffey JM. (1941) Lymphatics, lymph and lymphoid tissue: The physiological and clinical significance. Cambridge: Cambridge University Press.

Dubrovskii I, Sverdlik YA, Luchshev AI, Proshchalykin AI. (1992) The effect of massage on microcirculation in athletes' musculo-skeletal injuries. Fitness Sports Rev Int April:71.

Ebbeling CB, Clarkson PM. (1989) Exercise-induced muscle damage and adaptation. Sports Med 7:207–234.

Ebner M. (1956) Peripheral circulatory disturbances: Treatment by massage of connective tissue in reflex zones. Br J Phys Med 19:176–180.

Ebner M. (1962) Connective tissue massage. Theory and therapeutic application. Edinburgh: Churchill Livingstone.

Ferstat A, Davidson C. (1990) The effectiveness of massage on delayed muscle soreness induced by consecutive days of eccentric and concentric muscle activity. Unpublished undergraduate thesis. Perth, Western Australia: Curtin University.

Graham D. (1902) Treatise on massage. Its history, mode of application and effects. Philadelphia: JB Lippincott.

Graham, D. (1913). Massage, manual treatment, remedial movement: History, mode of application and effects, indications and contraindications. Philadelphia: JB Lippincott.

Hannaford P, Clews WS, Fardy E, Wajswelner H. (1988) Effects of therapeutic massage versus physiotherapy modalities on interstitial compartment pressure. In: Proceedings, 25th National Annual Scientific Conference. Sydney, Australia: Australian Sports Medicine Federation.

Hanten WP, Chandler SD. (1994) Effects of myofascial release leg pull and sagittal plane isometric contract-relax techniques on passive straight-leg raise angle. J Sports Phys Ther 20(3):138–144.

Hasson S, Barnes W, Hunter M, Williams J. (1989) Therapeutic effect of high speed voluntary muscle contraction on muscle soreness and muscle performance. J Orthop Sports Phys Ther June:499–507.

Hill DW, Richardson JD. (1989) Effectiveness of 10% trolamine salicylate cream on muscular soreness induced by a reproducible program of weight training. J Orthop Sports Phys Ther July:19–23.

Jacobs M. (1960) Massage for the relief of anatomical and physiological considerations. Phys Ther Rev 40:96.

Kaada B, Torsteinbo O. (1989) Increase of plasma β-endorphins in connective tissue massage. Gen Pharmacol 20(4):487–489.

Kamenetz HL. (1985) History of massage. In: Basmajian JV (ed): Manipulation, traction and massage, 3rd ed. Baltimore: Williams & Wilkins.

Ketchum LD. (1977) Primary tendon healing: A review. J Hand Surg 2:428–435.

Kisner CD, Taslitz N. (1968) Connective tissue massage: The influence of the introductory treatment on autonomic functions. Phys Ther 48(2):107–119.

Kleen EAG. (1921) Massage and medical gymnastics, 2nd ed. New York: WM Wood.

Krieger D. (1973) The relationship of touch with intent to help or heal, studies in-vivo haemoglobin values. In Proceedings of the American Nurses Association 9th Nursing Research Conference. Kansas City: American Nursing Association.

Krogh A. (1929) The anatomy and physiology of capillaries. New Haven, CT: Yale University Press.

Ladd MP, Kotte FJ, Blanchard RS. (1952) Studies on the effect of massage on the flow of lymph from the foreleg of a dog. Arch Phys Med 33:604–612.

Langen D. (1959) Study on the mechanism of action of massage of reflex zones in connective tissue. Psychother Med Psychol 9:194–201.

Lazarus RS, Speisman JC, Mordkoff AM. (1963) The relationship between autonomic indicators of psychological stress: Heart rate and skin conductance. Psychosomat Med 25:19–29.

Lowdon B, Mourad A, Warne P. (1991) Sports massage for competitive surfers. Sport Health 9(4):25–29.

MacKenzie J .(1923) Angina pectoris. London: Hodder & Stoughton.

Maggiora A. (1891) De l'action physiologique du massage sur les muscles de l'homme. Arch Ital Biol 16:225–246.

Mahoney L. (1957) Massage of reflex zones. Physiotherapy 43:74–76.

Major RH. (1954) A history of medicine. Oxford: Blackwell.

Mason ML, Allen HS. (1941) The rate of healing tendons. Ann Surg 113:424–456.

Mattson Porth C. (1986) Pathophysiology: Concepts of altered health states, 2nd ed. Philadelphia: JB Lippincott.

Maxwell S, Kohn W, Watson A, Balnave RJ. (1988) Is stretching effective in the prevention of or amelioration of delayed-onset muscle soreness? In: Proceedings of the 25th National Annual Scientific Conference of the Australian Sports Medicine Federation. Sydney, Australia: Australian Sports Medicine Federation.

McKechnie A, Wilson F, Watson N, Scott D. (1983) Anxiety states: A preliminary report on the value of connective tissue massage. J Psychosomat Res 2(2):125–129.

Mennell, JB. (1945) Physical treatment by movement manipulation and massage, 5th ed. Philadelphia: Blakiston.

Nekrasov A, Chuganov V. (1991) Acu-application Massage. A new resource in the training of track-and-field athletes (a doctor's advice). Soviet Sports Rev December, 26(4):169–171.

Noyes FR. (1977) Functional properties of knee ligaments and alterations induced by immobilization. Clin Orthop 123:210–242.

Noyes FR, Torvik PJ, Hyde WB, DeLucas JL. (1974) Biomechanics of ligament failure. J Bone Joint Surg 56A:1406–1418.

Pemberton R. (1945) Physiology of massage. In: AMA Handbook of physical medicine. Chicago: American Medical Association.

Prentice WE. (1986) Therapeutic modalities in sports medicine. St. Louis: CV Mosby.

Rawlins MS. (1930) Textbook of massage: For nurses and beginners. St. Louis: CV Mosby.

Scher S. (1988) Scarred stiff. Using massage to reduce muscular scar tissue. Triathlete 63:18–19.

Skull CW. (1945) Massage—physiologic basis. Arch Phys Med 261:159–167.

Smith LL, Keating MN, Holbert D, Spratt DJM, Cammon MR, Smith SS, Israel RG. (1994) The effects of athletic massage on delayed muscle soreness, creatine kinase, and neutrophil count: A preliminary report. J Sports Phys Ther 19(2):93–99.

Starling EH. (1894) The influence of mechanical factors on lymph production. J Physiol 16:224.

Stearns ML. (1940) Studies of the development of connective tissue in transparent chambers in the rabbit ear II. Am J Anat 67:55–97.

Tappan FM. (1978) Healing massage techniques. East Norwalk, CT: Appleton & Lange.

Tipton CM, James SL, Merger W, Tcheng TK. (1970) Influence of exercise on strength of medial collateral knee ligament of dogs. Am J Physiol 218:894–902.

Vailas AC, Tipton CM, Matthes RD, Gart M. (198) Physical activity and its influence on the repair process of medial collateral ligaments. Connect Tissue Res 9:25–31.

Wakim KG, Martin GM, Terrier JC, Elkins EC, Krusen FH. (1949) The effects of massage on the circulation in normal and paralyzed extremities. Arch Phys Med 30:135.

Wang GH. (1958) The galvanic skin reflex: A review of old and recent works from a physiologic point of view. Am J Phys Med 37:37–57.

Wiktorsson-Möller M, Öberg B, Ekstrand J, Gillquist J. (1983) Effects of warming up, massage and stretching on range of motion and muscle strength in the lower extremity. Am J Sports Med 11(4):249–252.

Woo SL, Matthew JV, Akeson WH, Amiel D, Convery FR. (1975) Connective tissue response to immobility. Arthritis Rheum 18:257–264.

Wood E, Becker P. (1981) Beard's massage, 3rd ed. Philadelphia: WB Saunders.

Massage for the Elderly and the Terminally Ill

Burke C, Macnish S, Saunders J, Galini A, Warne I, Downing J. (1994) The development of a massage service for cancer patients. Clin Oncol 6:381–385.

Dobbs BZ. (1985) Alternative health approaches. Nurs Mirror 160(9):41–42.

Doehring K. (1989) Relieving pain through touch. Advanc Clin Care 4(5):32–33.

Feltham E. (1991) Therapeutic touch and massage. Nurs Standard 5(45):26–28.

Graham D. (1913) Massage, manual treatment, remedial movements: History, mode of application and effects, indications and contraindications. Philadelphia: JB Lippincott.

Krieger D. (1973) The relationship of touch with intent to help or heal, studies of in-vivo haemoglobin values. In: Proceedings American Nurses Association 9th Nursing Research Conference. Kansas City: American Nurses Association.

Krieger D. (1976) Nursing research for a new age. Nurs Times 72:1–7.

Krieger D. (1979) Therapeutic touch: How to use your hands to help or to heal. Englewood Cliffs, NJ: Prentice Hall.

Krieger D. (1981) Foundations of holistic health nursing practices: The renaissance nurse. Philadelphia: JB Lippincott.

Levine S. (1982) Who dies? Garden City, NY: Anchor/Doubleday.

Montague A. (1978) Touching. Toronto: Harper & Row.

Pemberton R. (1945) Physiology of massage. In: AMA Handbook of physical medicine. Chicago: American Medical Association.

Pratt JW, Mason A. (1981) The caring touch. London: Heyden.

Regan G, Shapiro D. (1988) The power of touch. In: The healer's handbook. New York: Element Books.

Siegel BS. (1986) Love, medicine & miracles. New York: Harper & Row.

Skull CW. (1945) Massage—physiologic basis. Arch Phys Med 261:159–167.

White JA. (1988) Touching with intent: Therapeutic massage. Holistic Nurs Pract 2(3):63–67.

Infant Massage

Field T, Schanberg SM, Scafidi F, et al. (1986) Tactile/kinesthetic stimulation effects on preterm neonates. Pediatrics 77: 654–658.

Kuhn CM, Schanberg SM, Field T, et al. (1991) Tactile/kinesthetic stimulation effects on sympathetic and adrenocortical function in preterm infants. J Pediatr 119: 434–440.

Leboyer F. (1976) Birth without violence. New York: Knopf.

McClure VS. (1989) Infant massage: A handbook for loving parents. New York: Bantam.

Ottenbacher KJ, Muller L, Brandt D, et al. (1987) The effectiveness of tactile stimulation as a form of early intervention: A quantitative evaluation. Develop Behav Pediatr 8:68–76.

Prudence B. (1984) Pain erasure: New York: Evans.

Rice RD. (1975) Premature infants respond to sensory stimulation. Am Psychologic Assoc Monitor 6(II): 8.

Scafidi FA, Field T, Schanberg SM. (1993) Factors that predict which preterm infants benefit most from massage therapy. Developmental and behavioural pediatrics 14(3):176–180.

Schneider V. (1982) Infant massage. New York: Bantam.

Solkoff N, Yaffe S, Weintraub D, et al. (1975) Effects of handling on the subsequent development of premature infants. Develop Psychol 1:765–768.

Tiquia R. (1986) Chinese infant massage. Melbourne: Greenhouse.

Chapter 9

Massage for the Patient with a Respiratory Condition

In some parts of the United States, the practice of chest physical therapy is viewed with considerable skepticism, criticism, and a great deal of misunderstanding. In contrast, in many other parts of the world, especially Europe, Australia, New Zealand, and Canada, the techniques are widely accepted and have been used extensively for many decades (Frownfelter & Dean, 1996; Hillegass & Sadowsky, 1994; Irwin & Techlin, 1995; Watchie, 1995; Webber & Pryor, 1993). Perhaps because American society tends to be so highly machine conscious and technically oriented, physicians have been inclined to prescribe a *breathing machine*, rather than physical therapy, for patients in respiratory distress. Moreover, a physical therapist proficient in respiratory care techniques is not always available when such physical therapy is prescribed. This is a sad state of affairs, since many patients who suffer from respiratory distress could be significantly helped by some very simple and cost-effective procedures. At the very least, these techniques might be tried before much more expensive equipment and medications are ordered, and, of course, so much of the physical therapy involves teaching patients a variety of means to help themselves through such distress plus techniques to prevent further episodes. All of these valuable and very cost-effective treatments are lost if the patient receives only a machine and medication.

Statistics have shown a consistent increase in the incidence of chronic obstructive pulmonary disease (COPD). During a 10-year period (1950–1960), for example, deaths attributable to emphysema and chronic bronchitis increased more than fourfold (Carey, 1967). In an additional study (1950–1965), the mortality rate was shown to double every 5 years. Deaths increased almost eightfold, from 3157 patients in 1950 to 23,700 patients in 1965 (Weiss et al., 1969). More recent data suggest that about

Goals of chest physical therapy

- Prevent the accumulation of secretions
- Improve mobilization and drainage of secretions
- Instruct patients in home bronchial hygiene programs
- Promote relaxation to avoid muscle splinting
- Maintain and improve chest wall mobility
- Restore the most efficient breathing pattern
- Instruct and retrain the use of respiratory muscles
- Develop respiratory muscle endurance
- Prevent venous stasis
- Improve cardiopulmonary exercise tolerance
- Educate patients in every aspect of their condition so that they can take control of their own respiratory health

27% of adult males and 13% of females have symptoms of spirometric abnormalities indicative of COPD (Petty, 1978). It is very clear that the quality and duration of many lives are being affected by this disease. In effect, COPD is rapidly becoming one of the most important health problems of our time. This behooves health professions to upgrade their understanding and capacity to provide effective treatment.

A very effective treatment concept in widespread use around the world (chest physical therapy) has been meeting these needs; however, clinical experience has demonstrated that coordination of these procedures, in combination with the treatments given by other professionals (physicians, nurses, respiratory therapists, and so

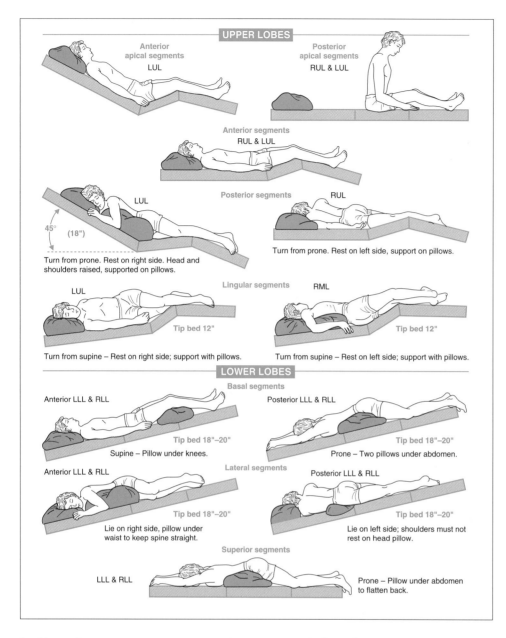

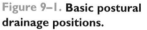

Figure 9–1. **Basic postural drainage positions.**
This figure depicts the postural drainage positions to drain various aspects of the lungs in the adult patient. (See legend for Figure 9–2 for abbreviations key.) (From White, G.C.: Basic Clinical Competencies for Respiratory Care: An Integrated Approach. Albany, NY: Delmar Publishers, 1988.)

forth) on the respiratory care service, promotes a unified approach to patient care that is more effective than the application of these techniques as separate entities (Miller, 1967).

The goals achieved by applying the physical principles and manual techniques of chest physical therapy are many. When a therapist fully understands these goals, skepticism and misunderstandings about chest physical therapy disappear. Several important treatment concepts are involved in chest physical therapy in order to accomplish the goals outlined above. The most important of these are the following: postural drainage, percussion, vibration and shaking, facilitation techniques, breathing exercise and retraining, relaxation techniques, posture correction and retraining, graded exercise, and endurance programs. A detailed discussion of all these areas is well beyond the scope of this chapter. Because our purpose here is to define and describe the contributions of massage techniques to

the treatment of patients with a respiratory disorder, the part played by methods such as percussion and vibration is presented in detail and other techniques are mentioned only briefly. The references cited earlier, together with other materials, provide excellent discussions of the general topic of cardiopulmonary physical therapy, including details of treatment techniques (Frownfelter, 1987; Frownfelter & Dean, 1996; Hillegass & Sadowsky, 1994; Irwin & Techlin 1995; Mackenzie, Imle & Ciesla 1989; Watchie 1995; Webber & Pryor 1993).

The removal of mucus (sputum) from the lungs and the proper use of the respiratory apparatus are major concerns of physical therapists' work in this area. Removal of adherent (and possibly infected) mucus requires the application of three basic techniques:

• Appropriate postural drainage

• Appropriate manual techniques to help loosen mucus

• Controlled breathing exercises and coughing to remove the mucus from the lungs

POSTURAL DRAINAGE

Postural drainage consists simply of allowing gravity to promote movement of lung secretions toward the bronchial tree and the trachea, where the patient's coughing helps expel them. Gravity both helps and hinders normal movement of lung secretions. Essentially, gravity tends to drain the upper lobes and pool secretions in the lower lobes. The constant movement of the cilia that line the respiratory passages, together with the normal cough reflex, usually ensure proper functioning of the respiratory system; however, disease or the effects of surgery may render the patient unable to expel retained mucus from the lungs. Mucus retained in the lungs is a prime nidus for infection that is costly to treat and can have serious, possibly fatal, consequences.

The technique of postural drainage requires a detailed understanding of the anatomy and physiology of the respiratory system. Placing the patient sequentially in a variety of positions makes it possible for gravity to promote cephalad flow of secretions. Positioning depends on the specific part of the lung involved. Three basic positions are used, namely, sitting upright, lying flat on the back, and lying on one side. In addition to the sitting upright position, the patient may also be "tipped" by raising one end of the bed or treatment table to an angle. Two basic tipping heights are used: a low tip is about 12 to 14 inches (30 to 35 cm), and a high tip is about 18 to 20 inches (45 to 50 cm). The high tip is used mainly to drain various parts of the lower lobes. It is the combination of positioning and tipping the patient that makes postural drainage so effective. Because a detailed description of all the postural drainage techniques is beyond the scope of this chapter, Figure 9–1 is provided and the reader is referred to other texts on the subject, including Frownfelter and Dean (1996) and Hillegass and Sadowsky (1994), excellent modern references in this area.

Certain diseases, such as cystic fibrosis, cause the production of large amounts of respiratory secretions. It is extremely important, especially in small children, that these secretions be removed daily; otherwise, the patient is likely to develop a serious chest infection. Figure 9–2 illustrates a variety of postural drainage positions suitable for the treatment of small children. (The positions illustrated in Figure 9–1 are not suitable for small children.) Watchie's book (1995) is another excellent source of information in this area.

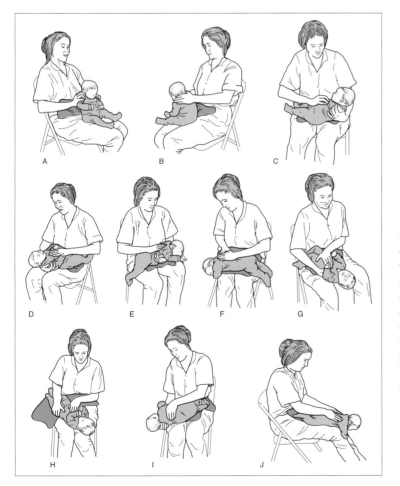

Figure 9–2. Postural drainage positions suitable for pediatric patients.
This figure depicts the postural drainage positions to drain various parts of the lungs of small children: (A) apical segments of both upper lobes (BUL); (B) posterior segment of left upper lobe (LUL); (C) anterior segment of LUL; (D) anterior segment of right upper lobe (RUL); (E) posterior segment of RUL; (F) superior, or apical, segments of both lower lobes (BLL); (G) anterior segments of BLL; (H) right middle lobe (also done on other side for lingular segment of LUL); (I) lateral segment of right lower lobe (RLL); also done on other side for lateral segment of left lower lobe (LLL); (J) posterior segments of BLL. (From Watchie, J.: Cardiopulmonary Physical Therapy—A Clinical Manual. Philadelphia: WB Saunders, 1995.)

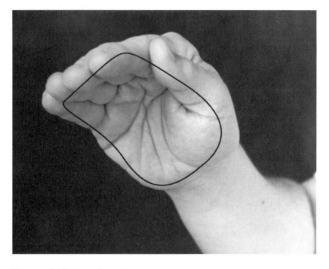

Figure 9–3. The hand in the cupped position used to perform the technique of clapping.
In this position a layer of air is trapped and compressed as the hand strikes the skin surface. A vibrating wave is set up and travels into the tissues, producing the mechanical effects that tend to loosen secretions. The line drawn on the hand represents the margins of the "cup."

PERCUSSION

The technique of clapping (or cupping) is used to help mobilize retained secretions adherent to the tracheobronchial tree. Percussion strokes send mechanical waves of vibration through the rib cage and into the lungs to shake loose adherent mucus plugs in the bronchial tree. (A mucus plug in a segmental bronchus could collapse a lung segment.) Percussion and vibration techniques, together with the proper postural drainage position, can help dislodge a plug and facilitate reexpansion of the lung

segment or lobe. Such techniques can also prevent mucus plugs from building up and closing off parts of the airway.

Percussion is performed with hands cupped (Fig. 9–3), fingers extended and held together, and wrists and arms very relaxed and loose. The hands strike the chest wall rhythmically and alternately, focusing on the area of the lung being drained. Cupping the hands provides a cushion of air between the hands and the chest wall, to mechanically deliver a shaking or vibratory movement to the lungs. This technique also serves to prevent unnecessary skin irritation or pain. Skin erythema (redness) can have several causes. If the therapist's hands are improperly cupped, a slapping or stinging effect may be produced, or too much force may be used over extremely sensitive tissues. Figure 9–4 illustrates the technique of clapping to the right lower lobe, with the patient in a high tip position. If the patient finds the technique uncomfortable, a thin towel, gown, or sheet may be placed over the area being treated. This does not significantly reduce the effectiveness of the technique but is usually much more comfortable for the patient. Figure 9–5 illustrates the use of a towel to cover the chest area during clapping.

Percussion is quite comfortable when the technique is applied properly; the rhythm and consistency of force and the direction of movement can have a relaxing effect. Generally, little force is needed for percussion; it is the cupping, not force, that is effective. The force of the percussion must be determined for each patient. For example, different amounts of force would be needed for a child, a large adult, or a frail, elderly patient who has recently had surgery. Conditions such as cystic fibrosis, atelectasis, and thick tenacious secretions may need more vigorous chest physical therapy and more percussive force to mobilize and remove secretions.

The therapist should have a plan for hand movements during percussion so that the hands do not wander

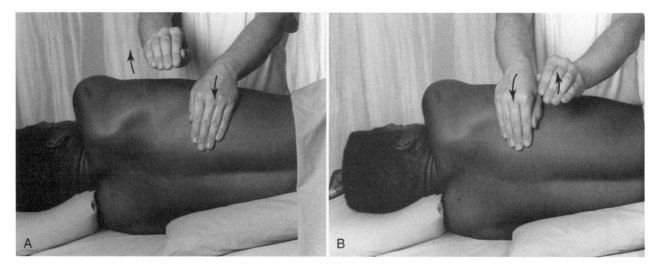

Figure 9–4. Clapping to the right lower lobe.
The patient is in the side-lying position with the foot of the bed elevated 18 to 20 inches (high tip). The wrist movements alternate during the performance of clapping to the right lower lobe.

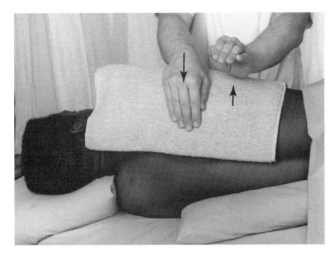

Figure 9–5. The use of a towel during the technique of clapping to the chest.
In this figure, the patient is in the side-lying position with the foot of the bed elevated 18 to 20 inches (high tip). A towel covers the anterolateral and posterolateral aspects of the chest during the performance of clapping.

aimlessly on the patient's thorax. One can work in a circular pattern or along the chest, but the pattern should be consistent throughout the treatment. Percussion should not be applied in one spot for any length of time as it becomes quite irritating. Once skin contact is made, the percussion should continue consistently for approximately 3 to 5 minutes, though the time varies according to the tolerance and needs of the patient.

Percussion should be applied only over the bony thorax. While the vibration wave spreads out into the tissues in all directions, it must be remembered that the lower margin of the lungs is adjacent to the eighth rib in the midaxillary line. When the patient is lying in the high tipped position, the pressure of the abdominal organs may push the lungs toward the neck. In short, if the objective of percussion is to affect the lungs, it is essential to perform the technique over lung tissue rather than the abdomen.

Care should be taken when applying percussion anteriorly and at the lateral basilar rib areas since the rib ends are attached loosely and sometimes not attached at all (i.e., floating ribs). The heel of the hand should not make contact with bony prominences such as the spine of the scapula, clavicles, or vertebral column or the female breast.

VIBRATION

Vibration is also used routinely with postural drainage, though it can be used with the patient in many positions. It is generally performed after percussion or alternating with it. Percussion is given to loosen adherent mucus plugs and to aid in their movement toward the bronchi and trachea, where the secretions can be coughed up or removed by suction.

Vibration is performed during the patient's *expiratory phase* of breathing. The chest is compressed simultaneously with the vibratory movement. Chest compression is extremely important in making vibration effective. The amount of chest compression is determined by several factors such as chest wall mobility, age of the patient, chest deformities, new postoperative incisions, chest trauma, or fractured ribs. In some cases the therapist may actually perform a "rib-springing" technique with the vibration, using a good deal of force in mobilizing the chest wall. This technique is possible only in a patient with a mobile thorax.

To accomplish the vibration, the patient is asked to "take a deep breath, pause for a moment, and then blow all the air out." As the patient begins to inhale, slight resistance is given to the movement of the chest wall. This encourages the patient to expand the lungs in the areas beneath the therapist's hands. The resistance offered to inspiration is gradually reduced as the peak of inhalation is reached. After a moment's pause, chest compression and vibration are performed as the patient exhales. To obtain maximum benefit, the patient is encouraged to breathe out for as long as he or she can, always within tolerance. Figure 9–6 illustrates the vibration technique.

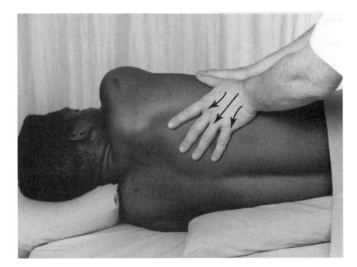

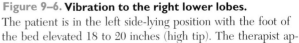

Figure 9–6. Vibration to the right lower lobes.
The patient is in the left side-lying position with the foot of the bed elevated 18 to 20 inches (high tip). The therapist applies the vibration stimulus only during the expiratory phase of the patient's breathing cycle.

The basic procedure illustrated in Figure 9–6 can be repeated several times; however, it is helpful for patients to breathe normally between each vibration session; otherwise they may become dizzy from too many deep inspirations. As the mucus loosens, the patient may wish to cough and clear the secretions. Suitable receptacles or tissues should be within easy reach. If the patient wishes to pause and attempt to cough to expel the mucus, it is often best to try this at the very end of an expiration. Certainly the patient needs to inhale and get some air behind the mucus, but the cough is likely to be more productive if given at the very end of the expiration, especially if the patient is unable to develop sufficient pressure behind the cough. It is as if the mucus is already on its way out and the cough at the end of expiration gives it the final push. This is important with very sticky mucus, because the patient can become exhausted very quickly from wasted efforts to clear mucus using an ineffective coughing technique.

To perform the vibration, the therapist tenses all arm and shoulder muscles in a co-contraction that virtually shakes the arm. He or she then transfers this shaking to the patient's chest wall. The vibration continues throughout exhalation. If a more aggressive form of chest compression and vibration (or shaking) is needed, the patient takes a deep breath and the therapist "springs" the ribs in compression three or four times during exhalation. If the patient is unable to take a deep breath on his or her own, intermittent positive-pressure breathing (IPPB) devices or a self-inflating bag technique may be used to promote deep breathing. The vibration technique is the same in both procedures. The patient is mechanically given a large breath, and vibration is performed from the peak of inhalation through the expiratory phase. Experience has demonstrated that atelectasis and pneumonia can be cleared more quickly when an ultrasonic nebulizer or heated aerosol is used one half hour before the chest physical therapy treatment, whether or not the IPPB or self-inflating bag technique is used.

The normal cough requires the patient to take a deep breath and to hold it briefly (closing the glottis and vocal cords). As the breath is held, the intrathoracic pressure is increased mainly due to the contraction of the abdominal muscles. The pressure is suddenly released (opening the glottis and vocal cords) in an explosive exhalation. The patient with an endotracheal tube cannot cough because the tube passes through the glottis and between the cords, preventing them from closing. Similarly, a tracheostomized patient has a tube below the cords and is unable to build up intrathoracic pressure by closing the glottis and cords. In either case, coughing, the major mechanism for clearing secretions, is not functioning. A cough may be simulated by using the self-inflating bag (with tracheostomy or endotracheal cuff inflated to seal off the airway), giving a large inspiratory volume, holding the bag for 2 or 3 seconds, then "popping" the bag open quickly. The therapist begins chest compression and vibration during the "hold" period of bag inflation and continues throughout the exhalation phase.

For some patients vibration may be indicated even when percussion would not be applicable. These include patients who have recently undergone surgery (including open heart surgery and thoracotomy—in which pain and splinting would be increased) and those who have hemorrhaged or fractured ribs. Generally, the same indications, contraindications, and precautions apply as for percussion. Lists of contraindications to a particular treatment are often difficult to interpret, since any one may not be a problem in *all* circumstances. In fact, the number of absolute contraindications is probably quite small. In many cases, it is appropriate to consider the items on the list as representing usual contraindications. Good clinical judgment is required to assess the risk for the individual patient. At the very least, in any given situation the therapist should certainly regard all items on the list as a definite warning to be extremely cautious and seek further medical advice.

Contraindications and Precautions for Percussion and Vibration Techniques

- Flail chest, fractured ribs
- Conditions prone to internal hemorrhage
- Conditions in which the ribs are fragile, such as metastatic bone cancer and "brittle" bones
- Frail, elderly, apprehensive patients
- Recent postoperative cases in which pain and muscle splinting would be increased
- Subcutaneous emphysema of the thorax and neck (The treatment could be ineffective since the percussion is absorbed by the subcutaneous layer of air.)
- Unstable cardiac conditions
- Lung emboli—Caution!
- Recent spinal fusion
- Recent burns, open wounds, or infection on the surface of the area

It must be emphasized that the contraindications to postural drainage, percussion, and vibration are relative. Priorities must always be considered. For example, if a patient has a poor cardiovascular function that is exacerbated by atelectasis, the atelectasis must be cleared. This situation obviously calls for proper medical judgment, advice, and support from a physician.

The indications for percussion are basically the same as those for postural drainage. Percussion may be routinely performed in conjunction with postural drainage, especially in patients with thick, infected secretions that are difficult to mobilize. A variety of devices, such as the ultrasonic nebulizer or heated aerosol, can be of tremendous benefit, especially if given just before postural drainage. This form of therapy helps liquefy secretions, making them easier to mobilize. IPPB treatments can also be administered in conjunction with postural drainage, percussion, and vibration, to distribute air peripherally. This increases the chances of getting air beyond the secretions and making the cough more productive.

Chest physical therapy has demonstrated its clinical effectiveness in treating a wide spectrum of respiratory problems whether the direct result of respiratory disease or secondary to some other medical or surgical condition—for example, spinal cord injury, cerebrovascular accident, myocardial infarction or neuromuscular disorders. These patients have common respiratory problems—poor ventilation and ineffective cough—and, as a result, retained, and often infected, lung secretions. Factors that contribute to these problems are muscle weakness or paralysis, poor co-ordination, lack of endurance, and abnormal breathing patterns.

Debilitated and dependent patients exhibit a marked decrease in general activity level, often including an inability to change basic body positions. In a bedridden patient, turning from side to side effects general postural drainage of each lung. Gravity becomes both a positive and a negative factor in lung drainage: positive in that the uppermost part of the lung is drained, negative as secretions accumulate in the dependent lobes. Thus, patients paralyzed on the right side are more likely to turn to the right because they have use of the left extremities. They find it difficult to turn to the left side and may well develop pneumonia in the right lung. Quadriplegic patients lying on their back are likely to develop bilateral posterior basal pneumonia or pneumonia in the superior segments of the lower lobes. The importance of frequent position changes for postural drainage cannot be overemphasized. These frequent changes for the paralyzed patient require a total team effort with the nursing staff.

Patients with neuromuscular disorders such as myasthenia gravis or Guillain-Barré syndrome require help in achieving or maintaining clear lungs so that they can maximize their rehabilitation. Shortness of breath is often caused by secretions in the airways. This is frightening to many patients and greatly limits their activity and progress. A program of bronchial hygiene, consisting of postural drainage, percussion, vibration, and breathing retraining, should be given before exercise. This will allow the patient

to tolerate more activity, because the airway is clear. The patient should rest after bronchial hygiene procedures as they are tiring.

Patients who receive chest physical therapy before and after surgery have demonstrated fewer respiratory complications and a shortened postoperative recovery period (Egbert et al., 1964). To gain expertise in chest physical therapy, therapists must be skilled in giving percussion and vibration, postural drainage, breathing exercises, exercise programs geared to the patient with respiratory problems, and other modalities of respiratory therapy. Though the trend today is toward ever more expensive, high-tech equipment, intelligent use of basic chest physical therapy concepts is a much more cost-effective approach in the long run, especially for patients who have chronic lung disease and wish to spend as much time as possible in their own homes.

References

Carey FE. (1967) Emphysema. The battle to breathe. U.S. Department of Health, Education and Welfare, Public Health Service Publication #1715.

Egbert LD, Battit GE, Welch, CE, Bartlett MK. (1964) Reduction of postoperative pain by encouragement and instruction of patients. N Engl J Med 270:825–827.

Frownfelter DL. (1987) Chest physical therapy and pulmonary rehabilitation: An interdisciplinary approach. Chicago: Year Book.

Frownfelter DL, Dean E. (1996) Principals and practice of cardiopulmonary physical therapy, 3rd ed. St. Louis: CV Mosby.

Hillegass EA, Sadowsky HS. (1994) Essentials of cardiopulmonary physical therapy, Philadelphia: WB Saunders.

Irwin S, Techlin JS. (1995) Cardiopulmonary physical therapy. St. Louis: CV Mosby.

Mackenzie CF, Imle PC, Ciesla N. (1989) Chest physiotherapy in the intensive care unit, 2nd ed. Baltimore: Williams & Wilkins.

Miller WF. (1967) Rehabilitation of patients with chronic obstructive lung disease. Med Clin North Am 5:349.

Petty TL. (1978) Chronic obstructive pulmonary disease. New York: Marcel Dekker.

Watchie J. (1995) Cardiopulmonary physical therapy—A clinical manual. Philadelphia: WB Saunders.

Webber BA, Pryor JA. (1993) Physiotherapy for respiratory and cardiac problems. Edinburgh: Churchill Livingstone.

Weiss, EB, et al. (1969) Acute respiratory failure in chronic obstructive lung disease. I. Pathophysiology. Disease-a-Month October.

Chapter 10

Connective Tissue Massage

Connective tissue massage (CTM; in German, *Binde-gewebsmassage)* is a total system of specialized massage techniques originally developed in Europe between the two world wars. It is a very interesting concept because it falls very nicely into the category of a treatment that produces a "remote site effect." This concept is well-known in many Eastern systems of massage and traditional methods of treatment. Intervention given to one part of the body is seen to have a profound effect on tissues apparently unrelated to the treatment site. Acupuncture, reflexology, and the more modern concept of trigger point stimulation share this conceptual foundation.

As our understanding of physiology increases, it is becoming clearer that there is a sound rationale for the use of these concepts, even though they may seem at first glance a little unlikely. CTM is a significant area of practice, deserving of a book in its own right. As with the other systems of massage described briefly in this text, the major intention is to introduce the reader to the basic concepts involved. Many massage textbooks address this topic, but the most comprehensive material on the subject in English is still probably the work of Elizabeth Dicke (1978) and Maria Ebner (1985). Other important sources of information in this area can be found in Bischoff and Elminger (1963) and Holey (1995a).

BRIEF HISTORY AND THEORETICAL FOUNDATIONS

CTM was first developed by a German physiotherapist, Elizabeth Dicke, in the late 1920s and early 1930s. Dicke was suffering from a circulatory impairment in the right leg that resulted in endarteritis obliterans of the limb. This painful condition was so severe that physicians proposed amputation. In an attempt to relieve the accompanying low back pain, Dicke discovered certain connections between the subcutaneous tissues in the posterior pelvic regions and

the affected leg. While she applied pulling strokes to the skin of her posterior pelvic region, she was aware of a sensation of warmth rushing into her leg. After 3 months of this massage (performed by a colleague) the severe symptoms began to subside. Within a year she was back to work as a physiotherapist, and much clinical study and evaluation followed this initial experience. Dicke, along with her colleagues, refined her original stroking technique to treat many pathologically involved tissues and organs. She went on to develop the method of *Bindegewebsmas-sage* (CTM) now widely used in Europe, and especially in Germany. Broadly speaking, Dicke and others claimed that this massage affects the autonomic nervous system and, by reflex action, corrects imbalances in the vegetative functions of the body. CTM is not just another massage stroke but rather a complete system of treatment that happens to use massage as a means of inducing reflex activity in various tissues.

REFLEX ZONES (HEAD'S ZONES)

It has been known since the late 1890s that visceral disease can cause changes in the skin in well-defined areas of the body. These areas are known as "Head's zones," after Head (1889), who first described them. Embryonically, the human body is derived from a series of 33 discs (33 mesodermal somites), each of which eventually gives rise to two nerve roots from the spinal cord, one on either side. In later stages of development these nerves continue to govern the activity of all structures derived from their original disc segment. These segments give rise to our concepts of dermatomes, myotomes, and scleratomes (areas, respectively, of skin, muscle, and bone that are supplied by a single nerve root). Various organs and sections of connective tissues are also supplied by each pair of segmental nerves. This gives rise to the notion of areas of representation on the posterior trunk (Fig. 10–1).

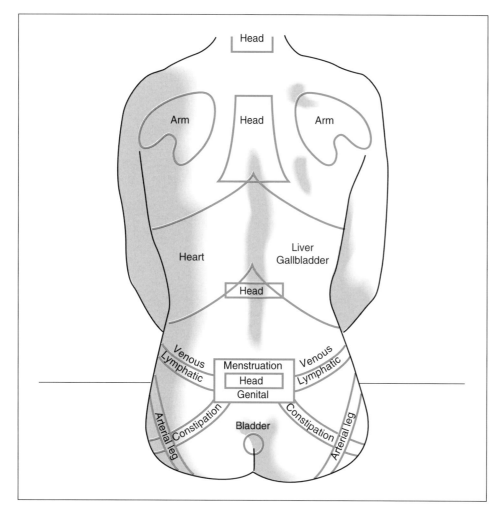

Figure 10–1. **Body areas in zones of the posterior trunk.**
The zones depicted are not complete. The intent is to show considerable overlap of zones and the functions they represent. There are zones for many parts of the body, including one for the head, zones for menstrual, genital, and colonic function, all overlying or radiating from the sacrum. These narrow bands or zones are generally described as being 5 to 8 cm wide. A stomach zone lies within the heart zone and may also be represented above the left scapula. (Modified from Ebner and Teirich-Leube.)

A key concept is that pathologic changes affecting any of the structures derived from a mesodermal somite (disc segment) may eventually give rise to symptoms in any related structures of the same segment. The fact that visceral lesions may give rise to changes in other areas is well known; for example, liver and gallbladder problems can be reflected in the right mid- to lower posterior costal segments (T 6–10) and in the right upper rectus region.

Changes that may take place in any of the related zones are detectable by palpation of the area. The connective tissues have characteristic local tension areas. There is a certain immobility of the different layers against each other where normally there would be a limited amount of movement between them (Hirschberg, Fatt, & Brown, 1986). Within each zone of influence of a spinal segment or segments, there is often a circumscribed area that is related to a particular organ; these are known as "maximal points." These changes can be detected by palpation of the area. Holey (1995b) and Holey and Watson (1995) describe the basic concepts of zone recognition and interrated reliability in the detection of these zones.

A key treatment concept in CTM is that, since visceral pathology is known to produce changes in the connective tissues of the skin in well-defined zones, treatment to the connective tissues of the skin in a defined zone might

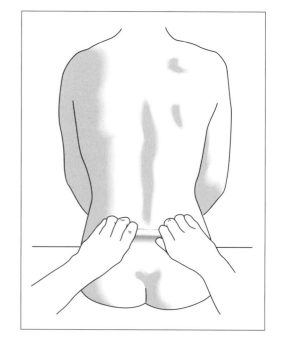

Figure 10–2. **A diagnostic stroke using a skin fold.**
The tissues are grasped to pull a roll of tissue into the hands. Lifting of skin folds is done to compare the two sides of the body. The fold of tissue must be large enough to distract the skin from the fascial layer.

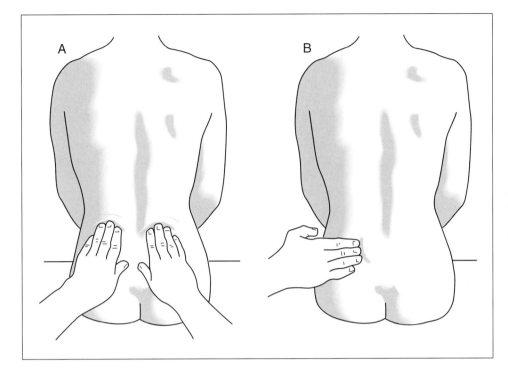

Figure 10–3. **Diagnostic techniques using the fingers to move the tissues.**
(A) Both hands are used to "push" a fold of tissue over the areas of interest. (B) The fingertips of one hand are used for the same purpose. Pressure may be exerted with one or more of the fingertips, the object being to feel the underlying tissue contours and tensions.

produce effects on other structures that are derived from the same mesodermal segment. This forms an important part of the rationale for the effects of CTM. For more detailed descriptions of the theory and practice of CTM, the reader is referred to Ebner (1962, 1965, 1968, 1978), Dicke (1978), Schliack (1978), and Ebner (1985).

Connective tissue changes on body surface areas are believed to correspond to lesions of the internal organs. These changes are often seen as flattened areas or depressed bands, which may be surrounded by elevated areas. The flattened areas are the areas of primary response and the connective tissue is tight, resisting distraction in any direction upon movement. The secondary elevated areas appear as areas of localized swelling and feel this way to the touch.

There are clearly two distinct types of stroke in CTM. One is a "diagnostic" stroke and the other a "treatment" technique. In effect, these two strokes are sometimes identical. Manual techniques are used to identify areas of connective tissue changes that may not be visible. These diagnostic techniques are used in a bilateral, symmetric fashion to compare the two sides of the body. Lifting of skin folds is performed with a deep enough fold to distract the skin from the fascial layer (Fig. 10–2).

In another technique the finger tips are used to move the skin over the underlying structures (Figs. 10–3, 10–4). The force of the finger tips is sufficient only to maintain contact with the skin and is directed in line with the reflex zones. These reflex zones have definite boundaries and locations (see Fig. 10–1).

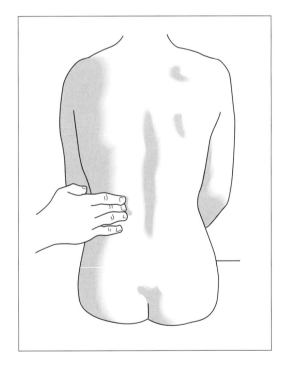

Figure 10–4. **Diagnostic techniques using the fingers of one hand to move the tissues.**
The fingertips of one hand are used for diagnostic purpose by pulling a fold of tissue under the third finger, followed by and reinforced by the fourth finger, the object being to feel the underlying tissue contours and tensions. (Note: This technique is also used for treatment using CTM, although some clinicians prefer to use the index finger reinforced by the middle one.)

Another diagnostic stroke pulls a fold of tissue under the third finger, followed by and reinforced by the fourth finger (see Fig. 10–4). Individual preference for a particular diagnostic technique determines which procedure is most effective for a given patient. All are equally acceptable. Resistance encountered during any of these manual techniques usually corresponds with a cutting or scratching sensation felt by the patient. The therapist may feel a tearing sensation if the movement is carried too far. The illustration of visceral reflex zones is included here to alert the therapist to those instances when traditional massage techniques reveal areas with no apparent peripheral pathology.

Anecdotally, this method of massage seems to have a profound influence on autonomic function. Applied skillfully, it can be directed to specific pathologic conditions with predictable results (Frazer, 1978); however, Reed and Held (1988) were not able to demonstrate changes in autonomic function in a range of healthy, middle-aged and elderly patients. Of course, there is likely to be considerable difference between the responses detected in patients who have a demonstrated problem and in those who are healthy.

All massage techniques require skill and experience on the part of the practitioner if they are to be maximally effective. Such skill must be developed under the supervision of an experienced therapist; it cannot be learned from a textbook. The basic concepts, however, can be learned from reliable sources. In this regard, Ebner's descriptions of the techniques are excellent. Bischoff and Elminger (1963), Teirich-Leube (1976), and Tappen (1988) also offer excellent descriptions and illustrations.

BASIC TECHNIQUE

The patient sits on a firm surface with the hips and knees at right angles and the feet supported on a stool. The whole of the back must be exposed, but the anterior aspect of the patient may be covered during evaluation and treatment. The therapist may sit or stand behind the patient, whichever is most comfortable or suitable. No lubricant should be used.

Treatment begins with an examination of the skin of the patient's back. Careful observation of the posture and muscles is undertaken, together with careful palpation of the cutaneous structures. Some zones may appear swollen, whereas others may seem drawn in. Diagnostic palpation may reveal tightness and tissue tension in certain areas of the back. These areas are often unilateral and fairly well-defined. The object of the examination is to map out the areas of abnormal contour and relate these to the patient's other signs and symptoms, but the evaluation itself may have a profound effect on the patient's autonomic nervous system (Kisner & Taslitz, 1968).

Following the initial examination, treatment proper may begin. Two types of strokes are usually performed—short and long. These strokes always start in the sacral, gluteal, or lumbar region, in that order. Strokes progress upward and outward to the affected zones as soon as possible. Ebner suggests that "the interrelation of all autonomically supplied structures makes it advisable to start every treatment in the sacral area, to make certain of a normal vascular reaction at the root of the autonomic supply tree. It is, however, important to progress as soon as possible into the affected segments." The strokes are produced by a tangential pull of the middle finger supported by either the ring or the index finger. Some practitioners prefer to use the index finger supported by the middle one.

CTM techniques can be practiced on most areas of the body, not only the back; however, it is common for treatment to be given to the back and to a more peripheral body part. While a detailed discussion of this technique for all body parts is beyond the scope of this text, several excellent works describe the basic concepts of CTM and its use in most parts of the body. Although last published in the mid 1980s, Maria Ebner's book (1985) on CTM remains arguably the most authoritative source on this topic in the English language.

EFFECTS

The patient usually feels either a cutting or a scratching sensation, or possibly dull pressure. These responses gradually fade as the patient recovers from the condition. Local and general responses are produced.

Local Responses

The most obvious response to CTM is the local response visible over the treated areas. After several minutes, bright red strips appear on the skin, tracing the areas where the therapist has applied pressure. This local erythema (redness) is the result of a triple response produced in the tissues. The pressure of the fingers on the tissues produces minor trauma to the area, and this releases various substances that trigger the reflex. Release of histamine, together with other substances, produces the marked vasodilatation of the area.

General Responses

The general response to CTM varies greatly, particularly depending on which areas are stimulated. General responses consistent with an effect on the autonomic nervous system last several hours after treatment: stimulation of the circulation, reduced blood pressure (with extensive treatment), shortness of breath, heart palpitations, headache, dizziness, perspiration, increased glandular activity, increased visceral organ function, and rebalancing of autonomic activity by stimulation of parasympathetic activity.

Treatment Indications

CTM has diagnostic and therapeutic implications and has been used clinically to treat the signs and symptoms of circulation disorders, rheumatic diseases, malfunctions of internal organs, autonomic and central nervous system disorders, respiratory conditions, and connective tissue disorders. CTM has been widely used in the treatment of autonomic disturbances of the cardiovascular system. Reflex sympathetic dystrophy (RSD) is an excellent example of such a condition, though our present understanding of this syndrome is far from complete (Fialka, Sadil, & Ernst, 1991).

Treatment Duration and Frequency

Following the initial examination at each treatment session, the treatment proper may begin. Each session usually consists of a general back treatment followed by specific treatment to various zones or parts of the back or other body areas. Treatment may be repeated daily for approximately 10 to 12 treatments. Some patients occasionally require longer courses of treatment (several weeks); alternatively, others may show significant improvement within a few days of commencing treatment.

Contraindications

The relatively few contraindications to CTM are certain cardiac conditions, certain generalized skin conditions affecting the back (e.g., psoriasis), cancer or tuberculosis, very hairy skin on the back (maybe too painful), open wounds, sores, or other skin lesions over the area to be treated.

SUMMARY

The use of CTM undoubtedly requires special knowledge and experience to be maximally effective. Like most, if not all, modern rehabilitation practices, CTM is likely to achieve the best results when used in combination with other techniques in a total treatment plan tailored to the individual patient. Although CTM is not now well-known or popular in North America, it is possible that it could enjoy a surge of interest, especially if combined with other treatment approaches.

References

Bischoff I, Elminger G. (1963) Connective tissue massage. In: Licht S (ed): Massage, manipulation and traction. Baltimore: Waverley Press.
Dicke E. (1978) Origin and development of the method. In: Dicke E, et al. (eds): A manual of reflexive therapy of the connective tissues. Scarsdale, NY: Sidney S. Simon, pp 11–143.
Ebner M. (1962) Connective tissue massage: Theory and therapeutic application. Edinburgh: E & S Livingstone.
Ebner M. (1965) Connective tissue massage. South Afr J Physiother 21(3):4–7.
Ebner M. (1968) Connective tissue massage: Therapeutic application. N Z J Physiother 3(14):18–22.
Ebner M. (1978) Connective tissue massage. Physiotherapy JCSP 64:208–210.
Ebner M.(1985) Connective tissue massage. Theory and therapeutic application, 2nd ed. Huntington, NY: Robert E. Krieger.
Fialka V, Sadil V, Ernst E. (1991) Reflex sympathetic dystrophy (RSD)—a century of investigation and still a mystery. Eur J Phys Med Rehab 2(2):26–28.
Frazer F. (1978) Persistent postsympathetic pain treated by connective tissue massage. Physiotherapy JCSP 64:211–212.
Head H. (1889) Die Sensibilitätsstörungen der Haut bei viszeral Erkrankungen. Berlin.
Hirschberg G, Fatt I, Brown RD. (1986) Measurement of skin mobility in the upper back. Scand J Rehab Med 18(4):173–175.
Holey EA. (1995a) Connective tissue zones: An introduction. Physiotherapy JCSP 8(7):366–368.
Holey EA. (1995b) Connective tissue manipulation—towards a scientific rationale. Physiotherapy JCSP 81(12):730–739.
Holey EA, Watson M. (1995) Inter-rater reliability of connective tissue zones recognition. Physiotherapy JCSP 81(7):369–372.
Kisner C, Taslitz N. (1968) Connective tissue massage: Influence of the introductory treatment on autonomic functions. Phys Ther 48(2):107–119.
Reed B, Held, J. (1988) Effects of sequential connective tissue massage on autonomic nervous system of middle-aged and elderly adults. Phys Ther 68(8):1231–1234.
Schliack H. (1978) Theoretical bases of the working mechanism of connective tissue massage. In Dicke E, et al. (eds): A manual of reflexive therapy of the connective tissues. Scarsdale, NY: Sidney S Simon, pp 14–33.
Tappen FM. (1988) Healing massage techniques: Holistic, classic, and emerging methods, 2nd ed. Norwalk, CT: Appleton & Lange, pp 219–254.
Teirich-Leube H. (1976) Grondbeginselen van de Bindweefselmassage. Uitgeversmaatchappij Lochem: De Tijdstroon, B. V.

Chapter 11

Specialized Systems of Massage

COLLEEN LISTON, Ph.D.

Alternative medicine encompasses a range of systems and incorporates various techniques of massage. The Research Council for Complementary Medicine (Australia) has been promoting vigorous research into the efficacy and use of techniques such as acupuncture, acupressure and shiatsu, reflexology, hypnosis, Eastern massage systems, and moxibustion for more than 10 years (Vickers, 1995). Surveys of Western medical practitioners in the Netherlands, Great Britain, New Zealand, the United States, and (most recently) Canada have highlighted a growing interest in and willingness to accept alternative or complementary medicine (Eisenberg et al., 1993; Hadley, 1988; Lynöe & Svensson, 1992; Verhoef & Sutherland, 1995; Wharton & Lewith, 1986)). This is particularly the case in the management of chronic pain and musculoskeletal dysfunction. The most widely accepted techniques are those that appear to be more efficacious, such as acupuncture, the deep pressure employed in acupressure or shiatsu, manipulations applied by chiropractors, or stretching like that used in myofascial methods.

This chapter and Chapter 12 look at some of the massage techniques that fall into the alternative or complementary medicine spectrum. The "body therapies," as many of the complementary techniques are called, include acupressure, acupuncture, applied kinesiology, chiropractic, deep muscle therapy, Feldenkrais, Hellerwork, Huna techniques, integrated psychophysical balancing, Lomi, massage (various systems), myotherapy, myofascial techniques, neuromuscular release or technique, orthobionomy, osteopathy, polarity therapy, point percussion therapy, postural integration, reflexology, reiki, rolfing or structural integration, shiatsu, therapeutic touch, Tragerwork, trigger point techniques, zone therapy, and others.

The proliferation of alternative practitioners within and without these established systems (which include massage to a lesser or greater extent) is evidence of dissatisfaction with established medical model methods of treatment and prevention (Jahnke, 1985). Not all systems can be included in this text. In this chapter we present trigger point massage, myofascial techniques, and reflexology and briefly discuss the lesser-known techniques of point percussion therapy and rolfing. In Chapter 12 we discuss Eastern systems of massage—acupressure, shiatsu, traditional Thai massage, traditional Chinese massage, and Huna massage.

Contraindications for all massage techniques were presented earlier. It is nevertheless important to note that, when autonomic responses may be elicited, such as with connective tissue massage, acupressure or shiatsu, or trigger point or myofascial techniques, contraindications include pregnancy (because of the autonomic response), serious cardiorespiratory conditions, and psychological disorders such as panic attacks.

TRIGGER POINT TECHNIQUES

Myofascial pain syndrome, often confused with fibromyalgia, is characterized by musculoskeletal pain that originates from a hyperirritable spot (Hey & Helewa, 1994; Waylonis et al., 1988; Yunus et al., 1988). These so-called trigger points—called "myofascial triggers" by Janet Travell and "myodysneuric points" by Dr. R. Gutstein—are sensitive points or areas that produce pain some distance away (Travell, 1981; Travell & Simons, 1983, 1992). Active trigger points produce referred pain when palpated: they "trigger" the painful experience. There may be localized sharp pain that may radiate to the referred, or target, area some distance away. Any or all of the signs or phenomena in the following list may be associated with sensitivity at the point:

- Movement restriction
- Muscle weakness
- Protective muscle spasm
- Lowered skin resistance
- Fibrositic nodules

- The "jump" sign on palpation
- Secondary trigger points in agonistic and antagonistic muscles (overloaded through "splinting" the injured muscle in compensation)
- Autonomic responses

Figure 11–1 illustrates the sites of common trigger points and associated muscle groups. The referred pain and motor, sensory, and autonomic responses are ameliorated

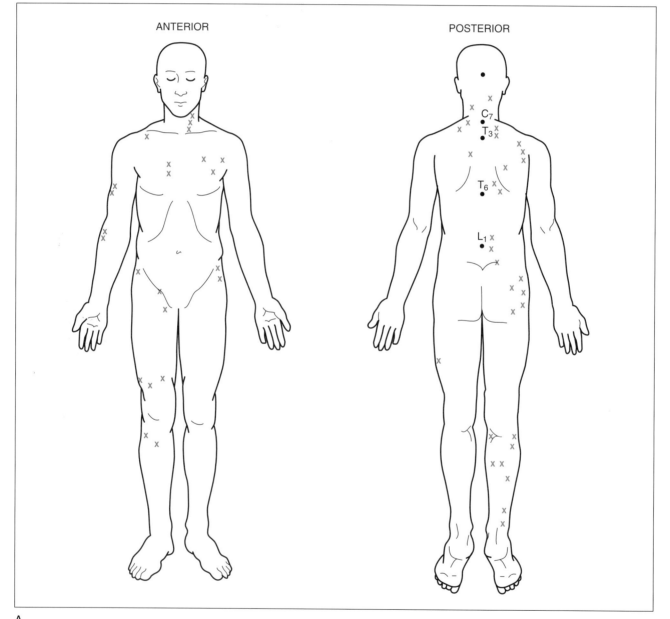

A

Figure 11–1. Common trigger points.
(A) The common sites of trigger points in the body. (B) The muscles associated with these points.

by releasing (desensitizing) the active primary point, so the treatment of trigger points can be a useful adjunct to treatment of chronic musculoskeletal conditions (Laing et al., 1973; Lundberg et al., 1984). Careful palpation and awareness of acupuncture points assist in the assessment of related soft tissues (Fischer, 1988; Goldenberg, 1989). The trigger point sustained pressure may be given with one finger, two or more fingers, a knuckle, an elbow, or by "strumming" (as in applying connective tissue massage)

with the fingers extended (Manheim & Lavett, 1989; Peppard, 1983; Travell & Simons, 1983).

A home program incorporating postisometric relaxation can be used to maintain gains after trigger point treatment. This should involve stretching gently to resistance, contracting against gentle pressure for 10 seconds, maintaining this range and relaxing, then gently, passively taking up the "slack" to gain greater range. The cycle should be repeated three to five times and may be used

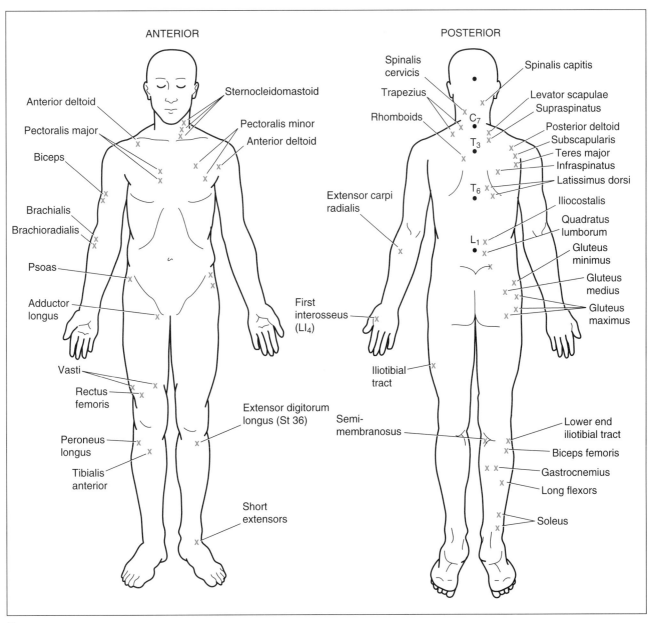

B

Figure 11-1. *Continued*

Treatment regime for trigger points

- Localize the trigger point. It will be found in tight or taut fascial or muscular bands. It may be in the skin (scar tissue), a ligament, a tendon, or even deeper, at the joint capsule or periosteal level. Knowledge of acupuncture points helps locate the point, as about 70% of trigger points are in corresponding sites.
- Treat more recent injuries and the generated primary trigger first; then work on older injuries. More secondary triggers will be associated with chronic injuries.
- Rapid icing with the edge of an ice block or parallel sweeps of vapocoolant spray given at the rate of 4 cm per second holding the can 50 cm away from the skin (Mance et al., 1986; Simons, 1985; Wolfe, 1988). Simons (1985) claims that Fluori-Methane sprays are safe.
- Apply gentle sustained stretch; with relaxation, the muscle lengthens.
- Apply 1 minute of sustained pressure (as for acupressure) over the trigger point. Increase the depth gradually or apply deep pressure intermittently, alternating with slight release.
- Ice or spray again.

with self-administered trigger point stimulation (Chaitow, 1981). Active trigger points may also be desensitized using some form of electrical stimulation (Alon & De Domenico, 1987) or other electrophysical agents.

MYOFASCIAL RELEASE TECHNIQUES

The type of gain in range referred to is achieved by myofascial release. Fascia, a type of connective tissue, has three layers—superficial, potential space, and deep. It assists in maintaining muscle force, and, whereas fasciotomy to release tight fascia results in a 15% loss of muscle strength, myofascial release techniques reduce constriction and pain without compromising muscle strength (Manheim & Lavett, 1989). Myofascial release, in conjunction with trigger point stimulation, is vital because the fascia tightens and shortens with inflammation (as the potential space swells), heals slowly (because of a poor blood supply), and is a pain focus (because of its abundant nerve supply).

Because the goal of myofascial release is optimal alignment of the body; proper assessment and reassessment of postural alignment are essential. Manheim and

Lavett (1989) provide postural assessment methods and a detailed description of techniques of myofascial release. During myofascial release the awareness of the effect of tension and release of tissues provides feedback between therapist and client and is a key factor. The application of the technique relies on the therapist's receiving feedback from the client's body. The response depends on the ability to interpret correctly the feedback about how long, how strong, and in which direction to give pressure. The technique is one of the body therapies that embraces the concept of integration and is akin to techniques such as rolfing and other forms of postural and structural integration.

For this technique the relaxed hands and outer fingers of the therapist are placed at each extreme of muscle attachments. The client is encouraged to relax. Firm pressure is applied using the body's weight to provide stretch along the fibers of the muscle for about 10 seconds and then is eased. The slack should be taken up and further stretch applied. After three to five repetitions the stretch should be released slowly and the client reassessed. This process may be repeated up to five times, depending on progress as gauged by the reassessment.

The following assumptions about myofascial techniques prevail:

- They are successful even though no relation to a neurophysiologic mechanism has been proven.
- Feedback ensures greater efficacy and comfort than traditional methods afford.
- There are no restrictions, either from the patient or the therapist, when feedback is correctly interpreted.
- Safety is ensured by the fact that client and therapist work together.

The role of myoglobin in myofascial pain and its dispersion (and associated pain relief) by massage techniques have been studied (Brendstrup et al., 1957; Danneskiold-Samsøe et al., 1982, 1986; Krusen et al., 1965; Simons, 1990). Ronald Melzack (1985) has reported on the similarity of the neural mechanisms involved in the relief of pain produced by acupuncture, acupressure, ice massage, and trigger point stimulation. This hyperstimulation analgesia is one of the oldest recorded remedies and should become a useful technique for relieving pain of musculoskeletal lesions, especially when chronic conditions have affected posture, gait, and other activities (Ehrett, 1988; Friction et al., 1985; Friedmann, 1989; Ingber, 1989; Kine & Warfield, 1986). The presence of type C nociceptors and adaptive shortening in the muscles and fascia contribute to the pain of chronic disorders (Reynolds, 1981; Rubin, 1981). Mobilization of peripheral nerves and breaking down of adhesions in the fascia that is continuous with nerve roots promotes pain relief. Attention to dysfunctional biomechanics, which may have been present before an injury or developed since, is an important component of treatment.

ROLFING

It is relevant to include a system of massage that combines deep pressure to trigger points in muscles with myofascial stretches along the muscles to achieve structural integration. Rolfing involves very deep massage strokes akin to those used in connective tissue massage. They are applied to trigger points using the thumbs, the elbows, the heels of the hands, and even the knees. Deep strokes and intense pulling on the soft tissues provoke acute and intense erythema—and often local bleeding. Severe discomfort for the client is an unfavorable side effect, and some may experience a cathartic response and intense negative psychological effects such as depression and anxiety. Rolfing is seldom used and should be chosen advisedly because less vigorous techniques claim a similar neurophysiologic effect and achieve the desired pain relief and soft tissue mobilization to integrate relationships between structures and return them to their normal alignment.

REFLEXOLOGY

Based on the principle of reflex points on the feet and (to a lesser extent) hands corresponding to organs and other structures, reflexology, or reflex zone therapy, dates back to folk law in China and India around 5000 years ago. Having not been used actively over many centuries, the Rwo-Shr method re-emerged in the Republic of China (Taiwan) this century (Adamson, 1994). There is evidence of its use in Egypt more than 2000 years b.c., and in Europe, a book on the topic was written in 1582 (Sahai, 1993). Two of the most influential contemporary contributors to the revival of interest in reflexology were Americans, an ear, nose, and throat specialist, Dr. William Fitzgerald, in the early 1900s, and a physical therapist, Eunice Ingham, in the 1930s. They undertook research into the therapeutic use of pressure and found that it relieved pain in areas of the body that corresponded to zones identified on the feet (Ingham, 1938/1984). Crystalline deposits were found at nerve ending sites in the feet and hands, and they were thought to reflect disease in the corresponding organ or area of the body. It is interesting to note that Fitzgerald claimed that the body could be divided into 10 longitudinal zones. This concept relates to the 10 main lines in traditional Thai massage. Furthermore, some authors suggest that the energy channels, or meridians, of acupuncture and the zones of reflexology correspond (Dougans & Ellis, 1991). One of Ms. Ingham's students, Doreen Bayly, introduced reflexology into the United Kingdom in the 1960s (Bayly, 1982). In 1973, The International Institute of Reflexology was founded in the United States, and there are other associations in various countries (Adamson, 1994).

It is claimed that applying pressure systematically to reflex areas on the feet clears "congested energy channels" and returns the body to homeostasis. That is, the natural healing powers of the body are summoned, toxins are cleared in the circulation of blood and lymph, and flow in the indefinable "energy channels" (Booth, 1994) is restored.

The same relaxing benefits of a full body massage are attributed to reflexology techniques. Indeed, Thomas (1989) reports reduced anxiety levels in elderly patients, and a calm feeling with a desire to sleep is described by Lockett (1992). In a randomized controlled study of 35 women with premenstrual syndrome Oleson and Flocco (1993) found that reflexology techniques decreased symptoms significantly ($P < .01$) as compared with that from a placebo. The women reported that the principal benefit was relaxation; many fell asleep during the 30-minute session. Greater energy on the following day was reported, and subjects continued to feel more relaxed 2 months after the study.

The soles of the feet and the palms of the hand are divided into zones. For example, the posterior medial heel corresponds to the prostate, whereas the posterior lateral heel relates to the ovary. Centrally, farther forward but still over the calcaneum, is the sciatic nerve zone. The medial border of the foot represents the spinal column: the cervical spine is at the base of the great toe and the coccyx at the upper part of the calcaneum. The great toe is related to the head, the pineal and pituitary glands, and the sinuses; the throat "lies" over the metatarsophalangeal joint. On the medial two toes are the eye zones; the fourth and fifth toes correspond to the ear. Over the metatarsal heads, from medial to lateral, are the thyroid and parathyroid glands, the bronchial tree, the chest, and the lungs, respectively. Beneath the thyroid and parathyroid are the stomach and then the pancreas zone. The heart, spleen, kidney, and central nervous system are in zones in the center of the foot, the liver along the lateral border below the metatarsal heads, and the ascending (right foot) and descending (left foot) colon down the remainder of the lateral border to the calcaneum. The bladder is represented in the medial arch, and the sigmoid colon along the anterior border of the calcaneum.

On the palms of the hands, the spinal column runs from the outer border of the proximal phalanx of the thumb (the cervical spine) to the wrist. Again, the representation mirrors that found on the feet, from the tips of the fingers to the proximal aspect of the wrist, where the ovary or prostate zone is situated. The various body parts represented on the sole of the foot and the palm of the hand are subjects of considerable research. Omura (1995), in a lengthy review of the topic, describes this concept in detail and is an excellent source of information. There are a number of different "maps" of the areas representing different body parts, and two of these are illustrated in Figure 11–2. Illustrations of the zones can be found in many texts and articles (Booth, 1994; Downing, 1974; Hillman, 1986; Lidell, 1984; Omura, 1994; Tappan, 1988).

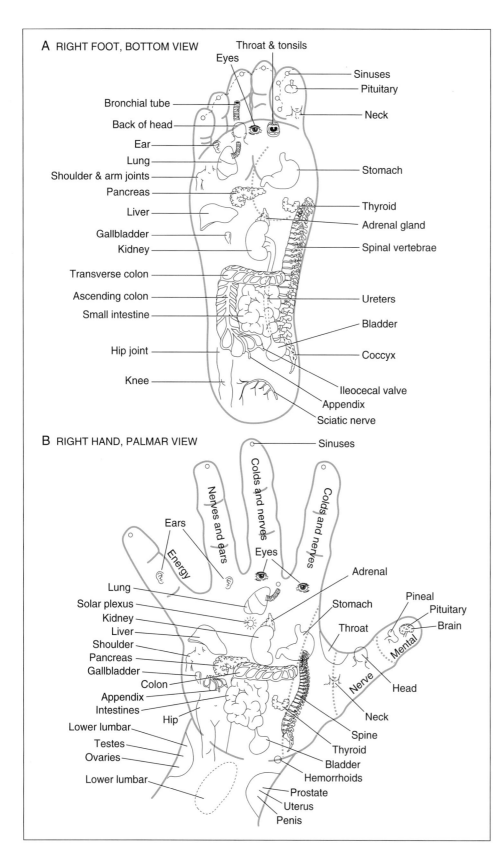

A RIGHT FOOT, BOTTOM VIEW

Throat & tonsils
Eyes
Sinuses
Pituitary
Bronchial tube
Neck
Back of head
Ear
Lung
Shoulder & arm joints
Pancreas
Stomach
Liver
Thyroid
Gallbladder
Adrenal gland
Kidney
Spinal vertebrae
Transverse colon
Ascending colon
Ureters
Small intestine
Bladder
Hip joint
Coccyx
Knee
Ileocecal valve
Appendix
Sciatic nerve

B RIGHT HAND, PALMAR VIEW

Sinuses
Nerves and ears
Colds and nerves
Colds and nerves
Ears
Energy
Eyes
Adrenal
Lung
Pineal
Solar plexus
Pituitary
Kidney
Stomach
Brain
Liver
Throat
Shoulder
Pancreas
Mental
Gallbladder
Colon
Nerve
Appendix
Head
Intestines
Neck
Hip
Spine
Lower lumbar
Thyroid
Testes
Bladder
Ovaries
Hemorrhoids
Lower lumbar
Prostate
Uterus
Penis

Figure 11–2. A "map" of various body parts on the sole of the foot (A) and the palm of the hand (B), used in reflexology.
(From Tappan, F.M.: Healing massage techniques: Holistic, classic and emerging methods, 2nd ed. Norwalk, CT: Appleton & Lange, 1988.)

Reflexology involves an initial assessment of the feet, to feel for tender areas and signs of thickening or tension. The therapist also checks for calluses, corns, hard skin, and signs of skin disruption secondary to peripheral vascular disease or diabetes. Individual reflex zones are given more attention if they are tender, but an overall reflexology session lasts between 30 and 40 minutes. The client should be seated in a reclining chair or with the feet elevated on a stool. The therapist sits in a comfortable well-supported position facing the soles of the feet. The thumb and index finger are most often used to move in the manner of a caterpillar, across the reflex zones.

A typical treatment begins with relaxation, using three techniques on each foot. First, the palms and fingers of each hand cradle both borders of the foot. Pressure is applied to push forward with the palm of one hand while pulling backward with the fingers of the other; then the pushing and pulling are reversed to rotate the foot alternately into inversion and eversion. Contact should be maintained at all times. Next, the metatarsals are held firmly with one hand, ensuring that the ball of the thumb is placed in the transverse arch. The other hand grasps the toes and flexes them over the thumb, working it sequentially along the base of the metatarsophalangeal joints from medial to lateral. The third technique used to accustom the client to having the feet handled and to promote relaxation is rotation of the ankle. Supporting the heel in the contralateral hand, the therapist holds around the outside of the lateral malleolus with the thumb to stabilize the leg, grasps the medial side of the toes and foot, and rotates it in alternate directions a few times, moving through dorsiflexion, pronation, plantar flexion, and supination. These three introductory techniques are repeated on the other foot.

The treatment involves alternately holding with one hand and manipulating with the other. The thumbs are used on the soles to press into the reflex zones, while the other hand and fingers work the foot over the thumb. Bending the joints of the thumb allows it to "walk" forward and backward over a point, much like the movement of a caterpillar. A hooking stroke with the thumb, akin to a short stroke in connective tissue massage, is used on tougher areas on the heel. In the forefoot, the phalanges and metatarsals can be rotated over the thumb. The index fingers can be used to "walk" along the toes and to flex and extend them.

Beginning with the toes, the therapist works systematically through the zones to the heel. In the hand, he or she works from the finger tips to the wrist. Specific techniques for each zone are suggested in texts on reflexology, especially Ingham's revised work. It is not within the scope of this text to provide prescriptive details; our intention is but to introduce the concepts and basic techniques.

POINT PERCUSSION THERAPY

To apply point percussion therapy, familiarity with both Western and Eastern techniques is required. In particular, a knowledge of traditional Chinese medicine facilitates understanding the rationale and mechanisms involved.

Principles of Therapy

Positioning of the Muscles and Soft Tissues

- Sustained stretch (for inhibition)
- Placement of postural muscles in middle to inner range, of phasic muscles in outer range or on stretch (both for facilitation)

Techniques

- To achieve inhibition, slow, deep and penetrating massage is used in a regular and soothing manner.
- To achieve facilitation, fast, light changing and stimulating massage is used.

In each case it is important to concentrate on the rhythm.

General Techniques

- General massage using effleurage
- Picking up (with one hand or both)
- Circular kneading (using the web space, four fingers or the whole palm, one hand, or both hands)
- Clapping using a slightly cupped, relaxed palm
- Shaking (for each muscle bulk)
- Squeezing (for each muscle bulk)

Specific Techniques

For localized sites such as trigger points or acupuncture points, the following specific treatment techniques can be applied to the points or areas of tightness:

- Cross fibers techniques (transverse deep friction using a thumb or index finger)
- Pressure techniques (using a thumb or index or middle finger reinforced with other fingers) by any of the following methods: press in and release, press in and rotate, press in and vibrate (upward and downward to each side of the point)
- Percussion using a tapping movement:
  One finger (the index or middle finger reinforced with other fingers) is used. The movement comes mainly from the wrist.
  Three fingers held together (thumb, index and middle fingers). This is a medium to strong tapping, and the movement comes from the elbow.
  Five fingers held together—with all the fingers held together, the tapping is very strong, with the movement coming from the shoulder and elbow.
  It is recommended to begin more gently, and progress to the stronger technique.
- Knocking achieved by using the fingers held loosely in a line. The movement is carried out in the line of the meridians or channels.
- Pinching with the thumb and index finger, either involving a pinch and release or a pinch and rotational or vibrating movement.
- Flicking, a specific technique for the fingers and toes from the sides of the fingers and toes to the tips on the anterior and posterior aspects of the nail roots to the tips.

General Sequence

An application of point percussion therapy for a child with cerebral palsy, aimed to inhibit muscle spasticity, could be undertaken using the following sequence:

1. The therapist assesses the child thoroughly, analyzes the findings in relation to spasticity, and plans a treatment program based on priorities.

2. If there is limited range of motion in a joint, the therapist assesses the focus of the restriction or tightness of muscles.

3. The spastic muscle is slowly positioned in a sustained stretch posture.

4. The therapist prepares the muscle by using a general massage technique. Effleurage, picking up, kneading, clapping, shaking, or squeezing may be used, depending on the body part.

5. The therapist selects and locates the acupuncture points according to the priorities in relation to spasticity (for example, points at or near the joint, muscle, tendon, or other soft tissue structures; points for analgesic effect; or stimulation of "energy flow" [chi] along the channels or meridians).

6. Using specific techniques to press the acupuncture points, the therapist performs deep frictions to any trigger points or area of tightness, concentrating on rhythm.

7. Percussion (using three fingers) is performed, moving downward along the meridians, and including all of those relevant to the area to be treated. Concentrating on the acupuncture points or area of tightness, the therapist applies percussion a few more times.

8. More stretching is applied as soon as the muscle relaxes.

9. Massage is applied to clear the "channels" and disperse tension.

10. Stimulation massage or percussion is directed to the antagonistic muscle group.

11. The sequence is repeated three to five times, depending on the condition.

12. The child is asked to contract the antagonistic muscle group or is positioned so as to facilitate contraction of the muscle.

Point percussion therapy may be used for intellectual stimulation (when applied to the head); for epilepsy and other systemic disorders; around specific joints; and on the trunk (Jia, 1984; Wang, 1991).

References and Bibliography

Introduction

Eisenberg DM, Kessler RC, Foster C, Norlock FE, Calkins DR, Delbanco TL. (1993) Unconventional medicine in the United States. Prevalence, costs and patterns of use. N Engl J Med 328:246.

Hadley CM. (1988) Complementary medicine and the general practitioner: A survey of general practitioners in the Wellington area. NZ Med J 101:766.

Jahnke R. (1985) The body therapies. J Holistic Nurs 3(1):7–14.

Lynöe N, Svensson T. (1992) Physicians and alternative medicine, an investigation of attitudes and practice. Scand J Social Med 20:55.

Verhoef MJ, Sutherland LR. (1995) General practitioners' interest in alternative medicine in Canada. Social Sci Med 41(4):511–515.

Vickers A. (1995) Research in complementary medicine and the work of the RCCM. Midwives, January: 14–16.

Wharton R, Lewith G. (1986) Complementary medicine and the general practitioner. Br Med J 292:1498.

Trigger Point Techniques

Alon G, De Domenico G. (1987) High voltage stimulation—an integrated approach to clinical practice. Chattanooga: Chattanooga Corp.

Chaitow L. (1981) Instant pain control. Northamptonshire: Thorsons.

Fischer AA. (1988) Documentation of myofascial trigger points. Arch Phys Med Rehab 69:286–291.

Goldenberg DL. (1989) Treatment of fibromyalgia syndrome. Rheum Dis Clin North Am 15(1):61–71.

Hey LR, Helewa A. (1994) Myofascial pain syndrome: A critical review of the literature. Physiother Can 46(1): 28–36.

Laing DR, Dalley DR, Kirk JA. (1973) Ice therapy in soft tissue injuries. NZ Med J 78(8):155–158.

Lundberg T, Nordemar R, Ottoson D. (1984) Pain alleviation by vibratory stimulation. Pain 20:25–44.

Mance D, McConnell B, Ryan PA, Silverman M, Master G. (1986) Myofascial pain syndrome. J Am Podiatr Med Assoc 76(6):328–331.

Manheim CJ, Lavett DK. (1989) The myofascial release manual. Thorofare, NJ: Slack.

Peppard A. (1983) Trigger-point massage therapy. Phys Sports Med 1(5):59–162.

Simons DG. (1985) Myofascial pain syndromes due to trigger points: Treatment and single-muscle syndromes. Manual Med 1:72–77.

Travell JG, Simons DG. (1983) Myofascial pain and dysfunction: The trigger point manual, Vol I. Baltimore: Williams & Wilkins.

Travell JG, Simons DG. (1992) Myofascial pain and dysfunction: The trigger point manual, Vol II. Baltimore: Williams & Wilkins.

Wolfe F. (1988) Fibrositis, fibromyalgia and musculo-skeletal disease: The current status of fibrositis syndrome. Arch Phys Med Rehab 69:527–531.

Myofascial Techniques

Brendstrup P, Jespersen K, Asboe-Hansen G. (1957) Morphological and chemical connective tissue changes in fibrositic muscles. Ann Rheum Dis 16:438–440.

Danneskiold-Samsøe B, Christiansen E, Lund B, Anderson RB. (1982) Regional muscle tension and pain ("fibrositis"). Scand J Rehab Med 15:17–20.

Danneskiold-Samsøe B, Christiansen E, Anderson RB. (1986) Myofascial pain and the role of myoglobin. Scand J Rheumatol 15:175–178.

Ehrett SL. (1988) Craniosacral therapy and myofascial release in entry-level physical therapy curricula. Phys Ther 68(4):534–540.

Friction JR, Kroening R, Haley D, Siegert R. (1985) Myofascial pain syndrome of the head and neck: A review of clinical characteristics of 164 patients. Oral Surg 60(6):615–623.

Friedmann LW. (1989) [Letter to the Editor.] Am J Phys Med Rehab 68(5):257–258.

Ingber RS. (1989) Iliopsoas myofascial dysfunction: A treatable cause of "failed" low back syndrome. Arch Phys Med Rehab 70:382–385.

Kine GD, Warfield CA. (1986) Myofascial pain syndrome. Hosp Pract 21(9):194–196.

Krusen FH, Kottke FJ, Ellwood PM. (1965) Handbook of physical medicine and rehabilitation. Philadelphia: WB Saunders.

Manheim CG, Lavett DK. (1989) The myofascial release manual. Thorofare, NJ: Slack.

Melzack R. (1981) Myofascial trigger points: Relation to acupuncture and mechanisms of pain. Arch Phys Med Rehab 62:114–117.

Reynolds MD. (1981) Myofascial trigger point syndromes in the practice of rheumatology. Arch Phys Med Rehab 62:111–114.

Rubin D. (1981) Myofascial trigger point syndromes: An approach to management. Arch Phys Med Rehab 62:107–110.

Simons DG. (1990) Familial fibromyalgia and/or myofascial pain syndrome? Arch Phys Med Rehab 71:258–259.

Travell J. (1981) Identification of myofascial trigger point syndromes: A case of atypical facial neuralgia. Arch Phys Med Rehab 62:100–106.

Waylonis GW, Wilke S, O'Toole D, Waylonis DA, Waylonis DB. (1988) Chronic myofascial pain: Management by low-output helium-neon laser therapy. Arch Phys Med Rehab 69:1017–1020.

Yunus MB, Kalyan-Raman UP, Kalyan-Raman K. (1988) Primary fibromyalgia syndrome and myofascial pain syndrome: Clinical features and muscle pathology. Arch Phys Med Rehab 69(6):451–454.

Zumo L. (1984) Cases of frozen shoulder treated by manipulation and massage. J Traditional Chin Med 235(4):213–215.

Reflexology

Adamson S. (1994) Best feet foremost. Health Visitor 67(2):61.

Bayly DE. (1982) Reflexology today. Wellingborough: Thorsons.

Booth B. (1994) Reflexology. Nurs Times 90(1):38–40.

Dougans I, Ellis S. (1991) Reflexology—foot massage for total health. Shaftesbury: Element Books.

Downing G. (1974) The massage book. New York: Random House.

Hillman A. (1986) Zone therapy. Nursing 3(6):225–227.

Ingham ED. (1984) Stories the feet can tell. [Revised as Stories the feet have told thru reflexology.], St. Petersburg, FL: Ingham Publishing Inc.

Lidell L. (1984) The book of massage. The complete step-by-step guide to Eastern and Western techniques. London: Ebury Press.

Lockett J. (1992) Reflexology—a nursing tool? Aust Nurses J 22(1):14–15.

Oleson T, Flocco W. (1993) Randomised controlled study of premenstrual symptoms treated with ear, hand, and foot reflexology. Obstet Gynecol 82(6):906–911.

Omura Y. (1994) Accurate localization of organ representation areas on the feet & hands using the bi-digital O-ring test resonance phenomenon: Its clinical implication in diagnosis & treatment—Part 1. Acupuncture Electro Ther Res Int J 19:153–190.

Sahai ICM. (1993) Reflexology—its place in modern healthcare. Prof Nurse 8(11):722–725.

Tappan FM. (1988) Healing massage techniques: Holistic, classic and emerging methods, 2nd ed. Norwalk, CT: Appleton & Lange.

Thomas M. (1989). Fancy footwork. Nurs Times 85(41):42–44.

Point Percussion Therapy

Jia LH. (1984) Pointing therapy. Shandong: Shandong Science & Technology Press.

Wang, ZP. (1991) Acupressure therapy. Point percussion treatment of cerebral palsy birth injury, brain injury and stroke. Melbourne: Churchill Livingstone.

Chapter 12

Eastern Systems of Massage

COLLEEN LISTON, Ph.D.

A number of systems of massage are closely linked and have been adapted by different cultures in many countries. In this chapter, their interrelationships are explored and the specific techniques presented. All are related to ancient Chinese culture, and specifically to Taoism. This philosophy recognizes health as a state of balance or harmony within the individual and between the individual and nature.

ACUPRESSURE

Acupressure is the application of pressure to acupuncture points situated along meridians, or lines, on the body that run from the internal organs to the skin surface. Although the history of acupuncture and herbal medicine can be traced back to Northern and Southern China more than 4000 years ago, it was around 300 B.C. that the first text on traditional Chinese medicine, the Huangdi Nei Ching Su Wen, usually referred to as the Nei Ching or The Yellow Emperor's Classic of Internal Medicine, was written by Huang Ti (Huangdi). In it, the meridians along which the life force, or energy, of the body (ch'i/chi/qi) flows, and their acupuncture points are presented in diagrams. There are about 1000 points, and stimulating them ensures that the flow of yin and yang (the opposing and complementary negative and positive energy) is maintained in balance (Beal, 1992; Ortego, 1994; Wanning, 1993).

Hyperstimulation analgesia can be achieved through acupuncture and acupressure, as well as through techniques already presented such as trigger point stimulation, myofascial techniques, reflexology, point percussion therapy, and connective tissue massage. This is because, histologically, the points and their immediate surrounding areas are associated with nerves, pressure, and stretch receptors (Weaver, 1985). Associated modalities, for example cupping and the use of transcutaneous electrical nerve stimulation (TENS), have similar effects (Anderson et al., 1974; Baldry, 1989; Fox & Melzack, 1976; Han, 1987; Lewit, 1979; Melzack, 1981, 1985; Travell & Simons, 1983, 1992). While it is beyond the scope of this text to provide detailed information concerning the neurophysiologic basis of acupuncture and associated techniques in pain relief (He, 1987; Kerr et al., 1978), there is abundant evidence of this effect via neurotransmitter links and responses to noxious stimuli in the thalamic nuclei and periacqueductal gray areas of the brain.

Originally, acupuncture was one of a range of external therapies, including moxibustion (burning of the herb *Artemisia vulgaris*, a type of chrysanthemum) and traditional Chinese (amma) massage (Armstrong, 1972; Cheng, 1987). Before the invention of material capable of being honed fine enough to actually puncture the skin, pieces of stone and bone were used to press points on the skin. The response to stimulation of some points corresponds to that associated with the "Head's zones" mentioned previously in association with reflexology and connective tissue massage. It is widely accepted that some acupuncture points correspond with the "*Head's* zones" and some with motor points. Fifty percent of acupuncture points are directly over nerve trunks, the other half are within 0.5 cm of the trunks, and 71% coincide with trigger points (Chaitow, 1981).

Today, acupressure is applied to the acupuncture points by means of pressure applied through the thumbs, fingers, or heel of the hand. Finger pressure to acupuncture points is administered with one finger—the middle one or the thumb. Limited circular frictions progressing more deeply to static pressure over the point are given for

Table 12.1	SOME ACUPUNCTURE POINTS, THEIR POSITION AND RELATED INDICATIONS	
POINT	LOCATION	INDICATIONS
B-40 (bladder 40 *Wei-Chung*)	Center of popliteal fossa	Leg cramp, low back pain, sciatica, knee joint pain, heat stroke
B-60 (bladder 60, Kunlun)	Midpoint between posterior margin of lateral malleolus and Achilles tendon	Low back pain, sciatica, ankle joint disorders, soft tissue sprains
GB-20 (gallbladder, 20 Feng-chih)	Midpoint of line from tip of mastoid to posterior midline groove between trapezius and sternocleidomastoid	Tension headache, migraine, stiff neck, vertigo
GB-21 (Gallbladder, 21 Chieng-ching)	Midpoint between the C7 and the acromion process	Shoulder pain, neck pain with rigidity, upper extremity motor problems
GB 30 (Gallbladder, 30 Huan-tiao)	Point at outer one-third of a line from greater trochanter to base of coccyx	Hip joint pain, soft tissue disorders of the hip, low back pain
LI-15 (Large intestine 15, Chien-yu)	Acromial depression in mid-deltoid with arm abducted to 90 degrees	Pain and motor problems of arm and elbow, shoulder joint and soft tissue disorders
SI-3 (Small intestine 3, Hou-chi)	Apex of the distal palmar crease on ulnar side of a clenched fist	Low back pain, neck pain and rigidity, upper extremity weakness
GB-34 (Gallbladder 34, Yangling Chuan)	Anterior to the neck of the fibula	Knee and lower extremity pain
LI-11 (Large intestine 11, Chu-chih)	At radial end of flexed elbow fold	Shoulder pain, elbow pain, soft tissue disorders of the elbow

1 to 5 minutes. Numerous texts are available that prescriptively give information about point location and indications for applying acupressure, particularly for orthopaedic conditions and pain relief. A plan of selection of points should take into account not only the symptoms but also the relative deficiency or excess in the meridian on which the point is situated. Further reading would elucidate both the underlying philosophy and the two frameworks, or diagnostic models, of the five elements and eight principal patterns.

Acupressure should not be given over contusions, scar tissue, or an irregularity in the skin (e.g., moles, warts, acne lesions). An adverse autonomic or psychophysiological response may occur in children younger than 7 years, whose autonomic nervous system is immature, and in those with severe cardiac conditions.

Points are named by their meridians, which are linked to their sources in internal organs. Two examples are the powerful acupuncture points used in anesthesia and in the treatment of pain: the large intestine (LI-) 4 and the stomach (St-) 36 (see Fig. 11–1b). LI-4 is found in the middle of the web between the metacarpals of the thumb and index finger. In Chinese it is delightfully called *Ho-Ku*, which means "meeting valley." The method of identifying points is by directions given in "body inches" (*cun*). Each person's *cun* is his or her own and should be used to identify points on the body. The middle phalanx of the middle finger or the distal phalanx of the thumb can be used as the unit *cun*.

For LI-4, the interphalangeal joint of the thumb is placed in the middle of the outstretched web of the other hand. By rolling up onto the tip of the thumb, the "meeting valley" point is found. It is hypersensitive and is readily detected.

A point finder can be used, or the simple method of identifying the "sore spot"! Stimulation of LI-4 is indicated in foreheadache, toothache, pain and paralysis of the upper limb, asthma, hemiplegia, facial paralysis, temporomandibular joint pain, and for anesthesia and analgesia in general. St-36, *Tsu-san-li* ("walk three more miles"), is one cun lateral and distal to the tibial tuberosity. It is highly sensitive and is also favored for anesthesia and analgesia. It can be useful for nausea and vomiting; lumbar pain; headache; edema; or aching of the hips, knees, or legs in general. Table 12–1 has been adapted from a number of the texts (Academy of Traditional Chinese Medicine, 1975; Chaitow, 1971; Tappan, 1988). It provides examples of useful points for a range of symptoms, injuries, and related problems that are common. A number of other points may be of use for the conditions and symptoms referred to in Table 12–1. They should be sought from the texts listed in conjunction with this section by those interested in using acupressure as a treatment modality.

SHIATSU

Shiatsu, meaning "finger pressure," is a form of body work that originated in Japan. It includes stimulation of points and rotation and stretching of joints (Nolan, 1989). The hands, thumbs, elbows, forearms, knees, and soles of the feet or toes are used. There is strong evidence of the influence of Chinese culture; some proponents include moxibustion in treatment regimens. Furthermore, the belief that human beings are dependent on the flow of energy or "life force" (*ki* in Japanese) is the basis for stimulation of points. Shiatsu, like most of the Oriental systems, approaches health holistically. The overriding concept is that there are dynamic relationships between the individual and the environment and the ascending, male, active principle, yang, being in harmonious balance with the descending, passive, female principle, yin, determine the flow of ki. Disruptions in this flow result in imbalance, disharmony, and illness, which can be detected through the *hara*, or lower abdomen. The "hara" is also the point from which the pressure of the body's weight comes from the person applying shiatsu. This simple, holistic approach is being acknowledged worldwide (Booth, 1993; Box, 1984; Dahong, 1984; Hare, 1988).

In shiatsu there are different emphases, including *namikoshi*, which reflects a Western approach with a physiological basis; *tsubo* therapy, which aligns closely with acupuncture; and Zen shiatsu, which incorporates the complexities of the meridians. All varieties have a common theme—to revitalize the body and mind.

Overall, there are three main techniques:

1. *Sustained pressure on a tsubo, or pressure point, at right angles to the body* is purported to tone the body by increasing the flow of blood and "energy" in the area.

2. *Passive and active stretching and squeezing for the joints* are meant to disperse blocked blood or "energy."

3. *Holding and gently rocking the body part, using little or no pressure* is intended to calm and counteract "agitated energy."

The technique is applied to the body through any of the parts mentioned earlier. With the therapist's body well

Sequence of a Shiatsu Treatment

- With the client lying prone on a mat on the floor or a broad wide low plinth, begin on the back, stretching to loosen it and to establish a rhythm. Apply pressure down both sides of the spine with palms and thumbs.
- Points on the sacrum and iliosacral joints are pressed; then the buttocks are squeezed and pressure is applied through the elbow to their upper curve.
- Press down the center of the back of each leg, first with the palms, then with the knees.
- Press on the ankle points; stretch the leg in each direction; then crook the knee in and the foot out to press down the lateral border. "Walk" the hands along the soles of the feet.
- Press along the top of each shoulder; rotate the shoulder blades; press the area between the shoulder blades; then loosen the shoulder muscles using the feet.
- Turn the client to the supine position, and open the chest by leaning the body weight through the hands onto the client's shoulders.
- Press along the spaces between the ribs; then press underneath on the back and sides of the neck, ending with a stretch to the neck achieved by gently elongating it by lifting the head upward and forward.
- Beginning at the top of the head, run the fingers through the hair, gently pull it, then finger massage the ears. Work with the finger tips on the face, including the temples, around the eyes, the nostrils, and the mouth, and across the jaw, concluding behind the midline of the base of the skull.

- The arms should be managed one at a time. Press down the inside with the palm facing up using a flat hand, then with the palm facing down, along the back of the forearm to the tip of the shoulder. Pull the fingers, concentrating on the point between the thumb and the forefinger (LI-4). End by shaking the arm to relax it.
- Work with both hands flat using a circular kneading technique on the "hara" in the lower abdomen, then press up gently under the lower borders of the ribs and thence down the midline, ending at the navel. Use a rocking motion to calm the "hara."
- Massage the legs one at a time, working from the groin to the feet. Press down the inside of the leg to the knee, then return to the groin and work down the front of the thigh. Manipulate the patella to loosen it; then press down the inside with one thumb and down the outside of the calf with the other. Dorsiflex and plantarflex the foot, pull the toes, and conclude by shaking the leg to relax it.

balanced the body weight is applied through the hands, the ball of the thumb (the part used most often), or another part of the arm or leg.

The techniques used in shiatsu are similar to those of traditional Thai massage and have much in common with the massage in Huna. Detailed information can be gained from specific texts and in particular from a general massage book that includes both Eastern and Western methods (Lidell, 1984).

TRADITIONAL CHINESE MASSAGE

Pressure and rubbing is known as "amma massage." This system of deep massage is a traditional part of Oriental medicine. Amma massage has been associated with blind practitioners and is used to normalize body functions and to encourage relaxation of the tired soft tissues of the body. It has a calming influence on the nervous system (Serizawa, 1973). There are 3 categories of Amma massage:

- Rubbing and pressure, much like kneading and frictions but applied with the knuckles

- Finger and palm work, as in picking up and wringing

- Passive stretches for the joints

Amma massage was used only to reinvigorate tired muscles and joints. Similar, so-called Swedish remedial massage techniques were introduced in 1868 during the Meiji restoration in Japan. The Japanese recognized the similarities of the two and combined them to develop their own system of six basic massage techniques that incorporated the rubbing, pressure, and finger work of Amma massage and some Swedish techniques, especially vibration and tapotement:

- Rubbing and stroking, using flat hands or the balls of the thumb and fingers and constant light pressure

- Circular motion massage, using the relaxed palm or the tips of the fingers but with the motion originating at the wrist, and light to moderate pressure

- Kneading massage, using the thumb; index and middle finger alone; or all four fingers together for tendons crossing joints

- Pressure massage, using the palms, the thumbs, or four fingers to apply 3 to 5 kg of pressure for 3 to 5 seconds. The body weight, not the fingers alone, should be used to apply the pressure. Pressure should always be directed toward the center of the client's body and should be increased gradually. It is similar to the pressure techniques applied in shiatsu.

- Vibration massage, in which the fingers or palms are placed firmly on the skin and vibrated rhythmically and gently. The rate of vibration is 10 to 40 times a second.

- Tapping massage, alternating hands to tap the client's body rhythmically with the palms, finger tips, and backs of the fingers or with the lateral border of the hand. The tapping is light and quick, at a rate of 13 to 14 times a second. The pressure should be around 1 kg. These techniques are closely related to those used in point percussion therapy (Jia, 1984).

TRADITIONAL THAI MASSAGE

The true origins of Thai massage are unknown, but, given its similarities to other Oriental systems, we can speculate that massage was, more than likely, introduced from India with the expansion of the Indian culture and of Buddhism into Thailand.

In the *Ayur Veda*, the classic Indian text of around 1800 B.C., recommendations for healing massage are recorded. At Wat Pho, a famous temple in Bangkok where traditional Thai massage is taught, Ajahn Chivakakomarapad, a Buddhist medical doctor, claimed in a stone inscription on the wall (Silajarug) that he knew the origins of all the lines of linkage in the human body. He presented around 72,000 lines, but ten main lines (Sen Pratarn) were the most important. Today knowledge of these ten lines is the basis of traditional Thai massage (Tapanya, 1993).

The imaginary lines in Thai massage closely match the meridians of traditional Chinese medicine along which *chi* flows and on which acupuncture points lie. Similarly, the 10 Thai main lines function as "energy" pathways or are described as the functional circulation in the body. These nonspecific systems function as balancing mechanisms for the body, linking a series of specific points on the surface with the deeper organs. In this way, the body's mental, digestive, nervous, circulatory, and reproductive processes, and, thus, nutrition, consciousness, and energy, are harmonized.

Illness and functional disorders are claimed to be the result of disruption of one or more of the ten main lines. It is suggested that pressure applied to a specific point along the relevant line may produce a physiological effect in the periosteum, fascia, muscles, blood vessels, or nerves that is perceived as a moving impulse. As a result, pain may be relieved, circulation improved, and muscles relaxed, and organ function may be improved.

The ten lines originate at the level of the umbilicus. They are listed in order:

1. *Itha* runs down the front of the left leg; up the back of the left leg; across the left buttock; up the left side of the back; up the back of the left side of the head; over the top of the left side of the head, ending at the left nostril.

2. *Pingkala* runs the same route as *Itha* but on the right side. Both *Itha* and *Pingkala* should be attended to for headache or neck or back pain.

3. *Smana* runs up the middle of the thorax through the neck and chin, and along the upper surface of the tongue. Chest, heart, jaw, and oral symptoms may arise from disruption along *Smana*.

4. *Kalathale* runs down both arms, through the fingers, through both legs, and through the phalanges. Symptoms in the arms or legs are related to *Kalathale*.

5. *Sahutsarungsi* runs down the inside of the left leg, across the base of the toes, up the outside of the left leg, across the left tibial crest, through the left nipple, and diagonally up to the left eye. The left leg and eye are governed by the functional circulation along *Sahutsarungsi*.

6. *Thavare* runs the same route as *Sahutsarungsi* but on the right side of the body. Symptoms in the right leg and eye are related to *Thavare*.

7. *Chunthapusang* runs up to the left nipple and up the left side of the neck, and ends on the left ear lobe. The left ear relies on uninterrupted flow along *Chunthapusang*.

8. *Ruchum* runs the same route as *Chunthapusang* but on the right side. *Ruchum* is the line for the right ear.

9. *Sukhamung* runs to the stomach, internal organs, anus, and urethra. The health of the internal organs depends on *Sukhamung*.

10. *Sikkhine* runs to the genital organs, and their functioning depends on *Sikkhine*.

The Technique

There are two classifications of traditional Thai massage. Thai massage in the Grand Palace is given using the hand, arm, or elbow. There is no stretching, and it is used only for therapeutic purposes. Thai massage for the people is

Major Elements of Thai Massage

- Pressing and releasing, the degree of pressure being judged in relation to the tolerance of the recipient. Pressure is applied along the main lines in a regular and rhythmic fashion at points around 5 cm apart, beginning at the origin near the umbilicus and proceeding to the end point.
- Picking up, where muscle is lifted away from the bone and squeezed
- Hacking, particularly to the calf muscles
- Stretching for joints
- Manipulation of joints, especially those of the fingers and toes

undertaken to maintain the functional circulation, for general health and well-being. The therapist's hand, arm, elbow, leg, and foot are used, and stretching is included, much as in shiatsu.

Thai massage is similar to both other Eastern techniques—and to Western ones. Given that the Swede Per Henrik Ling developed Western techniques associated with Swedish remedial massage from Chinese massage is not remarkable.

HUNA MASSAGE

Huna massage is a unique combination of massage techniques and healing traditions originating in Hawaii. It is based on the life principles in the millennia-old Polynesian philosophy, *Huna*, which has been described as "Kahuna magic" (Steiger, 1982). This body and mind work was formerly reserved for the shamans of Polynesia, who mastered the wisdom (Feinberg, 1990).

Huna is a Hawaiian word that, split up and put together in different ways, has several meanings: *huna* is "the secret or hidden knowledge"; *hu* is *yang*, the male principle, the giving and active part; *na* is yin, the female principle, the receiving and passive part; *una* is telepathy, a way to communicate; and *hua* is seeds or fruit.

Huna tradition, with the body work to balance the male and female principles, aims to cleanse away old patterns and old habits and prepare "the soil" for new crops. A philosophy that teaches how to sow in proportion to what harvest is desired is a tradition to which many cultural and social groups relate. The seven principles of *huna* philosophy are simple, dynamic, proactive, optimistic, and of great current interest. This philosophy clearly illustrates how we create our own experiences and circumstances in life, via our thought patterns and belief systems. It also teaches us how to change undesirable patterns of thought and action so they can inspire us and serve our intentions and goals in life. It is a very effective tool for creating our consciousness and growth.

Characteristics of this form of massage are beauty and rhythm, because it is performed as a dance. The simple dance steps provide the basis for rhythmic movements of the arms, which feel like waves moving lovingly across the body. The arms being used at full length ensures very good contact. The dance gives a deep feeling of joy and is a formidable grounding whereby the giver and the recipient together have the opportunity to "recharge their energy."

The music accompanying the massage is mainly Polynesian—beautiful, cheerful, and stirring. By means of dance, music, and touch all levels of consciousness are activated: physical, emotional, mental, and spiritual. The massage itself incorporates deep effleurage and kneading along the trunk and limbs together with passive stretching of the joints, in a manner similar to the application in shiatsu.

Courses teaching *huna massage* are designed for people who seek self-development and self-healing and those who want to do professional body and mind work. In Scandinavia, the training is built up in seven modules, each a complete unit. This makes it possible for anyone to take the modules at his or her own pace and as required. In New Zealand and Australia a module is presented twice a year that has been adjusted to the needs of these countries. Apart from basic instruction in *huna* massage and the principles of *huna* philosophy, special techniques such as pregnancy massage, joint massage, draining, astral dancing, and body reading are included.

The old Hawaiian traditional method of massage, using the hands and emphasizing special breathing techniques, is combined with release techniques, which include the Eastern philosophies of polarity, energy points, and energy flows (or chakras). The links between the Chinese traditions of maintaining balance in the energy level for optimal health are an integral part of the *huna* philosophy. Like many of the techniques described in Chapters 11 and 12, the massage aims to enhance energy and teach intuitive guidance, in order to train the senses to transform and direct energy.

References and Bibliography

Acupressure

Academy of Traditional Chinese Medicine. (1975) An outline of Chinese acupuncture. Peking: Foreign Language Press.

Anderson DG, Jamieson JL, Man SC. (1974) Analgesic effects of acupuncture on the pain of ice water: A double-blind study. Can J Psychol 28:239–244.

Armstrong ME. (1972) Acupuncture. Am J Nurs 72(9):1582.

Baldry PE. (1989) Acupuncture trigger points & musculo-skeletal pain. New York: Churchill Livingstone.

Beal MW. (1992) Acupuncture and related treatment modalities. Part I: Theoretical background. J Nurse Midwif 37(4):254–259.

Chaitow L. (1979) The acupuncture treatment of pain. Northamptonshire: Thorsons.

Chaitow L. (1981) Instant pain control. Northamptonshire: Thorsons.

Cheng X. (1987) Chinese acupuncture and moxibustion. Beijing: Foreign Language Press.

Fox EJ, Melzack R. (1976) Transcutaneous electrical stimulation and acupuncture: Comparison of treatment for low back pain. Pain 2:141–148.

Han JS. (1987) The neurochemical basis of pain relief by acupuncture. A collection of papers 1973–1987. Beijing: Chinese Medical Science & Technology Press.

He L. (1987) Involvement of endogenous opioid peptides in acupuncture analgesia. Pain 31(1):91–121.

Kerr FW, Wilson PR, Nijensohn DE. (1978) Acupuncture reduces the trigeminal evoked response in decerebrate cats. Exp Neurol 61:84–95.

Lewit K. (1979) The needle effect in the relief of myofascial pain. Pain 6:83–90.

Melzack R. (1981) Myofascial trigger points: Relation to acupuncture and mechanisms of pain. Arch Phys Med Rehab 62:114–117.

Melzack R. (1985) Hyperstimulation analgesia. Clin Anaesthesiol 3(1): 81–92.

Ortego NE. (1994) Acupressure: An alternative approach to mental health counseling through bodymind awareness. Nurse Practitioner Forum 5(2):72–76.

Travell JG, Simons DG. (1983) Myofascial pain and dysfunction: The trigger point manual, Vol I. Baltimore: Williams & Wilkins.

Travell JG, Simons DG. (1992) Myofascial pain and dysfunction: The trigger point manual, Vol II. Baltimore: Williams & Wilkins.

Wanning T. (1993) Healing and the mind/body arts. Am Assoc Occup Health Nurses 41(7):349–351.

Weaver MT. (1985) Acupressure: An overview of theory and application. Nurse Practitioner 10(8):38–42.

Shiatsu

Booth B. (1993) Shiatsu. Nurs Times 89(46):38–40.

Box D. (1984) Made in Japan. Nurs Times April:39–40.

Dahong Z. (1984) Skilful hands bring relief. World Health May:15.

Hare ML. (1988) Shiatsu acupressure in nursing practice. Holistic Nurs Pract 2(3):68–74.

Lidell L. (1984) The book of massage. The complete step-by-step guide to Eastern and Western techniques. London: Ebury Press.

Nolan B. (1989) Sorting out your yin and yang. Nurs Times 85(35):58–60.

Traditional Chinese Massage

Serizawa K. (1973) Massage. Tokyo: Japan Publications.

Traditional Thai Massage

Tapanya S. (1993) Traditional Thai massage. Bangkok: Duang Kamol.

Huna Techniques

Feinberg R. (1990) Spiritual and natural etiologies on a Polynesian outlier in Papua New Guinea. Soc Sci Med 30(3):311–323.

Steiger B. (1982) Kahuna magic. Rockport, MA: Para Research.

Appendix

Closed-Chest (External) Cardiac Massage

Closed-chest cardiac massage is included here because it is a technique that all persons involved in direct patient care of any type should know for emergency treatment of cardiac arrest. The technique somewhat resembles the shaking and vibration procedures described in Chapter 9; however, it is performed only over the sternum and much more slowly.

If a quick check of the pulse at the carotid arteries on either side of the trachea confirms that the heart has stopped, the patient should be placed supine on a solid support such as the floor or a firm plinth or stretcher (whichever is quickest). The patient's head should be tilted back to ensure a patent airway. This can usually be achieved by placing one hand under the neck and lifting the cervical spine upward (Fig. App.–1), allowing the head to fall into extension. If the airway is obstructed internally, it must be cleared before any other procedures are performed. The reader is referred to national or local Heart Association guidelines for currently recommended procedures for clearing an obstructed airway.

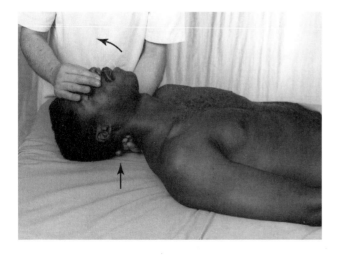

Figure App–1. Hand positions to ensure patency of the airway for artificial respiration.
The patency of the patient's airway is ensured by lifting the cervical spine upward while the patient is lying supine. This causes the head to fall into extension and prevents blockage of the airway, provided there is no internal blockage. The nostrils may be pinched together lightly to close them off when blowing into the patient's lungs.

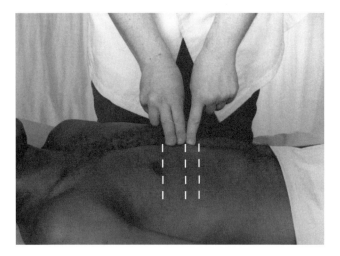

Figure App–2. Locating the area over the sternum where pressure is applied during external cardiac massage.
The index finger of the hand farthest from the patient's head locates the xiphoid process as the other hand is placed on the sternum, two finger breadths from the xiphoid.

Before compression can begin, the rescuer must determine where to place his or her hands on the patient's chest. A simple way to do this is to place the index finger of one hand on the xiphoid process. Two fingers of the other hand are then placed next to this finger (Fig. App.–2). The first finger is removed and the flat hand placed on the chest next to the two fingers, on the same side as the patient's head. It is very important that no pressure be applied to the ribs or abdominal contents. Pressure is applied directly to the lower third of the sternum.

Since the sternum is a relatively narrow structure, the heel of the palm of only one hand is positioned in direct contact with the skin while the other hand is used to reinforce it (Fig. App.–3). The fingers are spread and raised so that pressure is applied only to the sternum and not to the ribs or abdomen. Vertical pressure sufficient to depress the sternum 1 inch (2.5 cm) or a little more is applied and quickly released. If the patient is a child one hand may be used with less pressure. If an infant (less than 1 year old) is being resuscitated, the finger tips may be used, and much less pressure, at a rate of at least 100 times per minute.

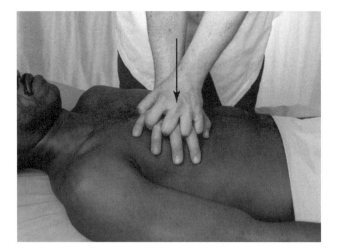

Figure App–3. Hand positions for external cardiac massage.
Pressure is applied using the heel of the palm of one hand reinforced by the other. Sufficient pressure is applied to displace the sternum by approximately 1 inch (2.5 cm). Pressure must be applied only to the sternum, to avoid damaging the ribs or abdominal organs.

It is assumed in cardiopulmonary resuscitation (CPR) training that respiratory support will be required with all cardiac arrests. Therefore, a single rescuer must perform both artificial ventilation and circulation stimulation. The lone rescuer should apply compression at the rate of 60 to 80 strokes per minute, giving two quick breaths to the patient after each set of 15 compressions. The rate of 60 to 80 per minute provides at least 60 compressions per minute plus the ventilatory interruptions. When two rescuers are available, one performs compression at the rate of 60 to 80 per minute as the other delivers a breath after each fifth compression; they alternate positions as necessary. A rate of 80 to 100 compressions per minute should be used on children from the age of 1 to 8 years. The patient's nostrils may be lightly pinched to seal off the nasal passage during the inflation cycle of the ventilation (see Fig. App.–1).

In all situations, an advanced life support or emergency medical team must be summoned at the earliest moment and CPR efforts should be continued until the team arrives or until effective circulation and ventilation have been restored. When the patient is a child or when cardiac arrest is associated with hypothermia prolonged resuscitation efforts may be justified and should be continued even after long periods of unconsciousness.

Unless much care is taken to perform these procedures properly, fractures of the ribs and sternum, and laceration and rupture of soft tissues, such as liver, spleen, pancreas, lungs, and blood vessels, can easily occur. Although there are, of course, individual variations, most medical standards for CPR and emergency cardiac care recommend that all health care workers involved in any capacity in direct patient care be certified in basic life support techniques and be well-informed about the CPR plan of the facility in which they work. It is usual, nowadays, for a basic CPR certificate to be valid for 1 year. For certification, a qualified CPR instructor must verify that the person has demonstrated knowledge of when to perform CPR. Sufficient psychomotor skills for correct timing and technique for both one- and two-person rescues must also be demonstrated. The practice necessary to develop these skills and the repeated demonstration of them should be performed on a training mannikin under the supervision of a certified CPR instructor.

Index

Note: Page numbers in *italics* refer to illustrations; page numbers followed by t refer to tables.